To clothe the fiery thought

In simple words succeeds,

For still the craft of genius is

To mask a king in weeds.

— RALPH WALDO EMERSON —

The Nurse~ Herbalist

INTEGRATIVE INSIGHTS *for* HOLISTIC PRACTICE

Dr. Martha Mathews Libster

GOLDEN APPLE PUBLICATIONS

Cover/Book Design: Mark Gelotte www.markgelotte.com
Copy Edit: Rose Foley
Foreword: Dr. Marlaine C. Smith

Printed in the United States

Library of Congress Control Number: 2011942980

Libster, Martha Mathews 1960-
Includes bibliographical references and Index
ISBN 9780975501849

1. Nursing–United States–History 2. Medicine–Botanic
3. Holistic medicine 4. Herbal medicine
5. Family–Health and Hygiene 6. Self–Care
7. Spiritual healing 8. Spirituality–The Goddess 9. Medical policy
10. Health policy I. Libster, Martha Mathews author

— Dedication —

This book is dedicated to each and every plant, flower, tree, bud, and blade of grass that teaches us to find our true green nature and to comfort and heal with plants as partners. This book is also dedicated to the essence of the Green Woman in everyone and to those readers who seek a deeper relationship with healing plants. To you, I offer my insights on nursing and healing inspired by the vibrancy of the green world and my meditations on the love of Mother in Nature. I hope that this book will assist you, who follow the plants into a world of beauty and peace, in emerging transformed as gentler healers.

— Acknowledgments and Gratitude —

There are many who have made this work possible for which I am most grateful. My deepest gratitude goes to all of the clients and students who asked the questions that have compelled me to write this book. Thank you to everyone who has tried my gentle remedies over the years and allowed me to witness and tell stories of those experiences so that others can learn from them. Thank you to my herb teachers: Grandpa, Oma, Elizabeth, Sandra Jean, Roger, Duke, Norman, and Zezi, and the numerous others who have "talked plant" with me along the way.

A special thank you to my editor, Rose, and book designer, Mark, for helping to manifest this message. Your love of the creative process matches my own, step by step.

I am most grateful to beloved Harold, my plant-lovin' husband, and my four-legged Sheeva whose steadfastness and support for me and my writing projects seem to know no limit. I also am grateful to the Creator for the opportunity to do my work with plants and continue my studies in Mother Nature.

Every effort has been made to deliver a book on nurse-herbalism that is accurate. While many have helped in the process, the content of these chapters is my responsibility and any errors most definitely my own.

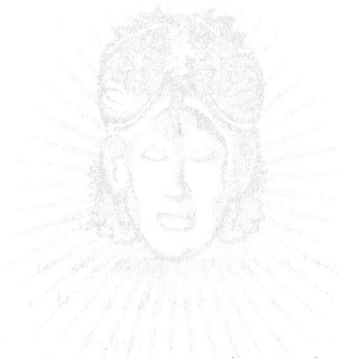

Notes about the Artwork from Martha (Author) and Mark (Designer)

"Tess"

We refer to the image of the Green Woman who appears on the cover and throughout this book as "Tess" – short for quintessential. The five elements represented in nature are quintessential for the alchemical process of self-transformation. As we were designing this book, we realized that while there are numerous images of the Green Man in Celtic literature and culture there are few to none of the Green Woman. Martha met some jewelry vendors from Bali at a conference. On their table was an exquisite wooden mask of a Green Woman. The vendors said that the mask was carved from hibiscus wood by the hand of a man in Bali known for his beauty and healing presence. The mask (shown below) is the face of a woman emerging from hibiscus leaves and flowers. Two frogs sit on her head. We adopted Tess as our prototype for the image of the Nurse-Herbalist in this book. We had many conversations and discussions with reviewers about having a Green Man appear in the book as well. Everyone agreed that the image of the Green Man is well known and that this book *The Nurse-Herbalist* should carry the image of the Green Woman alone. The Green Woman represents the enduring feminine energy that is nursing and which is rising in cultures across the globe.

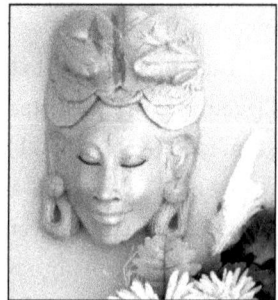

Five Elements Paintings

The paintings that appear at the beginning of each chapter on the elements were painted by Nicholas Roerich (1874-1947), a renowned Russian mystic and painter known most especially for his use of color. Martha has been a student of the works of Nicholas and his wife Helena Roerich for almost thirty years and uses the paintings presented in this book in her presentations on the five elements of care with permission of the Roerich Museum in New York City. The E-Book version of *The Nurse-Herbalist* is in color and captures the beauty of the elements represented in the five Roerich paintings: Ether, Fire, Air, Water, and Earth. Roerich's painting, The Five Treasures, is also included to represent all five elements.

Roerich was also an anthropologist, botanist, and humanitarian nominated for the Nobel Peace Prize for The Roerich Peace Pact treaty signed at the White House, in the presence of President Franklin Delano Roosevelt, on April 15, 1935, by all the members of the Pan-American Union. The Peace Pact banner includes the image of a red circle representing culture. Within the circle of culture are three red dots representing the unity of science, art, and religion. The motto accompanying the Peace Pact banner is *Pax Cultura, Peace through Culture.*

The treaty is still active. Many peoples and associations around the world continue to promote awareness of the Pact, the Banner, and their underlying principles. The pursuit of refinement and beauty was sacred for Roerich. He believed that peace on Earth was a prerequisite to planetary survival and the continuing process of spiritual evolution, and he exhorted his fellow man to help achieve that peace by uniting in the common language of Beauty and Knowledge. Woman is depicted in his paintings as the carrier and defender of the Banner.

For more information on Peace through Culture, the Peace Pact Banner, and to view a grand collection of Roerich paintings go to the website: www.roerich.org.

PAX CULTURA

Welcome to the beautiful green world!

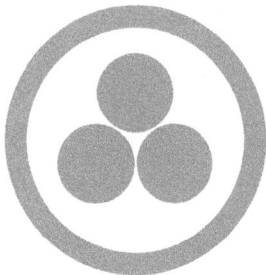

CONTENTS

FOREWORD

Marlaine C. Smith, RN, PhD, FAAN

The Nurse-Herbalist by Martha Libster is a revolutionary publication for the professional discipline of nursing. As an advanced practice nurse, herbalist and nurse historian, Libster asserts that the knowledgeable, skillful integration of plants for the purposes of health and healing is within the domain of nursing. She makes this claim from an historical analysis of the practice of western nursing in the 18th and 19th centuries, the correspondence of nurse-herbalist practice within the articulated focus of the discipline, and a grounded understanding from her extensive experience of how to integrate herbs into a practice that is authentically nursing. Just as touch and dietary therapies are considered to be nursing modalities, so is the knowledgeable use of plants for self care, comfort and symptom management. This work calls us to re-claim a lost and abandoned legacy for the discipline and practice of nursing in the post-modern era. This will mean re-introducing plant therapies as nursing therapeutics through promoting the study of and experience with botanical remedies including engaging in a relationship with nature and plants. In contrast to the biomedical approach of prescribing or using herbs to fix health problems or cure disease, the nurse-herbalist partners with plants to promote healing within patterns of sleep and rest, mobility, pain, energy, emotions and thought, hormone balance and nutrition.

It is time for nurses to appreciate the patterned consciousness of plants and to be open to the gifts they offer. We don't use plants or herbs, we participate knowingly with them in repatterning the human-environment energy fields for health and healing. With about a third of the American public using some form of herbs for self care, it is essential for all nurses to understand more about the therapeutic value of plants.

This has been a missing piece for holistic nursing. Many nurses have considered herbalism "off limits", within the realm of naturopathic practice. Generally nurses know very little about how people are using herbal remedies except to assess for drug-herb interactions. This book re-forms the way that plants are situated in nursing, giving us permission and encouragement to learn, grow and experiment with using herbs in creative ways.

This book is organized by weaving together threads of essential knowledge to create an epistemic tapestry for the practice of nurse herbalism. Seemingly unrelated threads such as nursing theories, tenets of Traditional Chinese Medicine, the healing traditions of the French Daughters of Charity and nurses in the Shaker and Mormon communities, foundations of primary health care, evidence-based practice and legal and regulatory issues in herbalism form this tapestry. Readers are guided in the preparation of self for practice as a nurse-herbalist. The five elements: earth, air, water, fire and ether provide a structure to present the preparatory material for a nurse-herbalist's practice. For example, in *Entering the Earth Element* the reader learns to create sacred space for her practice as a nurse-herbalist and to create a practice plan. In *Awakening the Air Element* Libster addresses coming to know and understand plants through a variety of conceptual maps from evidence-based practice to traditional Chinese medicine. *Welcoming the Water Element* focuses on water and flow for delivering plant medicine. From hot water bottles to preparing teas, infusions, decoctions, soups, syrups, extracts, compresses, plasters, poultices, infused oils, salves and ointments, inhalations and steams, and baths, this chapter introduces us to these gentle, powerful caring-healing traditions that have until now been lost to nursing. In *Fanning the Fire Element* we learn about the regulations, statutes and guidelines in the practice of nurse-herbalism. *Effecting the Ether Element* focuses on our sacred relationship to Nature manifested with plants. This chapter includes a fascinating discussion of the alchemical process that occurs in making plant medicines where the consciousness of the maker and plant co-create transformation and healing. *Appendix A: The Nurse's Herbal* gives "last but not least" new meaning; it includes a glossary and comprehensive compendium of remedies related to health patterns.

I am so grateful for this book. I know of no one else who could have written it. It is the work of a master who truly knows her subject matter. Libster possesses a stunning depth of knowledge, expertise and experience in both nursing and herbalism; with this she speaks confidently and credibly about the knowledge, competencies and Self formation needed for nurse herbalism. She is a nursing scholar who integrates 25 years of experience as an herbalist with a clear understanding of the scope of the discipline of nursing. In addition she brings a breadth of knowledge in traditional medical systems, counseling and consultation, and the political-legal environment surrounding herbal remedies.

The reader can look forward to being guided by a wise teacher who shares her knowledge and experience through personal stories and "integrative insights", those realizations that have informed her practice over the years. The book contains experiments, experiential exercises that engage the reader in reflections and interactions on and with plants. This book is an absolutely essential volume for the library of all holistic nurses, and it is my hope that someday soon it will be required reading for all nurses.

Marlaine C. Smith, RN, PhD, AHN-BC, FAAN
Dean and Helen K. Persson Eminent Scholar
Christine E. Lynn College of Nursing
Florida Atlantic University
Past President Society of Rogerian Scholars

THE NURSE-HERBALIST

Introduction

Herbalism, the study and application of medicinal plants, is a nursing tradition. The modality of herbalism is not a passing fad that some nurses may choose to occasionally use *with* conventional nursing practice. Herbalism *is* nursing practice. Herbal remedies—like touch, compassionate communication, diet therapies, and creating a healing environment—are essential elements of nursing and midwifery care. Historically, nurses have championed, promoted, and protected the American public's safe use of herbs for centuries.[1] Nurse-herbalists partner with plants to explore the clinical applications of providing human comfort with plants as a catalyst for change. They are guided by principles and practices from science and the healing arts, demonstrating their commitment to providing counseling and care that flows from the center of a living ethic. Nurse-herbalists' work is informed by knowledge, experiences, and beliefs about healing plants as well as by the insight that comes from their personal relationships with plants. They use herbal remedies today when caring for clients in their community hospitals, public health facilities, hospices, outpatient clinics, schools, and skilled nursing and psychiatric facilities. All of these concepts are presented throughout this book as an opportunity for your

---

1   Martha Libster, *Herbal Diplomats: The Contribution of Early American Nurses (1830-1860) to Nineteenth-Century Health Care Reform and the Botanical Medical Movement.* (Thornton, CO: Golden Apple Publications, 2004).

consideration and exploration. Step by step, element by element—fire, air, water, earth, and ether—this comprehensive textbook guides you in the creation and implementation of your own nurse-herbalist practice plan rooted in the knowledge, experiences, and insights gleaned herein.

People are most often familiar with the television portrayal of nurses as hospital workers and supporters of physician practice. Therefore, they may assume that nurses' uses of herbs, historically and contemporarily, reflect the way herbs are used by physicians. Nurses, however, have their own history of herbal practice that is distinct yet complementary to that of physicians and other community and traditional healers. It is important that nurses who partner with plants mindfully actualize that distinction so that nurse-herbalist science and healing tradition is not only preserved but advanced. I know the necessity of this work because I am a nurse-herbalist who has partnered with plants in the care and comfort of people, families, and communities for twenty-five years. My research continues to be focused on that goal of defining and distinguishing nurse-herbalism.

Though sometimes arduous, I love this work. Plants are my joy and inspiration and the perfect chalice for carrying the love of my heart to those in need of healing, light, and understanding. Plants are also my teachers. In this book, you will learn what they have taught me as a nurse and as a person. I am their student, called time and again to enter their green and flowery world, only then to re-enter the world of people in need of healing where I share what I know about plants. The first thing I know is that it is possible for people to have a personal relationship with a plant, even a single plant, that will bring them so much understanding of the beauty of the Creator and the creation— human, animal, and plant—that healing can occur at all levels of being. It is possible to heal spiritually, mentally, emotionally, and physically from an experience with a single plant. I know this because I have been healed many times and I have witnessed others' healings from plants, many times. Some of those stories are included here. I hope that they make you smile.

I also hope that they help you to remember your own personal connection with plants and how you think about and relate to them. How have you learned to care for yourself and others over the years? What do you believe and think about healing plants? Do you recommend plants—such as the juice of an orange—when someone asks you how to care for a cold? Do you drink orange juice yourself because you think that it is a "good source of vitamin C"? Have you ever thought about how plants manifest in your life and in the lives of your clients? This book is a guide for deep reflection on your experience of healing plants, flowers, and trees and for creating your own unique nurse-herbalist practice plan. It is a guide for nurses who "stop and smell the roses" and mindfully enter the plant world in a new way. Many have forgotten our history with roses and the nursing profession's momentum of healing with flowers and plants, not to mention their own history of plant partnerships. It is time to restore our healing tradition. People need it. We need it.

Throughout this book, you will find instructions for developing yourself as a nurse-herbalist. There are opportunities for reflection, herbal experiments, and readings that complement the content you read. They are included to deepen your understanding of the nurse-plant relationship and for your own healing and delight as you make your way through the elements of care represented in this guide.

As technology-based practice has grown, as manifested primarily in the reliance on pharmaceutical drugs, herb use has waned and, in some industrialized countries, fallen out of use by professional nurses, particularly those who practice in hospitals. *The Nurse-Herbalist* shows how nurses can create a practice in which herbalism is re-integrated with nursing. The premise of this book is that humans rely on plants for their existence and therefore partnership with plants is essential to holistic nursing comfort and care. The scope of herbal practice varies from nurse to nurse but general re-establishment of partnership with plants is fundamental nursing and midwifery art and science.

Unlike urban communities and highly industrialized nations, nurses and midwives in rural communities and developing nations often continue to partner with plants. While herbal remedies may be perceived by some as crude, outdated medicine and therefore lesser care, there are countries around the globe as well as cultural communities within industrialized nations that continue to apply herbal remedies. Nurses in those communities are often quite versed in medicinal plant use. Developing nurses' knowledge and capacity to continue to utilize healing traditions in nursing, such as herbal remedies, is a global health need.

This book addresses that need. *The Nurse-Herbalist* details ways in which herbalism can be integrated with contemporary nursing science, art, and practice in support of global health while furthering the profession's long-standing values and history of successful practice that contributes to the promotion of health and peace.

According to the last World Health Organization (WHO) study in the 1980s on the subject of traditional healing, 80 percent of the world's population still used their traditional methods of healing, including the use of medicinal plants.[2] In my international experience, this statistic is accurate today if not a bit low, particularly in rural areas where medicinal plants grow. However, reporting is a bit more complicated than it might seem. Herbal application is often so common that when asked about their health practices, people may not even think of the cup of coffee or tea they drink each morning as an "herbal remedy" per se, which in fact it is. In addition, communities are quite reticent to reveal their herbal beliefs, knowledge, and practices to others who may not understand, let alone value, their cultural beliefs and healing practices.

Nurses also may not think about the plant-based dietary recommendations, remedies, and topical applications they use and recommend in client care as "herbalism" either. But nurses, as well as the public, continue to employ herbs in care. For example, a compress of the distillate of the bark of the witch hazel tree (*Hamamelis virginiana*) is often used by nurses in care of postpartum women to astringe swollen peritoneal tissue and relieve discomfort. Though often under-acknowledged, even a large percentage of the pharmaceutical drugs administered and prescribed by nurses, midwives, and advanced practice nurses are developed from the knowledge of the chemical structures of medicinal plants and sometimes even derived from actual plant material. Acknowledgment and participation in nurse-herbalist practice, as will be outlined in this book, are often a matter of degree rather than an overall question of practice. Herb use is nursing practice and science but the degree of use—the art of nurse-herbalism—is determined by the individual nurse.

For the purposes of this book, I use the term "nurse-herbalism" to identify nurses' practice of partnering with plants in providing holistic

---

2 Norman Farnsworth and others, "Medicinal Plants in Therapy," *Bulletin of the World Health Organization* 63, no. 6 (1985): 967.

Herbal Experiment: Creating a Safe Place for Reflection

Before beginning herbal experiments of any kind, you must have a "safe place" for doing your scientific work – within and without. Find a physical space in your home or elsewhere where you can close your eyes and know that you will be completely safe and not be interrupted or disturbed. Take a comfortable position and close your eyes. Place your fingers on your radial pulse and notice the rhythm of your pulse. Then move your awareness to the center of your chest and your heart – the heart that beats as pulse. Using your memory and imagination, find and/or create a place in your mind in which you are completely safe … and by yourself. Carefully note all sounds, shapes, colors, smells, sensations, and tastes associated with your safe place. Take your time. Notice any plants in your safe place.

After your creative reflection, try to synthesize this reflection of creating a safe place into one word that represents the essence of the safe place. Note the name of your safe place in a journal dedicated to nurse-herbalism and your plant experiences and experiments. Be sure to explore any plants that you found in your safe place. You might ask an herbalist about the plant or read about it. Record what you learn about the plant in your journal. You can re-create this safe place at any time of the day and anywhere you go. Lock it in to your memory now for future reflection.

care. The use of a hyphenated term should be interpreted as emphasizing the connection between herbalism and nursing, which is the focus of this book, and not construed as suggesting any separation between them. Nurse-herbalism is the study of and experience with plants and their therapeutic application that is evidence-based, culturally and clinically relevant, client-focused, and wellness oriented. Nurse-herbalism has existed for centuries. This is not a nostalgic ideal; its presence is demonstrated in publications that include primary sources that I have found in my research in the archives of communities such as those of European and American nurses dating back to as early as the seventeenth century.

Nurse-herbalism, as will be shown throughout this book, also exists in present-day practice of nurses around the globe. There is evidence that nurses apply medicinal plants in the care and comfort of others because plant remedies are accessible, inexpensive, empowering, and effective. Plants not only play an important role in the healing arts. Plants provide us with food, spiritual inspiration, and oxygen and therefore are intrinsic to life itself. Plants are also essential to the design of a holistic nursing practice that is to support and nurture life. This book is organized according to the spheres of holistic nursing and elements of nurses' nature care—spiritual (fire), mental (air), emotional (water), and physical (earth) —recorded in nursing history.[3] Nurses, who integrate whole-plant remedies such as juices, extracts, compresses, poultices, teas, syrups, soups, plasters or baths in their care of clients, are demonstrating the art and science of an enduring holistic nursing tradition.

Ten years ago, I wrote a book titled Delmar's *Integrative Herb Guide for Nurses*[4] based upon my experiences in herbal art and science from wildcrafting and botanical identification to cultivation, harvest, and plant processing, formulation, herbal applications in the care of clients, and even a few years in spagyric experimentation. The book has been used as a reference and textbook in at least fifteen countries by nurses, herbalists, health practitioners, and the public. It is, as I have been told many times, unique in that it is a book specifically *written by a nurse-herbalist about nurse-herbalism*. Since writing the *Herb Guide*, I have researched the history of nurse-herbalism, particularly of that in the United States and Europe. I have worked and taught with traditional healers in Turtle Island (United States and Canada), Hawaii, Africa, and Central America, and continued to develop the science and art of nurse-herbalism and its translation in contemporary practice settings. I have also continued to develop the integration of Traditional Chinese Medicine (TCM) practice and nursing, some of the results of which are shared in this book.

Because nursing is a unique discipline unlike others in which healing plants may be a focus such as medicine, herbalism, naturopathy,

---

3   Martha Libster, "Elements of Care: Nursing Environmental Theory in Historical Context," *Holistic Nursing Practice* 22, no. 3 (2008).

4   ———, *Delmar's Integrative Herb Guide for Nurses* (Albany, NY: Delmar Thomson Learning, 2002).

or pharmacy, the application of plants in nursing care and comfort is truly unique. This book seeks to define the unique qualities of nurse-herbalism by focusing on herbalism in terms of nursing scope of practice, nursing scientific theory, principles of holistic nursing, and the art of demonstrating nurses' nature care with plants as it has been conveyed throughout history. This book also includes stories from my twenty-five years of clinical experiences, lessons learned about practice, scientific understanding, and *integrative insights* from my nursing practice and research, most particularly in nurse-herbalism.

"Integrative insight" is the phrase that I have used since writing the *Herb Guide*. The phrase was inspired by my scientific and creative work with plants. To learn about the ways in which a particular plant heals, I employ a number of ways of knowing which lead to integrative insight. I apply plants in practice with different people, grow plants and/or harvest them in the wild, make different remedies from the plants, and taste and apply the plants to my own body. I also read botanical research on the constituent parts of plants as well as any clinical trial research done with the whole plant or its constituents. The depth and breadth of understanding that occurs as a result of the experience with a plant in which body, soul, and mind actively invite learning and remain mindfully receptive to outcomes that will often challenge any preconceived human notions of the natural world we may have is a cornerstone for integrative insight. Plants can teach us many things; yet they are non-verbal. Their "instruction" is perceived by us through different ways of knowing such as insight. Psychological science informs us that this way of knowing and communicating occurs in the non-verbal world—at the level of the subconscious and unconscious mind with all of its sense experience, patterns, and symbolism. Openness to integrative insight and a commitment to reflective practice are the invitation for a synergistic understanding of the plant world, an enlightening human-plant relationship, and a rich understanding of the healing potential that can emerge as a result of a shared space and shared consciousness with members of the plant kingdom.

The focus of this book is not encyclopedic or exhaustive; rather it is pointed to what I know best—my clinical work and research in partnership with some specific plants that I have come to know quite well because they have a very real affinity for the work and service that nurses provide people and communities. Nursing's tradition has focused mostly on herbal teas; topical applications, such as compresses, poultices, distillates, baths, and floral waters; and other solutions such as syrups and alcohol extracts. *The Nurse-Herbalist* focuses on the integration of these traditional remedies with which we have had a successful history of application in care and comfort.

The impetus for this book has been to more fully respond to my readers' and students' requests. For decades, I have heard nurses say that they would use herbal remedies in practice if they could just figure out how to do it legally, ethically, and safely. In 2000, when I published the *Herb Guide*, I thought that would help. It did to a certain extent. While many have found the *Herb Guide* to be a good practice reference, it did not seem to thoroughly address the needs of nurses who wanted help in actually creating a nurse-herbalist practice that is congruent with scope of practice and the tenets of nursing science. This book addresses this in much greater detail.

WONDERING ABOUT
ST. JOHN'S WORT'S STORY

Plant-human relationships inspire stories and stories inspire integrative insights. I will discuss integrative insight further on but think it important that the plant stories begin here. Plants have much to teach. They are wonder-full in that their stories sometimes evoke in us a wonder about this natural world that we call Earth. This story about St. John's Wort has had me in a state of wonder about the plant and nature herself for years. This is how the story goes.

Many nurses I have spoken with over the years have strong ties to the plant world and have been really perplexed as to how to fully integrate plants into a twenty-first century nursing practice that often requires such extensive focus on high-tech devices and drugs as well as systems of care that can seem so far removed from the earth elements—fire, air, water, and earth—the common bond that links human beings with the green and flowered world. I can really relate. Even after I had practiced for eight years (from 1984 – 1986 and 1989 – 1995) in holistic community clinics where I freely used herbs in my nursing care, I moved to Colorado and worked in a hospital where my education, botanical knowledge, and experience were really put to the test.

Many years ago, an herbal teacher of mine had taught me what the scientist Paracelsus and other renowned teachers of plant medicine, including twentieth-century American herbalist John Christopher, maintained: that "the plant medicines we need grow outside our backdoor." The theory seemed fairly abstract to me when I first heard it and I remember thinking that I would tuck it away in my mind and someday, somehow I would be shown evidence of the truth of the statement or not. A number of theories such as this are taught today as a routine part of herbal education. The back door theory was proved for me in a vivid experience when I was working as a nurse on a postpartum labor and delivery unit in a suburb of Denver, Colorado, in the 1990s.

Over the course of a number of weeks, physicians had delivered several babies on the unit by performing a fourth-degree episiotomy on the mothers. This really concerned everyone because it was not typical to do so many fourth-degrees and the women who had to undergo the procedure were so uncomfortable after delivery. I was also concerned because I knew that fourth-degrees were often avoidable. Over the years, I observed the results of deliveries performed by a British-educated nurse midwife who massaged the perineum of her laboring mothers with St. John's Wort (*Hypericum perforatum*) oil to help relax the cervix. My observation was that the oil most often prevented the need for any episiotomy, let alone an extensive one. I had also prepared and used the oil in my nursing practice for many years in the healing of wounds and injuries to the nervous system and in trigger point therapy for clients with fibromyalgia. I knew the healing properties of the plant and thought that it would really help those women. As they came into my care at the hospital, I could not help but wish that I knew how to convince our labor and delivery team to consider another approach such as that used by the midwife I had worked with. At that time, I was knowledgeable about nurse-herbalism but not so much about nurses' roles in creating change in hospital systems. Even though I cared so much about the women, I found myself very intimidated to speak up about my nursing knowledge. One morning, I was parking my car behind the hospital (we parked near a field), and I looked up in the hazy sunlight to see an entire field of small, yellow flowers. Every year, I had wildcrafted

9

St. John's Wort flowers to make oil and tinctures for my clients, family, and friends. But that year, there had been no flowers. My herbal colleagues and I could find no plants in the mountains at all. It had been a very peculiar year in that regard. As you might imagine, when I went to investigate the flowers in the field, I found that the yellow flowers were indeed St. John's Wort. There was a huge field of the flowers growing literally outside the back door of the hospital just as the herbal teachers had said the herbs that we need do. Never before had I seen such a demonstration of a theoretical proving. The medicines we need really do grow outside our back door. I have seen it many times since then.

What was particularly interesting about this situation with St. John's Wort was that I had tried to find the flowers in the mountains as I had done in years past. There did not seem to be any flowers for harvest on the feast of St. John, June 24th, as there should have been. By July, when I discovered the field of plants outside the hospital in that suburb of Denver, it appeared to us as if all of the plants had magically come down from higher elevations to grow right outside that hospital unit where I had prayed for assistance from that very flower. It was such a powerful spiritual experience in understanding the consciousness and life force of healing plants, as well as my own connection with the plant world, which I had actually been aware of since early childhood. I remember speaking to the nurse manager about the presence of the St. John's Wort. But even with her support, we could not figure out a way at that time to create the change that we knew could help the doctors and nurses as well as the women facing episiotomy. I vowed to dedicate my life to figuring out a way to create that very system change and to tell this story—St. John's Wort's story—wherever and whenever I could.

While elated at my personal plant connection, I was quite distraught at the outcome in the hospital. Unfortunately, the labor and delivery staff never could take advantage of the healing power of the St. John's Wort. My husband, friend, and I harvested what we needed for our remedies and left the rest. When I went back the next year to the field behind the hospital, there was not a single St. John's Wort plant to be found. Although they had appeared at the hospital's back door wanting to help us, the door was not yet open to them. Since that time I have worked to open those doors for plant partnerships, but it is not easy. This experience and many others like it are the reason I refer to nurse-herbalism as plant partnership. My experiences have shown me that plants are sentient life and that their healing effects are expressed *in relationship* with people—a dimension of healing yet to be more fully explored in health science. Because they are sentient, I try to be conscious about the language I use when referring to them. For example, I often say that nurses "apply" plants in the care and comfort of clients rather than saying that we "use" plants in practice.

My readers' questions have made me realize that although nurses go to continuing education workshops or take courses on herbal medicine, they often leave those educational experiences without the knowledge of how, when, where, and why to partner with plants in the creation of a nurse-herbalist practice. *The Integrative Herb Guide* addressed the professional, legal, and ethical issues involved in the practice of nurse-herbalism to a certain extent, but it was not a how-to guide for designing a practice and therefore did not fully address important concerns of nurses who were ready for the challenge of creating change in their professional practice circles to include herbs from simple single-herb remedies (simples) to formulations.

This book, *The Nurse-Herbalist: Integrative Insights for Holistic Practice*, has a two-fold purpose. First, this book seeks to educate and address the professional needs and concerns of those who are called spiritually and professionally to partner with plants in their scientific and creative endeavors in nursing comfort and care. In so doing, the second purpose is to dispel any lingering myths and misconceptions, ambiguity, and intimidation associated with herb use in nursing and midwifery perpetuated over the centuries that would impede the opportunity to freely experience the joy and healing that is available to those who enter the natural beauty of the plant world receptive to the potential for integrative insights that can guide holistic practice. I hope to accomplish this in this book that speaks to the heart of the matter by giving you experiments in which you can apply the content immediately in your own practice.

It is possible to make your use of herbs in nursing care congruent with nursing scope of practice and any ethical, moral, social, and professional obligations. Professional congruence is a key. The context for nurse-herbalism is nursing care. This means that the language used in describing herbalism, the treatment of clients from assessment to evaluation and scholarship all relate to nursing science and art. This book provides examples and case studies and reflects the way in which I practice and teach nurse-herbalism—as professional nursing. I advocate for *nurse*-herbalism and differentiate it quite clearly from the practice of medicine, pharmacy, and herbalism. The practice described here is rooted in nursing scholarship, experience, policy, creative practice, theory, and science. *The Nurse-Herbalist* also further delineates the work that I started in the *Integrative Herb Guide* to reveal "integrative insight" as an open door to health and herbal diplomacy.

INTEGRATIVE INSIGHT

The plant world is so very full of beauty, color, fragrance, and extraordinary design. Entering the healing world of plants can inspire integration and insight. Integration is the ability to *embody* or make something a genuine part of our whole being. Being embodied is easy when we interact with a world that is beautiful and fragrant and there is no danger that would cause us to raise our defense mechanisms. Integration is also a quality of heart that supports the desire to broaden one's consciousness to move beyond preconceived agendas that preclude us from including and affirming others who have their own ideas, feelings, and experiences. Insight is the understanding, sensitivity, heightened awareness, and humanity that become possible as a result of this broadened state of consciousness. Plants are able to inspire integrative insight in us because, as I will show through numerous case studies and examples, they are sentient, living beings with consciousness and energy fields that interact with our own. The whole-plant remedies used in nursing care are quite different from pharmaceutical drugs because they are alive!

Because plants are alive, there is a living ethic that accompanies the work with healing plants. It begins with acknowledgment that plants are sentient. They are receptive and responsive. Some people, scientists to shamans, have concluded from their study of plants that they are also intelligent and feeling. Many of the accounts for how I, too, have come to know about the sentient nature of plants are recorded in this book. Throughout my nursing career, I have partnered with plants in helping people. But long before that, actually all of my life, healing plants have been by my side, in my thoughts and dreams, and connected with my spirit. They have healed me and are my source of inspiration for creating ways to help others. The beauty of the plant world raises me up when human suffering stifles my senses. Exploring them has given me some of the greatest scientific experiences and existential awakenings of my life. Therefore, I must caution you that this guide for nurse-herbalist practice is written not only from a human perspective. The "voice" of the plant world as I experience it is given an equal platform. For example, you will learn not only of the human regulations that govern your practice but also the laws that protect plant populations. You will be encouraged to commune and communicate directly with plants in suggested nurse-herbalist "experiments."

Plants require our attention and protection because they are a vulnerable population. Because they are non-verbal, we must attune to them. Plant attunement is a foundation for integrative insight. In return for attuning to plants, they provide us with opportunities for healing. Plant remedies affect body, mind, emotion, and spirit. This is why this book is a guide to *holistic* practice, one in which the heart and soul of people-plant partnerships are accessed in designing a practice to heal all.

A Plant Profile of Heal All

Although plants do not use a voice, they often communicate quite clearly with those who are willing and able to tune in to their patterns of non-verbal communication. Plants communicate through behavior. Our ability to perceive and interpret that behavior is what determines whether communication occurs or not. We use our senses to interpret non-verbal behaviors that manifest as patterns of movement, sound, and energy. If you are having trouble imagining plant communication, start with human babies. Babies do not use formal language yet parents interpret their behavioral cues and vocalizations so that they can understand or communicate with their infant. As time passes since the day of birth, parents begin to recognize a pattern in their baby's cries, movements, and energy levels. For instance, a mother might recognize that her infant is beginning to get sleepy because the baby starts to yawn, rub its eyes, and make short puffing sounds.

A major difference between plant and infant communication is that plants do not vocalize. Therefore, one must become quite adept at observing their behavioral patterns over time. As we work with plant patterns, we begin to understand the plant's presence and their abilities to help us in healing. The first step in mastering plant communication is to engage all of one's senses and use them to recognize and affirm the presence of plants. Plants are present everywhere! They are in the houses we live in, the food that we eat, and the medicines we use. They are part of our celebrations and rituals: holly at Christmas, horseradish at Passover, bay leaf in victory, and rose petals at baptisms. These examples represent the human perspective. However, partnering with plants in healing requires full communication as an open two-way channel.

Think about the presence of plants from their perspective that is without a connection to human events of any kind. Become aware of the presence of plants by becoming an active participant in their world. Use your senses to validate the patterns of their presence. This is a highly subtle process because this work is done in the non-verbal world, the realm of the subconscious and unconscious mind. The process involves attuning one's self deliberately, consciously, and enthusiastically to plants.

Start with observation and simple acknowledgment of the plants in your environment and then as you grow in your plant communication connections you will understand more about this subtle world of plants and their power to heal. You will come to experience first-hand that the healing power of plants is much vaster than simply providing substance for human remedies. They are sentient life with a story to tell. That story is as healing, in my experience, as their chemical constituents and the chopped up fibrous material we put in capsules. They have the ability to heal—one and all—in a way that is quite unique. The best way to understand their healing ways is to be with the plants and to listen to the stories of people who have insight into their world.

This story I will tell you about the presence of plants starts in the country of the Wiyot People in Northern California. It is the story of a beautiful low-lying plant commonly known as "Heal All" or "All Heal" (*Prunella vulgaris*). The plant covers much of the hillsides in Wiyot country. It has been one of my favorite herbs since I first met it in the late 1980s. I don't really have "favorite" plants per se because I truly love them all, but I had an affinity for or recognition of this plant right away. Maybe I knew in some part of my mind or being that someday I would be writing their story in a book teaching about partnering with healing plants? I am a historian storyteller and it is the right time to tell this Heal All's story.

I think that I always liked Heal All so much because of its gentle beauty and its versatility in terms of its healing properties. The "signature" of the purple flower, (that is the reference to the geometric congruence with a human body part or system), is the throat or, more specifically, the trachea. This means that the flower head actually looks like a trachea. In medieval plant science, Paracelsus developed a theory called the Doctrine of Signatures in which it was presumed that there was a connection between the structure, color, and smell of a plant and the body part or system it could be used for in healing. I have given the tea of the aerial parts (leaf and flower) of Heal All to children and adults with sore throats and they have felt "*all* better." I also have given the tea to those with stomach upset and applied salve made from the flower in the healing of wounds.

When I went to Mohawk country in upstate New York in 2005 to visit one of the wisdom-keepers for Turtle Island (United States and Canada), she and I went on a medicine walk together. We came upon Heal All at one point and she said that it was "one of her favorite plants." I told her that it was also one of my favorites. We then shared stories about the ways in which we have harvested and prepared the medicine from the plant and how we have applied the plant in the care of others. When I went to Northern California, I thought of the wisdom-keeper because Heal All was growing everywhere!

Other than the local herbalists, the people I spoke to about the presence of Heal All did not seem to notice it. Its ubiquitous presence begged the question if there was some reason that the geographic area needed the qualities of the All Heal plant. I found that it really did. In 1860, there had been some white men who had massacred most of the Wiyot people on that land. In a meeting with one of the tribal leaders I mentioned the All Heal. I told her the story of All Heal as I had come to know it. She smiled and we talked about the plant's ability to heal all of the wounds of people and wondered about the plant's presence on the land as a way of healing the place as well. On two occasions I, as a white woman, had been given the opportunity to communicate and connect with an Indian elder because of All Heal. The plant represented not only potential for human medicine but also an encounter with the land that could ultimately heal through the transmutation of the prejudice that resulted in historical records of death and destruction.

Our readiness to perceive and seek to understand the presence of plants seemed to be a match for the plant's readiness to communicate and teach us their healing power. It was the foundation for opportunity. Recognizing the importance of Heal All to the healing of land as well as people occurred as a result of communication over time with a plant that is living medicine. I define that communication as meaningful and recognizable experience of patterned energetic exchange that does not include verbalization.

The story seems so simple, but in truth, I have witnessed so many missed opportunities for communication as human beings ignore and even dismiss the healing *presence* and patterns of plants. It also seems a bit surreal as to the power of the presence of Heal All in my life and the lives of others. Perhaps that is how it got its powerful name—*Heal All*? But plant-human communication is an acquired skill. Experiencing plant patterns in the subtle world is a skill rather than a phenomenon. That skill has to do with the ability to enter the green world, the plant world, where the vibration of existence is very different from that of humans. That vibration is gentle, quiet, and delicate in comparison with the human world. This description holds true even when referring to the presence of gnarly vines or to trees with the toughest of barks. One must change vibration to enter the world of plants. Vibration change and communication occur as a result of change in consciousness. This skill is not unknown to people. The ability to change vibration can be observed in adult to infant communication. But just as I witness that some people do not really seek to enter the world of an infant and appreciate and validate them for who they are, many do not appreciate the sentient world of plants, even when representatives end up on the dinner table or outside the back door. Human relationship with plants is most often unconscious if not nonexistent.

The holistic nurse-herbalist heals in many ways and is not simply a master of dosing out plant supplements. Understanding and communicating with plants and sharing their stories are fundamental to nurse-herbalism. It is in the story, the history, that we learn the healing power and properties of plants. This is a book about realizing opportunities to master skill in partnering with the world of healing plants. Nurses of previous generations have had this relationship with plants. They have cultivated and treasured their knowledge of healing plants. Their knowledge has been preserved in receipt (recipe) books, domestic guides, and sick room management books.[5] Nurses have so many opportunities today to carry on the nurse-herbalist tradition in rural and international nursing services, hospice and home health agencies, parishes, tribal nations, school health, and private practices.

The plant kingdom is a vibrant, colorful, aromatic, and quiet world of sentient life that has provided some of the most simple and yet powerful remedies, which nurses have used in professional caregiving practices throughout the centuries. Plant remedies are an extraordinary chalice for healing expression and therefore require a different experience in education and scientific exploration. This book is an introduction to that practice that takes place in gardens, fields, and forests with the plants themselves, for they are the most appropriate teachers. This book will guide you element by element—fire, air, water, and earth—to commune with plants as you create a holistic practice that adheres to the laws of man, nature, and plants, and of professional nursing standards. The book also prepares you to engage the plant world and interact with people in other disciplines such as horticulture and ethnobotany in order to create and sustain an informed practice that resonates with the joy and beauty of the plant world. *The Nurse-Herbalist* seeks also to inspire you to enter the ether, the fifth element of nature care, where you may experience a change in consciousness and experience integrative insight, peace, and loving kindness because of powerful plant partnerships.

Welcome to the vibrant world of the seeds and sound, fruits and fragrance, leaves and colors, flowers and flavor, roots and textures that will amaze you. Connect through your senses to them and the plants will lead you where you need to go and to what you need to learn. Enter the garden, meadow, forest, desert, ocean or river and you will find them— the plants—awaiting connection and quietly and eagerly ready to show you what they can do to help and heal—all.

---

5   Libster, *Herbal Diplomats: The Contribution of Early American Nurses (1830-1860) to Nineteenth-Century Health Care Reform and the Botanical Medical Movement.*

REFERENCES

Farnsworth, Norman, Olayiwola Akerele, Audrey Bingel, Djaja Soejarto, and Zhengang Guo. "Medicinal Plants in Therapy." *Bulletin of the World Health Organization* 63, no. 6 (1985): 965-81.

Libster, Martha. *Delmar's Integrative Herb Guide for Nurses.* (Albany, NY: Delmar Thomson Learning, 2002).

———. "Elements of Care: Nursing Environmental Theory in Historical Context." *Holistic Nursing Practice* 22, no. 3 (2008): 160-70.

———. *Herbal Diplomats: The Contribution of Early American Nurses (1830-1860) to Nineteenth-Century Health Care Reform and the Botanical Medical Movement.* (Thornton, CO: Golden Apple Publications, 2004).

CHAPTER ONE

Preparation for Plant Partnership

What is your connection with the green world? Partnering with plants in creating a nurse-herbalist practice will be rooted in that very connection. Take out a blank journal and write down the plants for which you have a memory. What plants stand out for you? Start with infancy and childhood and end with the present moment. Plants are associated with human life events and so some of those plant memories may be happy memories and others may not. Be mindful of the memories associated with this list of plants as they can influence your experiences when studying nurse-herbalism and performing the herbal experiments in this book. Memories can inspire and they can hinder the learning process. I have seen this many times. Because partnership with plants in nurse-herbalism is a non-verbal process, all associated non-verbal functions such as memory become important in the choices made for designing a practice. Your plant memories have already helped to form your beliefs, specifically health beliefs about medicinal plants and herbalism. They contribute to the professional framework or foundation for which you have and will continue to be a nurse-herbalist.

One of the first steps in designing a nurse-herbalist practice is to create or adopt a professional framework. I suggest that nurse-herbalists create a "space" or framework for the organization of their thoughts and beliefs about partnering with plants just as they would choose the best room on a unit in which to place a newly admitted client coming to a hospital or infirmary for care. A professional model for practice can provide that framework. *The Nurse-Herbalist* presents three practice models—consumer, herbalist, and integrative—that can be used as an organizing framework for nurse-plant partnerships. While nurse-herbalists can employ all three models, sometimes within the same client interaction, the integrative model is ultimately the best support for creating a holistic practice. This chapter detailing the consumer and herbalist models focuses on the development of the nurse-herbalist's ability to partner with healing plants to catalyze change and help people solve tough problems by employing the nursing process. The integrative model is described in the next chapter. It includes three views or paradigms of health and healing that support the integrative process: biomedical, traditional, and holistic nursing. These three models and paradigms discussed in these two chapters provide the framework for the demonstration of caring professional practice that each nurse-herbalist expresses during the nursing process—from assessment to evaluation of outcomes that can ultimately lead to what I have come to know as *integrative insight*!

PRACTICE MODELS

What is your current practice model? If you can definitively answer this question, then please know that the information and suggestions that follow are meant only to enhance your practice. The practice models I include here are broad and inclusive enough that I think you will be able to find congruence with them and your current model. I like to learn new things and add to my repertoire of guidelines and techniques because I work with such a variety of clients. In my experience there is no "one size fits all" approach to care and therefore having a repertoire of guidelines and theoretical frameworks is helpful in creating a more thorough, holistic, and effective practice that really helps people. For those who do not have a practice model or defined approach to care, I hope that you will find this section helpful and perhaps even a bit liberating.

I have learned over the years, especially in my work with plants, that practice structure, such as guidelines and models, is helpful, especially when I am called to solve the really tough problems. The beauty of science is its organization of thought, which allows for pattern recognition, communication of discovery, and evolution of understanding of the natural world. Plant identification and taxonomy is one example in the plant science world. Another example of the usefulness of practice models is from the practice realm—gardening.

I had really never had any problem growing herbs in my gardens in Montana or Colorado, but when I moved to North Carolina where the moist heat was so intense in the summer months and some of the soil had been farmed to death over the years, I found myself reaching for a guideline. When I chose biodynamic gardening, I realized that I was learning a model for care just as is found in nursing science. All my life I had never had to do soil testing. I just watered plants when they looked like they were thirsty and monitored the amount of sun my plants were exposed to. The only problem I ever remember having was when I attempted to transplant *Arnica montana* from its wild mountain habitat to my garden located at a lower altitude. It never worked for me but that was OK. In North Carolina though, I had trouble with a number of plants. I seemed to overwater even when the ground and the plants appeared dry. Plants grew upward but not outward and I realized early on that planting root vegetables such as carrots and radishes in early March was too late for any kind of successful harvest. Just as practice models had helped me throughout my nursing career, the biodynamic gardening model (as well as native farmer friends) helped me understand plants and soil in a whole new way.

Practice models are a framework for scientific process. They help us organize our thoughts, identify problem-and-solution patterns and priorities for care, and communicate our practice with clarity to our colleagues as well as recipients of our care. Each practicing nurse-herbalist educates the public not only about healing plants but also about the care nurse-herbalists provide. The science and art of herbalism is quite broad. Practice models can guide the practitioner in the integration of herbalism and nursing, and provide focus for community or consumer health education. Practice models can also help in the promotion of quality care. The framework and organization they provide helps in identifying areas of care that are strong and effective in helping people and those areas that need shoring up. People have learned to expect and request "quality care" from nurses but their only frame of reference for that care may be the images of hospital nursing they see on television, which are distorted if not detrimental. The public today does not have a frame of reference for what quality nurse-herbalist care is and therefore it is the responsibility of the nurse-herbalist to clearly convey what professional nurse-herbalism is and is not. What nursing is and is not has been a topic of concern in nursing for centuries[1] so I realize as a historian what the task requires. Nurse-herbalists must face the challenge of defining their role in community. Raising one's awareness of the foundations for the construction of practice, such as the application of practice models, is one way to become a clear conveyer of professional quality care.

Consumer Model: *Herbal Dialog About Information and Resources*

The focus of the consumer model for the nurse-herbalist is education, resources, and information rather than clinical intervention. Some nurses choose only to educate and inform patients about herbs; they do not perform their assessments with the intention of providing herbal interventions. In the consumer model of care, the goal is to hone the client's specific question about herbs, assess the resources that they have to answer their question, and help them obtain herb information and resources that they need to be an informed herb and herbal product consumer.

One of the most common points of herbal information that people living in industrialized countries need is the understanding of the differences between traditional herbs and herbal products. Nurses are in an excellent position to explain the important distinctions between the two.

"Herb" is a broad term most often used to refer to plants used for culinary and medicinal purposes. The word "herb" has traditionally referred to whole plants or whole plant materials whereas "herbal products" is a term that has emerged as a result of industrialization or processing of the plant. Nurses as well as their clients may only know of herbalism as represented by the herbal supplements sold in pharmacies and health food stores in capsules. They often relate herbalism only to

---

1   Florence Nightingale, *Notes on Nursing: What It Is and What It Is Not* (Edinburgh: Churchill Livingstone, 1980 Original publication 1859), 3.

	HERBS	HERBAL PRODUCTS
Source	Gardens, Herb Companies, Wildcrafting	Herb or Pharmaceutical Company
Production	Whole Fresh or Dried Plant	Made of Whole Fresh or Dried Plants. Also made of Plant Constituents
Dosage	Use traditional guidelines	May be based on clinical trials or national materia medica and pharmacy documents
History of Use	Long-term evidence to draw on. Tradition and Folklore recorded in herbals*, recipe/receipt books, diaries, oral history	Short-term evidence. Because of production technology, herbs may be sold in new forms undocumented in history and folklore.

*An herbal is a collection of descriptions of medicinal plants that typically includes common and scientific botanical names, growth patterns, medicinal and culinary properties and applications, toxicity, and history. A Nurses' Herbal is found in Appendix A of this book.

the plants that are ingested and have no experience of applying herbs topically or taking them in the numerous forms that make up the body of herbal science and art of medicine making. Nurses and midwives have traditionally applied herbs in the care of clients, most often as teas and topical applications. Nurses, such as those in the American Shaker and French Daughter of Charity communities, also made and used simple herbal products such as syrups, pills, waters, liniments, and tinctures.[2] An herbal tea made from the flower of a plant, such as chamomile, harvested from a garden would not be referred to as an herbal product or supplement. A chamomile ointment would be. Whole herb chamomile that the consumer can use in making an herbal compress or a steam might be sold in a grocery store but a chamomile compress cannot. An onion is an herb as well as a vegetable. An onion poultice is referred to as an herbal application as opposed to an herbal product. Onions are products sold in the marketplace but onion poultices are not. Neither onions nor onion poultices are referred to as herbal products. Nurses and nurse-herbalists can help the consumer understand the nuances of terms by informing

---

2   Martha Libster, *Herbal Diplomats: The Contribution of Early American Nurses (1830-1860) to Nineteenth-Century Health Care Reform and the Botanical Medical Movement* (Thornton, CO: Golden Apple Publications, 2004).

them about how plants are actually applied in healing practice.

The root of the consumer model is information and resources for further herbal support. Those using a consumer model draw primarily on herbal publications. The consumer advocate may have no direct knowledge of a plant or herbal product in question and no knowledge of herbal applications. In fact, the client may have more botanical knowledge than the nurse. In the consumer model, having direct knowledge or relationship with a specific plant is not imperative to be able to educate the public about herbal information and resources. There are thousands of plants on the planet and I am often introduced by clients to plants that they have in their own sphere of influence. For example, upon moving to North Carolina, people joyously shared their love of rabbit tobacco (*Gnaphalium obtufifolium*) with me. I had not grown up with rabbit tobacco when I had a cold, but they had. Plants bring people together. We share plant stories of healing as a way of getting to know each other and welcome people to our small space on the planet.

If a client moves from questions about herbal information into wanting to know how to apply those herbs in their own health practice, the nurse would then need to refer the client to a knowledgeable herb practitioner. The nurse using the consumer model would not "lead" or advise the client at any time. This is the model used by health sciences and consumer health librarians. They provide wonderful information and resources but do not cross the line into the realm of diagnosis and intervention.

Nurses who have never been educated in nurse-herbalism often feel most comfortable engaging in the consumer model of practice. I have seen those using this practice model become trusted advocates for clients making health decisions. I have also seen some people use the consumer health model to misinform the public, if not instill fears, especially about the application of healing herbs. I have heard a number of students and colleagues over the years state that they will "not give information to anyone about herbs until the herbs have been thoroughly researched and proven safe." While they may be well meaning on one level, they do not realize that their statement is culturally biased, that they are conveying only their belief in how health care is conducted rather than listening to the client. There are a number of scientific, ethical, and professional reasons why this statement about research is an inappropriate thing to say to a consumer/client seeking information and resources.

First, many of the herbs people tend to use more commonly in self-care *have indeed* been researched and therefore the statement is scientifically inaccurate and a gross generalization. I often let people know when I hear them say this that I worked as the director for the information hotline service of the Herb Research Foundation back in 1997 and there were file drawers full of research often including clinical trials on so many herbs. The question then is for them to define what they mean by "thorough" research and "proven safe." This is language used in common social discussions about health science, but scientists who perform research do not and cannot fully "prove" safety as the Food and Drug Administration (FDA) can attest. Different language is used when referring to the scientific process. Quality science acknowledges its limitations.

Research is a tool of the scientist. It is one way of knowing about the object of discovery, which in this case is an herb or herbal product. Waiting for proof through research before providing information about healing herbs could mean that one would never give herbal information and resources. This could lead to a violation of the American Nurses Association (ANA) Nursing Code of Ethics, which states that: "Patients have the moral and legal right to determine what will be done with their own person: to be given accurate, complete, and understandable information in a manner that facilitates an informed judgment."[3] Not providing information on herbs simply because of a lack of research is equivalent to withholding information about a particular intervention in nursing care because there is no research. There are many remedies and interventions used in all of the health sciences that have not been studied let alone "proved" by formal research. A study done in the 1990s by the United States Office of Technology Assessment found that only 20 percent of *common* medical interventions at that time had been shown effective through research.[4]

Given the body of knowledge regarding health modalities that have little or no research base, it could be posited that herbalism poses less of a

---

3   ANA Code of Ethics – See Website http://www.nursingworld.org/MainMenuCategories
     /EthicsStandards/CodeofEthicsforNurses.aspx
4   Walter Brown, "The Placebo Effect," *Scientific American* 278, no. 1 (1998).

risk for those who value research in health decision making. Many of the herbs that are commonly known and people have applied in the care of themselves and others have centuries of traditional evidence supporting their application in humans. One might ask the question if there is a reason for conducting research when there is already a centuries-old body of evidence of safe human use in some cases. Many practices such as traditional healing and nursing involve the application of more than one modality, making the use of the "gold standard" randomized controlled clinical trial neither feasible nor ideal. Demanding that all herbs be studied, such as in a clinical trial, is not only unnecessary, it is unaffordable and exponentially time consuming. Therefore, it is best if nurses follow ANA ethical standards of practice as well as consumer health advocacy models and provide the best evidence and information they can from a number of sources representing multiple ways of knowing.

Consumers often ask questions about simples or single whole herb remedies, such as raspberry leaf tea for toning the uterus during the third trimester of pregnancy, elderberry syrup for allaying symptoms of influenza, and calendula salve for diaper rash, rather than complex formulations. They typically refer to the plants they are interested in by common names. Nurses who discuss herbal simples with their clients typically learn about them from each other. One study conducted in certified nurse-midwives (CNMs) showed that 69 percent of those who used herbs to stimulate labor learned from other CNMs. Sixty-four percent of the nurse-midwifery education programs included instruction in the use of herbs for labor in their curricula and 92 percent included informal discussion,[5] but CNMs continued to rely on each other for herbal education just as has been the historical format for education across centuries. One of the simples I often introduce to nurses and nurse-midwives is the preparation and application of a lemon compress for use in patients with fever.[6] Nurses often comment to me that while they may not feel as comfortable working with herbal formulations or supplements, they have no concerns about simples, such as lemon compresses made from whole herbs, which they can

---

5   Barbara McFarlin et al., "A National Survey of Herbal Preparation Use by Nurse-Midwives for Labor Stimulation.," *Journal of Nurse-Midwifery* 44, no. 3 (1999).
6   See Nurse's Herbal Appendix A of this book for recipe for lemon compress.

learn and apply in the care of clients very quickly.

Clients also ask questions about herbal products that contain multiple ingredients. These formulations may be based upon traditional recipes used in many people over time or they may be the result of the ingenuity of an herbalist, phyto-pharmacy scientist, or research and development team. In a consumer health model, formulations represent greater challenges to clients and their caregivers than do simples. The reason is that every herb in a formulation should be indicated for a person, energetically as well as from a phyto-therapeutic and biochemical standpoint. A formulation, for example, could be a concoction of herbs known to support a specific system such as the cardiovascular system. There are many herbs that fall into this category from a Western standpoint. But an herbalist has other criteria than this system's approach that they use when formulating for a client. Formulation will be discussed in more detail later on but it is important to identify here that those nurses and nurse-herbalists using a consumer health approach focus on single herbs when giving information, particularly if the client is using a formulation. This is because the focus of the consumer model is primarily education rather than intervention. Formulations that might be likened to herbal recipe patterns are supposed to match the client's pattern of need. Discussing formulations leads the conversation directly down the pathway to intervention. Focusing herb information giving on the subject of simples or the individual herbs in a formulation is the consumer model approach that I recommend to help the nurse or nurse-herbalist maintain their role as a client educator and resource. The following is a simple guideline for herbal counseling using a consumer practice model:

1. Identify and be clear that you know what herb or herbs the client is asking about. Read the labels of bottles, ask to see whole herbs, and show a joyful interest in plant remedies that promotes dialog about herbs so that the client feels supported rather than interrogated. Remember the rabbit tobacco…you, too, can learn about herbs from clients.

2. Focus on single herbs in your educational plan. It is possible to find information about individual herbs but

much more challenging to find information about specific herbal products. Assessing the effectiveness and validity of a formulation in general or for a particular client requires a significant knowledge of herbalism. The situation with herbal education is not unlike what nurses do with education about medication. For example, if a patient is taking pain pills following a surgery, nurses explain what is in the pill that is a combination narcotic and analgesic. Explaining the effects of the drug, the nurse breaks down the information into two parts: information about the action of analgesics and information about narcotic drugs.

3. Refer the client to a knowledgeable practitioner if they:[7]
    a. Plan to take the herb or herbal product for more than 30 days.
    b. Are pregnant and are treating a condition with an herb or herbal formulation. This does not refer to drinking a beverage that contains small amounts of common herbs.
    c. Are a parent considering giving herbs to an infant younger than 15 months of age. The liver of an infant is immature.
    d. Are taking prescription drugs on a daily basis.

None of these conditions necessarily preclude a person from taking or applying an herb. They just require more in-depth consideration.

The consumer model can also be used by nurse-herbalists when they do not know a client very well. Examples of when I use this model are when caring for clients in a hospital setting, when people ask questions during a public lecture, and in social situations. The consumer model allows for the promotion of herbal dialog and education without putting the client and nurse-herbalist at great risk. The consumer model provides the space for the talking *about* care rather than the specifics of caring

---

7   Martha Libster, "Guidelines for Selecting a Medical Herbalist for Consultation and Referral: Consulting a Medical Herbalist," *Journal of Alternative and Complementary Medicine* 5, no. 5 (1999).

interventions for that person or persons that happens when a healing relationship and the nursing process have been initiated. If a client seeks more specific care, then a referral should be made for herbal care.

Herbalist Model: *The Presence of Plants and Systems*

Nurses who partner with plants also practice from an herbalist model when they are educated and actively engaged in herbalism, the study of the application of medicinal plants. The focus of herbal education is the healing plants. Herb teachers often refer to healing plants as the best teachers about healing plants! This is why herbal teachers bring plants and plant materials to the classroom. Some lessons in herbalism, such as when studying with traditional healers, do not involve the use of books or even classrooms. Lessons are conducted outside with the plants in their natural habitats or cultivated gardens. Any reputable herbal education program or course of study can be beneficial to the nurse-herbalist *if* the nurse-herbalist becomes engaged with the world of plants through that course of study. Herbal education typically strikes a balance between plant education and application to human health. There are continuing education courses and programs as well as professional and educational publications that focus solely on plant applications and never invite understanding of or interaction with healing plants. This is associated with the biomedical approach, which I will discuss later on.

Nurse-herbalists develop their botanical knowledge in relationship with plants. I grew up with plants as a big part of my experience in the world so I am quite biased toward anything that supports the human-plant relationship. The baby book my mother kept as a history of my life includes a photo of my older sister feeding me marigolds when I was but one year old. Marigold is one of my favorite herbs today. And on my third birthday, as my grandmother told the story, I ordered "Artichokes!!" from the restaurant maître d'. I was *called* to nursing but *I am* a plant-loving herbalist. I prefer to learn by relating the object of study to the presence of plants. In my being I cannot separate the human, animal, and plant worlds so when I learn or teach, I ultimately find myself including all life forms. Perhaps this has something to do with my upbringing as well as who I am. I spent my childhood playing outdoors. A fun afternoon for me was sitting in a raspberry patch talking with my friends and playing with the dog while eating raspberries. Later on in my career, I "lived and breathed" herbs while managing an herb program and gardens. Growing plants is one way of knowing plants. Studying medicinal plants from books alone is not adequate for entering into the science and art of herbalism. This view is shared by most herbalists today and was the prevailing belief of early Americans about herbalism and the practice of medicine prior to rapid industrialization. Nursing programs may include textbooks that discuss herbs but that type of learning experience is not sufficient. The nurse-herbalist must seek out the full educational experience with plants offered in herbal education.

Herbal education may be guided by a traditional model or philosophy, such as Ayurvedic herbalism or Unani medicine, or it may be conveyed as is typical in many American educational programs and publications using a systems model approach: that is explaining which herbs are applied in the case of problems with anatomical or physiological systems such as the nervous, digestive, or respiratory systems. Herbal knowledge is also taught under the broader frameworks of nutritional or medical science or phytotherapy. All such programs have the potential to endow the nurse-herbalist with a medicinal plant perspective. However, I recommend two frameworks for the study and use of herbs in nursing practice. First is to study the plants applied for the care of persons with particular *health patterns*. The health patterns include sleep and rest, mobility, pain, energy, emotions and thought, hormone balance, and immune response *(See Appendix A)*. The herbal tradition I recommend for study that most closely complements health patterns and nursing science is Traditional Chinese Medicine (TCM). I will give a comparison of TCM and nursing in the next section on the integrative model.

Herbalists study the concepts recorded in the writings of Greek and Roman physicians who were renowned for their knowledge of plant medicines. The teachings of Dioscorides, Hippocrates, and Galen, to name a few, are still discussed today in herbal education and historical texts. Medicinal plants have been used within a theoretic or scientific framework for centuries. Herbalists study the humoral theory of physicians such as Hippocrates and Galen. "In Hippocratic teaching the healthy body was one in which the four 'humors' of blood, bile, phlegm, and choler were equally balanced. . . . Careful observation of a plant's specific action disappeared, and was replaced by Galen's theoretical approach which assigned every plant to its proper station in an orderly scheme."[8] Herbalists study a system of plant use defined by renowned physicians such as Avicenna (980–1037) and, much later, Culpeper (1616–1654) who included the science of astrology in determining which plant was used for a particular patient. "The Arabs were experts in astrology, which they had developed to a precise science . . . both the patient and the medicinal plant were subject to astrological influences. . . . Culpeper consulted the motion of the planets when prescribing for his patients."[9] Many herbalists today study the science of astrology not only for the purpose of matching the plant with the patient but also for the purpose of understanding order in nature. Plants and stars are both believed to be linked to the natural order of the universe. Historically, herbalists have understood the effects of astrology (the position of the stars, the moon, and the planets at the time of harvest or medicinal use) on the properties of herbs given to patients. There are also some herb manufacturers who integrate astrological principles when growing, harvesting, and creating their products.

Another historical theory that is learned by clinical herbalists is the Doctrine of Signatures often associated with the work of Paracelsus, a Swiss-German physician (1493–1541). The Doctrine of Signatures states that each plant has a signature, something in the way it looks or how it grows, that lets the user know the healing purpose of the plant. For example, the potatoes mentioned before have "eyes" and are therefore used in the healing of the eyes. Also, the shape of *Panax ginseng* root looks like the shape of the human body. This signature of the whole body suggests that ginseng's properties may support the whole person. And indeed, ginseng is traditionally used to promote energy or "qi" in the whole body. The signature of violets is that they hide from the sun and love the shade; therefore, they have been found to be of benefit to the migraine sufferer whose individual "signature" or "pattern" is sensitivity to light and they desire to seek the solace of a darkened room.

In the Doctrine of Signatures, there is a matching of signatures

---

8   Barbara Griggs, *Green Pharmacy* (Rochester, VT: Healing Arts Press, 1991), 15-16.
9   Ibid., 25, 97.

or patterns of the patient with the patterns associated with a plant. One of the plant remedies I use most often according to the Doctrine of Signatures is grape *(Vitis vinifera)*. The signature of the grape is associated with the lungs: the large stem representing the main stem bronchus and the grapes the alveoli. Green grapes are cooling to the lungs and red or purple grapes warm the lungs. I find that I most often have reason to cool the lungs when the client's sputum is yellow or green, which are symptoms of heat, or they have a dry burning cough such as after undergoing diagnostic procedures in which physicians prescribe chemical bowel cleansing liquids.

Some may consider this theoretic system "primitive." If they mean primitive in the sense that it is "relating to the earliest stage of development,"[10] this is not the case. If they mean that the Doctrine of Signatures is "of a people or a culture that is nonindustrial and often non-literate and tribal,"[11] this is not really the case either. "Time-honored" and "accessible" would be far better descriptors for theories such as the Doctrine of Signatures, or those theories used in Ayurveda (traditional medicine of India) and TCM that continue to be referenced by the clinical herbalist when deciding on the proper remedy for the individual. The Doctrine of Signatures and other theories used in plant medicine are part of an adaptive system of knowledge used by intelligent people. In the case of the Doctrine of Signatures, numerous health practitioners, especially in Germany and Switzerland, continue to develop their understanding of nature and how it may apply to the healing of human body in regard to the Doctrine of Signatures.

Paracelsus was an unusual physician in his time because he valued the medicinal plant knowledge of the country healers. He worked and studied with them. He also was very biomedically oriented in that he believed and taught that the action of a plant remedy "did not depend upon its qualities such as moistness, but on its *specific* healing virtue, which was determined by its chemical properties."[12]

Although herbalism, like all healing arts, is a caring practice, herbal education does not specifically address the science and art of

10 Merriam Webster, *Merriam Webster's Collegiate Dictionary*, 10th ed. (Springfield, MA: Merriam-Webster, 1999).

11 Ibid.

12 Kremers & Urdang as cited in Griggs, *Green Pharmacy*: 50.

nursing. The nurse-herbalist sometimes chooses to maintain separation between the two worlds. It is possible to separate our herbal practice, assessment, diagnoses, treatments, and clients from our nursing practice—physically speaking—but it is much more difficult to draw strong boundaries between one's philosophy of care that infuses any healing art, herbal, nursing or otherwise. This is what seems to me to be the biggest point of conflict that drives a person to either integrate nurse-herbalism more fully or stop practicing as a nurse all together. I have heard nurse-herbalists say that they feel something missing when they care for patients without the presence of herbs. On the other hand, many have said to me that they feel "more" like a nurse when they are practicing as an herbalist. It is this kind of authentic reflection and struggle that can spawn constructive change in the profession. I, for one, have been moved by it to create change.

In the late 1990s, Beverly Malone, who was the president of the American Nurses Association at that time, came to Denver to speak at a Colorado Nurses Association meeting. During the question and answer period, I stepped up to the microphone and asked her why she thought nurses were leaving nursing to practice modalities such as massage and herbalism. Her response to me was something like, "I do not know but we need people like you to teach us and write about this." I published my first book *Demonstrating Care: The Art of Integrative Nursing*[13] soon after that, but I still do not feel satisfied that we understand why there is this professional splitting that goes on rather than the welcoming of unification, especially when modalities such as herbalism are such an enduring part of nursing heritage. My historical research shows that modalities such as massage and herbalism are healing traditions in nursing. It is sad for me to learn of highly talented, experienced nurses who feel that they must leave the profession just so they can practice the caring modalities that they love and believe are congruent expressions of their nursing philosophy. I was blessed to have had the opportunity to practice for six years in a community clinic where I could use all of my talents in the care of clients. I have also had excellent education and support in being an agent of change. So I started the process back in

---

13   Martha Libster, *Demonstrating Care: The Art of Integrative Nursing* (Albany, NY: Delmar Thomson Learning, 2001).

the '90s to manifest the vision of nurse-herbalism. I believe that the herbalist model is part of the platform for change that is ultimately necessary in the process of bridging and integrating nursing and herbalism more fully.

Herbal Change Agent

In addition to competence and compassion, practice as a nurse-herbalist in private practice or in out-patient care requires a certain level of skill and comfort with independent decision making, leadership, self-determination, and the will to create change. I learned many years ago that creating change in physician-dominant, in-patient hospital systems would be very difficult because of the nursing profession's historical role in that system for the last century. I learned through my historical research of nineteenth-century nursing that this was not always the case and that nurses had held roles in in-patient settings prior to the later part of the century in which they were able to determine patient care. Political, economic, sociocultural, and religious issues were just some of the variables for the strengthening of physician dominance at the time. There is extensive evidence, at least in the United States, the primary geographical focus of my research, that nurses were quite autonomous in years past and able to construct their practice and influence care given in hospitals. Nurses were change agents and reformers as well as caregivers. In my historical study, *Herbal Diplomats*[14], I reconstructed the histories of three communities of nurses, and in so doing defined nurses' professional roles during the period and explained the nurses' use of herbs in practice and in health reform. The three communities studied were the Sisters of Charity, the Shakers, and the Church of Latter Day Saints (Mormons). One historical example of this is taken from a nursing text or "advice book" written in 1840 by Sister Matilda Coskery, a nurse identified by physicians, nurses, and community leaders as an "oracle" in psychiatric care. She wrote in a section of her book on "Teas, Tonics, Etc.":

Make them strong and in a clean vessel, have the water boiling. ...

In warm weather do not make too much at a time & keep it in a

---

14   Libster, *Herbal Diplomats: The Contribution of Early American Nurses (1830-1860) to Nineteenth-Century Health Care Reform and the Botanical Medical Movement.*

cool place. Nurses are often careless in these things, thinking they are only simple matters, thus, they prepare them negligently, & are irregular in giving them—or give them after they are sour & mouldy, & this makes the stomach sick, or getting them irregular does no good. The Dr thinks it is the fault of the tonic & changes it for something stronger, perhaps brandy or some other thing that does real harm- He loses confidence in that tonic, names it to his students and Medical friends who likewise discontinue it, in all these cases that fall into their hands, some stronger thing is given, when the thing itself was right, in right hands. How often, these, seemingly small things, are the beginnings of the death-bed & in many, many cases, Life and Death is (in) the hands of the nurses, more than in the Physicians.

> Coskery (1840), "Advices Concerning the Sick" as cited in Libster and McNeil, *Enlightened Charity*.[15]

This excerpt from Sister Matilda's book provides an approach to the design of a practice in nurse-herbalism if one reads it not only for herbal and nursing knowledge and new ideas for care. It provides insight for the nurse-herbalist who must also understand professional practice issues and one's role in a health care system. She explains quite well what the impact of proper attention to the preparation and administration of teas can be not only on patient outcomes and nursing care but on decision making by physicians and their students. She also demonstrates the power that nurses have to create changes in the in-patient setting, even with simple interventions such as tea preparation, which was by that time, an intervention that the Sisters and their French counterparts, the Daughters of Charity, had used expertly in the care of patients for more than two hundred years.

The word "change" provokes anxiety in some people simply because of its connotations. People frequently associate change with some type of negative or uncomfortable event in which something is relinquished such as a personal habit, object, practice, belief, thought or action. Change may be perceived as that which happens in life that is against one's own

---

15 Martha Libster and Betty Ann McNeil, *Enlightened Charity: The Holistic Nursing Care, Education and Advices Concerning the Sick of Sister Matilda Coskery, (1799-1870).* (Farmville, NC: Golden Apple Publications, 2009), 198.

will or desire. However, people actually serve as the agents of change in their own lives by the decisions that they make. Decisions lead to change. Change does not necessarily require that a person relinquish something. Change can also be about adding something to one's life or a simple shift or movement from one point to another. Let's take, for example, a watercolor painting of a landscape set in an oak frame. If you were asked to "change the painting," you might not even consider painting over it or throwing the painting away, although that would fulfill the requirement for "changing" the painting. You might readily consider other possibilities for creating change, such as changing the frame to a walnut frame or decorating the frame in some way that is complementary to the painting. Most change actually begins with re-framing. There are at least three approaches to re-framing: "adding to," relinquishing, or "moving things around."

Change Experiments

Experiment #1. Try this change experiment with some friends and family. First have each person select a partner to work with. Have each one face their partner and study the appearance of the partner for 30 seconds. Then have the partners turn back to back and give them the following simple instruction: "Change Your Appearance in 3 Ways." After one minute, have the pairs turn around to face each other and give them a few minutes to discover what changes were made. After everyone finishes the experiment, have them sit down and record on a board the number of changes in which the person either gave away, added to, or moved around something in their appearance.

Having done this experiment with groups on numerous occasions, I have found that most people translate "change" to mean relinquish or remove. People take their glasses off rather than move them to their pocket. They remove an earring rather than move the earring to their button hole. Even more rarely do people pick up an object in the environment around them and add it to their appearance as a form of change. Change, whether taking away from, adding to, or shifting a "picture," is the beginning of the process of transition. Change always involves movement that serves as a catalyst for the process of transition. William Bridges, author of *Managing Transitions*, defines transition as a "psychological process for coming to terms with a new situation that change brings about." (p. 3) He describes three stages to the transition process:[16]

1. Letting Go of old ways and identities. (I call this breaking the habit.)
2. Neutral Zone – After letting go of old habits but before the re-patterning has taken hold.
3. Renewal – Coming out of the transition with new energy, new identity, renewed sense of purpose.

Experiment #2: Imagine your nurse-herbalist practice as it is today. What would you change—that is relinquish, add or move around? Write down your vision for change.

Change – Relinquish:

Change – Add:

Change – Move around

Where are you in the process of transition?

Letting Go:

Neutral Zone:

Renewal:

As you participate in these experiments, you are reflecting upon the change and transition process that is part of everyday life. Change is so common that we often forget that it is our response to change and our ability to transition that can define us as people. Illness, injury, and death are major examples of change and transition in the health care world. Creating change is never an easy process, but nurses are actually experts in creating and sustaining changes and transitions with patients and communities moving through healing crises such as illness, injury, and death.

Nurses have a history of leading large social change such as health reform movements in their communities and nations. Before the Civil War, Americans were engaged in a number of attempts to reform such social structures as religion, the banking system, slavery, and health care. Herbs were at the center of health care reform for some Americans.

---

16   William Bridges, Managing Transitions: Making the Most of Change. (Cambridge, MA: Da Capo Press, (2003).

Nurses and midwives were very successful agents of change in their communities' health care "systems" during that period of time.[17] Social changes are made by citizens who act on a vision with the hope of bringing it into manifestation for the good of community. Nurses have held the vision for the inclusion of healing plants in care for many reasons. Herbs are accessible, inexpensive, empowering, and effective.

As you develop your nurse-herbalist practice, pay attention to your perception of change and transition and what impact herbalism has on social change. A renowned American herbalist, Michael Moore, taught me that "herbs are catalysts." Indeed, herbs are change agents, too! Partnering with plants in health care presents an opportunity today for health reform to our nation just as it was given nearly two hundred years ago. Taking time to reflect on your own perception of change and transition can help you help others deal with change and transition in their own lives. It is important to cultivate this particular observation and counseling skill as a change agent who works with catalyzing herbs. Regardless of their application, plant remedies can create powerful shifts or movements in energy flow, circulation, digestion, respiration, or growth in people. These changes are often subtle, occurring gently over time, and are best noted through holistic assessments of body, mind, emotion, and spirit. Herbs catalyze changes defined in herbalism as adaptogen[18], stimulant, cathartic, carminative, sedative, tonic[19], diuretic, demulcent[20], hallucinogen, alterative[21], aphrodisiac, counterirritant, vermifuge[22], febrifuge, emmenagogue, emetic, and vulnerary[23] actions to name just a few.

Reflection and re-framing can catalyze an ability to *perceive* the positive experiences that change and the process of transition bring. Perception is influenced powerfully by consciousness, habit, and momentum. Here is an experiment to demonstrate the power of perception:

---

17   Libster, *Herbal Diplomats: The Contribution of Early American Nurses (1830-1860) to Nineteenth-Century Health Care Reform and the Botanical Medical Movement.*
18   A substance that increases overall, nonspecific resistance to stress.
19   A substance that improves overall general health.
20   A substance that soothes by providing a protective coating and relieving inflammation of the membranes.
21   A substance that gradually changes the metabolism and elimination in the body to improve general health. Formerly known as blood cleansers.
22   A substance that expels parasites from the body.
23   A substance that promotes wound healing.

Experiment #3: Count the F's you see in Figure 1

> # FINISHED FILES ARE THE RESULT OF YEARS OF SCIENTIFIC STUDY COMBINED WITH THE EXPERIENCE OF MANY YEARS.

Figure 1

I have shown this experiment as a slide at conferences and asked people to simply count the F's that they see. On the count of three, I ask them to call out the number of F's that they see. People call out numbers from two to six. There are six F's in the sentence and yet few people actually see the six F's. This experiment really causes people to think about perception and the mind. This experiment shows that we may not always see what is right in front of us. The lesson of this experiment can be applied to herbalism as well. How many plants are there in front of us that we just step on not even perceiving that we have just crushed some medicine beneath our feet until someone—a healer, teacher or other change agent—points them out to us?

Forces of Change

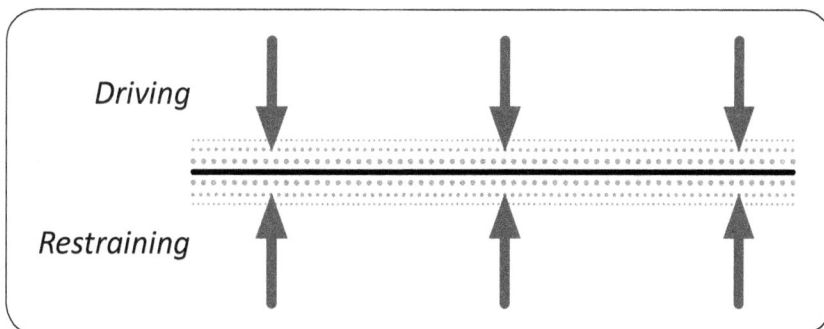

Figure 2

This is a simple diagram of the forces of change that Kurt Lewin elaborated on in his work as a social scientist. Driving forces can be persons, ideas, attitudes, actions, incidents, customs, and interactions that incite a desire or will for change. Change is movement and driving forces move us toward change. Restraining forces represent persons, ideas, attitudes, actions, incidents, customs, and interactions that maintain a certain state or habit. This figure can be interpreted to show balance or status quo. The driving forces for change are equal to the restraining forces. Conflict occurs when opposite forces overlap. The desire to dispel tension resulting from conflict as overlapping forces will often instigate rapid change. For change of any kind to occur, the picture must shift. Restraining forces must decrease or driving forces must increase. There must first be a desire or reason for change.

Illness and disease are a result of changes in the body. Change is also involved in wellness. Health as a process is often described as a continuum from wellness to illness. Change is a constant in the health process. Healing modalities such as nursing care and herbal remedies and applications catalyze change. If the changes catalyzed by herbal remedies and applications are viewed as beneficial, the plants are often called "medicine." Herbalists partner with plants that people may not acknowledge as medicine. There are forces that shift perception of plants typically eaten as food toward recognition as medicine.

Changing Food into Medicine

From the definition of medicine, "a substance or preparation used in treating disease; something that affects well-being,"[24] just about any substance on the planet could be a medicine, if it is used to treat disease or affect someone's well-being in some way. Water, for example, is a substance that can be used in treating disease. It also affects the well-being of a person because people cannot exist without water. Does this mean that water is medicine? Nurses use water in the care and treatment of those who are ill. People who have tasted the natural spring waters found around the country might attest to the fact that water can indeed be medicine. When does water become medicine and not just a fluid we need to drink every day to survive?

Something becomes medicine when people decide to call it medicine. That which is called medicine is different for various cultures. Water becomes medicine at Lourdes, France, because many people have seen the water heal the lame and the dying. Foods from grains such as

---

24   Webster, *Merriam Webster's Collegiate Dictionary*.

oatmeal to fruits and vegetables such as pomegranate and cabbage can also be medicine. Water and foods are named "medicine" when they are intentionally *used* for medicinal purposes and found to be healing. They become a medicine because people assign them healing properties. All plants have the potential to be medicine but people may not value a plant as medicine until it has brought them healing in some way. Assigning the title of "medicine" to a plant is an honor that people bestow on a plant. There are five common types of people-plant applications:

1. Ornaments—Aesthetic Application
2. Foods—Nourishing Application
3. Medicine—Care and Cure Application
4. Abused substance—Excessive Application
5. Weeds—No application

When a plant is given the label of "medicine," it then becomes an object of power. Plants that can heal are valued in societies because they have the potential to heal and extend life. The plant is no longer an ornament, a pretty object growing outside the back door. It is no longer a food used to nourish the body alone; it can be a commodity and a resource used to cure and heal. The plant becomes a source of revenue because it is valued for its healing properties. Countries that use plants as medicine often have regulatory bodies whose job it is to determine standards for the plant medicines. This subject is explored in greater detail in Chapter 4. Determining standards includes being able to identify how a plant is used. It may be quite simple for a society to determine when a plant is considered a weed. The age-old definition of a weed is "a plant for which no use has been discovered yet." Humans do not use the plant deemed a weed, and it is either ignored or destroyed. One medicinal plant that comes to mind is Kudzu (*Pueraria lobata*). I have used the root in nursing care for more than two decades; but when I moved to North Carolina where the plant grows everywhere, I discovered that the majority of natives believe the plant to be "a damn weed"! While the Edwards family[25] in the southwestern corner of the state knows the health benefits of Kudzu to plants and humans, others spend years and hundreds of thousands of

---

25   http://kokudzu.com/KudzuCowFarm.aspx

dollars trying to eradicate the weed. I have taught many people how to heal problems in their gastrointestinal tract with kudzu pudding, but North Carolinians have been a bit more hesitant to explore the medicinal side of their invasive weed.

At the other end of the spectrum, plants that are abused, such as opium poppy *(Papaver somniferum)* and marijuana *(Cannabis sativa),* are clearly able to be identified by members of a society. Such plants may be highly valued (and expensive) for their ability to create a certain effect on the body and mind, such as euphoria, but are considered plants of potential abuse because they may be linked to addictive behavior or excessive recreational use in humans. Plants used as ornaments and foods are clearly identifiable as well. Ivy *(Hedera sp. L.),* for example, is used as a house plant, and raspberries *(Rubus idaeus L.)* are eaten as fruit.

The ability to discern when a plant is a medicine and not a food is often more difficult. Some plants are used only as foods or medicine, but some can serve both purposes. How a plant is used does not determine its categorization as a food or medicine because some plant medicines can be eaten just as plants are used for food. How a plant looks or how much it costs is not a determining factor as to whether it is a medicine or food. The main difference between plants used for food or medicine lies in the *intent* of the user.

When a plant becomes a medicine, valued for its ability to heal, it may be used for care and/or cure. Potatoes *(Solanum tuberosum)* are one example. People in some countries eat potatoes —the tuber or root of the *Solanum* plant—as a staple food. Potatoes are sold as food and valued as food. Some people, such as those of Irish or Mexican heritage, also know the medicinal value of potatoes. Herbalists may recommend the medicinal use of the potato, based on their recognition that part of the personality of the plant is demonstrated in the appearance of the root (the potato) and its numerous "eyes." Traditional healing for the human eye has often included putting potato on the outside of the eye. After peeling, the inner part of the potato can be used to heal sties that appear on the eyelid, for instance. "Potato" becomes "potato medicine" when it is used with the intent to care for and cure the eye. Potato can be part of a healthy diet and contribute to the healthy lifestyle of a person, but it is "medicine" when it is used for the care of a specific health concern.

Grapes *(Vitis vinifera)* are another example. Grapes would be considered only a weed by those who have the vines growing in their yard when they cannot identify the plant as grape. Red, purple, and green grapes are eaten as fruit. The leaves also are included in Greek and Middle Eastern cuisines. Grapes also have anti-inflammatory and pain-relieving properties because of constituents such as ferulic acid, salicylic acid, ascorbic acid, and quercetin. Traditionally grapes, fresh or dried (raisins), have been used in relieving discomfort related to arthritis and migraine. Grapes also are used in producing wine, which has a number of medicinal benefits. Wine was historically administered by nurses to their patients as *Spiritus fermentae*. Grapes, as wine, also can be used excessively. The grape in the form of wine is a good example of a plant that can be *used* medicinally in the same way it would be used as a food. Wine is taken by a patient as medicine in the same way it is taken as part of a meal. The difference is in the intent or purpose of the user.

Herbal Experiment: When Does Food Become Medicine?

Pick or purchase a fresh lemon (*Citrus limon*). Wash it thoroughly. Use all of your senses to experiment with the lemon. Smell, feel, and taste the outer peel, the inner peel, the juice, and the pulp of the fruit of the lemon tree. Cut three slices of the fruit and place in tea cup. Pour boiled water over the lemon and cover with a lid. Infuse for 5 minutes and sip. What are the qualities of this tea? Is this tea "medicine"? Record your reflection.

Every time nurse-herbalists teach about a plant or herbal medicine, or share a new remedy with someone, they are acting as agents of change. They change perceptions, paradigms, and beliefs about health and healing (not to mention herbalism) just by being part of a community and speaking out about the opportunities for healing that plants offer. Like medicine, the ways in which herbs and nurse-herbalists who speak about them are perceived by people and communities are determined by numerous social, cultural, religious, and personal beliefs, customs, attitudes, and habits of thought. Nurse-herbalists, in their role as community educators and healers, can be diplomats between the worlds of humans and healing plants. There are many people and communities whom I have met who eschew herbal remedies and there are also those who have deep personal and professional connections to plants. It is best not to attempt to convert people to consider healing plants, but rather to invite people to learn about the healing qualities and beauty of the plant world. Studying history, sharing stories, educating and promoting open communication about herbs and herbalism along with a good cup of tea can help broaden consciousness catalyzed by change that is the essence of life.

NURSING PROCESS AND SOLVING TOUGH PROBLEMS

Successfully catalyzing and managing change and transition with clients, families, organizations, and communities is a skill that requires a sense of comfort with *process*, which is defined as "continual forward movement" and "a natural phenomenon marked by gradual changes that lead toward a particular result."[26] Becoming comfortable in dealing with process has a lot to do with becoming comfortable in dealing with change and transition. Nurses are faced with process in their daily work; we deal with outcomes management and evidence-based practice, people experiencing life changes—birth, death, and illness. More specifically, nurses are educated, experienced, and, in many cases, expert in helping people solve the tough problems often associated with those life changes. That is the work called nursing care. Nursing's most basic practice model for problem solving and nursing care is referred to as "The Nursing Process." In my experience of teaching nursing theory and science to graduate and undergraduate students, I have often sensed a resistance to learning nursing process and a desire to get on with the process of caregiving, i.e. intervention. But I have found the nursing process to be very helpful in doing nursing—assessing, diagnosing, planning, implementing, and evaluating care with people. The five phases of the process can be used as checkpoints when sorting through tough problems. The nursing process is also helpful in professional life. I have

---

26 Webster, *Merriam Webster's Collegiate Dictionary.*

also found the nursing process to be helpful in distinguishing nursing practice from other disciplines. This is particularly important when creating and maintaining a new professional practice. The five phases of the problem-solving nursing process are:

1. Assessment – The nurse-herbalist observes and identifies behaviors while suspending judgment about the client or their behaviors. In addition to the physical, emotional, mental, and spiritual assessment of the client, the nurse-herbalist assesses all aspects of the environment, which includes the driving and restraining forces (people, issues, and things influencing the client behaviors) to the change that is envisioned.

2. Diagnosis – The nurse-herbalist synthesizes the assessment and names the pattern of observed behaviors. The nurse's diagnosis serves also as a summary of the needs identified during assessment.

3. Plan – The nurse-herbalist assists the client in finding meaning in life challenges, establishes priorities and desired outcomes, and sets measurable short-term and long-term goals using all necessary and available resources. Measurable goals may be subjective or objective. An example of a measurable subjective goal might be that the client's pain will go from a 10/10 to an 8.5 within one to two weeks as measured by a 10-point pain scale. Plans of care must validate the client's health beliefs, practices, and culture.

4. Intervention – The nurse-herbalist implements the plan of care in accordance with the wishes of the client. The nurse-herbalist implements the plan of care and the specific interventions associated with that plan at a pace that harmonizes with the client's patterns, lifestyle, and beliefs. Skills related to intervention and implementation as well as theoretical applications to support this process are discussed further in Chapter 3.

5. Evaluation – In this phase, the nurse-herbalist reflects and reviews the pattern, changes made, and client progress

toward short- and long-term goal fulfillment. The nurse-herbalist affirms all movement toward resolution using client reports and story, chart review, and personal reflection of both client and self. The effectiveness of the plan is reviewed with the client, and changes and progress are examined. If necessary, the plan for change is revised and further assessment of behaviors may be done.

Learning the nursing process helps people develop a new level of comfort and mastery in managing the challenges associated with change and transition. It is also a practice model used in caring for clients as they solve simple or tough problems. While it is a stable model for constructing care with clients, the nursing process is also energetically dynamic. The five-part process is really just a scaffold for guiding clients through problem solving and change.

In my experience, having a structure such as the nursing process that I can use in guiding discussions with clients emphasizes the professional nature of the relationship and the difference in approach to problem solving between professional and social relationships. In social relationships, people often listen to each other's problems. They might just listen and never assist with solving the problem. Social relationships do not dictate that people intervene. People in social situations also listen to another's problems often with the intent to intervene or help—often as quickly as possible. Friends listen to someone's account of a problem and then offer a solution that is often based on their own experiences. These are all typical of social convention and the network of self-help that exists in communities that share information about the application of herbal remedies.

While the self-help network is very important, there is a different approach to care that I would stress here as that which often first distinguishes the professional, holistic nurse-herbalist from the consumer network. That different approach is the use of the nursing process as a framework for care. It is not only a different intention but a scientific process, the nursing process that sets the nurse apart from the social network approach to problem solving. Here is a common example of what I often observe: A person at a party says, "I have a headache" or "I am having trouble sleeping." It is quite common for the host, who might even be a health professional, to offer an over-the-counter medication—or an herbal remedy if the person is so inclined. There is often no assessment or diagnosis. The person skips right over the first phases of the nursing process to intervention. But then the guest might respond, "Thanks, but I think that my headache is just a sign that I am hungry because I have been too busy today and I skipped lunch." The host then offers the guest a turkey sandwich from the buffet, again without assessing the guest's needs and desires, and the guest responds, "Oh thanks, but I am vegetarian." In a professional situation, however, the nurse-herbalist employing the nursing process would not offer an intervention without doing an assessment. What happens in the social situation is much akin to hit or miss. The client may or may not be helped, but that isn't always the purpose of the interaction. Sometimes people are simply seeking support from the social network and not necessarily solutions.

When clients seek solutions, they then appreciate a knowledgeable practitioner who demonstrates a caring, validating approach in which the focus is the client's problems and solutions. The nursing process model as a focused, organized framework for interaction accelerates the process of finding solutions and demonstrates a desire to understand the client's world.

Nurses have been identified as experts and "set apart" in their communities for centuries.[27] Records do not indicate that nurses of earlier centuries used the nursing process per se. But infirmary notes and diaries demonstrate that they did really think through what they were doing. They evaluated their choices of care and communicated frequently with clients about progress and plans. In my research, it was herbal knowledge and its skillful application to comfort and care and creating healing environments that set apart many early nurses. Nurses' relationships with healing plants were expressed from a different dimension than that of the social networks where many had knowledge of herbs. It is the way in which nurses apply herbs that sets them apart as nurse-herbalists, not just *that* they simply use herbs in practice.

Nurses are not as free today to partner with plants in some practice settings as they were one hundred years ago. Nineteenth-century nurses

---

27 Libster, *Herbal Diplomats: The Contribution of Early American Nurses (1830-1860) to Nineteenth-Century Health Care Reform and the Botanical Medical Movement.*

did not separate herbal remedies from the caring services they offered. Experienced nurses typically practiced with a high degree of autonomy, often propelling them into positions as community leaders because of their healing and botanical knowledge and experience.[28] Some nurses today choose to practice herbalism with its associated assessment strategies, scientific theories, herbal formulations, and plans of care but do not identify themselves in their work with herbs as "nurses" nor do they associate what they do with the practice of nursing per se. This is the root of the herbalist model. Those nurses who choose to or are required to keep the two practices separate often do so because of the dictates of their workplace environment and policies rather than their own beliefs and vision. It is important for nurses to continue their tradition in nurse-herbalism in any practice setting should they choose to do so. Although nurse-herbalists can utilize the consumer model of care in most any workplace, they must be able to practice the kind of care that they believe best defines professional nursing or they can become discouraged. I have met many such nurses and midwives who have either separated their herbal and nursing practices and/or don't use their knowledge in public and only use a consumer model in practice. Reasons and advisability for following the consumer (information and education) and herbalist (separatist) models in a holistic nurse-herbalist practice are discussed throughout the book. There are many practice environments, however, in which nurses *are* able to bring herbalism and nursing together more fully using an integrative practice model of nature care that honors both healing traditions. Applying the nursing process in practice is one important step in building a holistic practice in nurse-herbalism. Establishing an integrative model of nature care for implementing the nursing process is another.

---

28 Ibid.

REFERENCES

Brown, Walter "The Placebo Effect." *Scientific American* 278, no. 1 (1998): 90-5.

Griggs, Barbara. *Green Pharmacy*. Rochester, VT: Healing Arts Press, 1991.

Libster, Martha. *Demonstrating Care: The Art of Integrative Nursing*. Albany, New York: Delmar Thomson Learning, 2001.

———. "Guidelines for Selecting a Medical Herbalist for Consultation and Referral: Consulting a Medical Herbalist." *Journal of Alternative and Complementary Medicine* 5, no. 5 (1999): 457-62.

———. *Herbal Diplomats: The Contribution of Early American Nurses (1830-1860) to Nineteenth-Century Health Care Reform and the Botanical Medical Movement*. Thornton, CO: Golden Apple Publications, 2004.

Libster, Martha, and Betty Ann McNeil. *Enlightened Charity: The Holistic Nursing Care, Education and Advices Concerning the Sick of Sister Matilda Coskery, (1799-1870)*. Farmville, NC: Golden Apple Publications, 2009.

McFarlin, Barbara, Mary Gibson, Jann O'Rear, and Patsy Harman. "A National Survey of Herbal Preparation Use by Nurse-Midwives for Labor Stimulation." *Journal of Nurse-Midwifery* 44, no. 3 (1999): 205-16.

Nightingale, Florence. *Notes on Nursing: What It Is and What It Is Not*. Edinburgh: Churchill Livingstone, 1980 Original publication 1859.

Webster, Merriam. *Merriam Webster's Collegiate Dictionary*. 10th ed. Springfield, MA: Merriam-Webster, 1999.

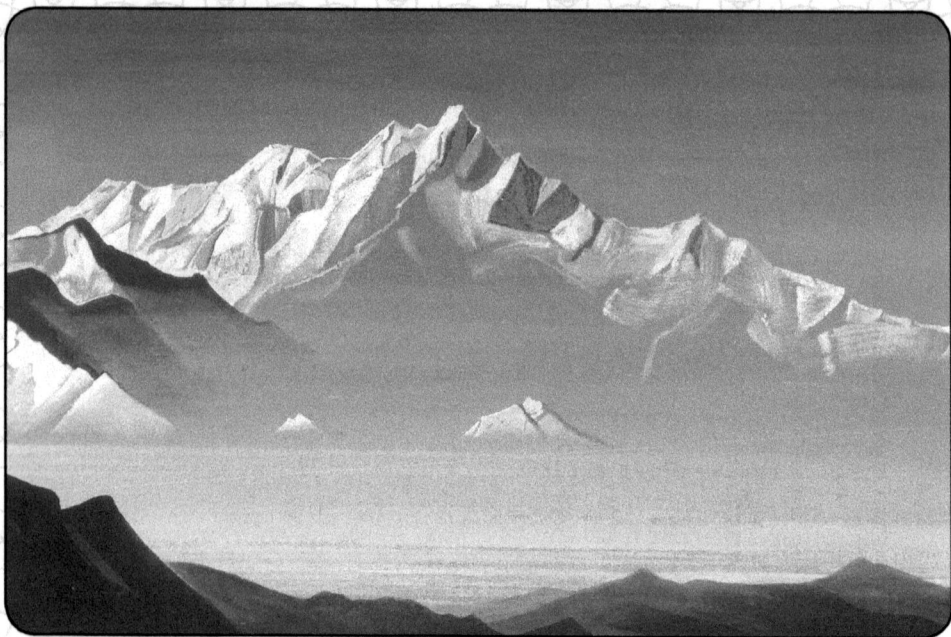

Mountain of Five Treasures (Two Worlds)
Nicholas Roerich, 1933

CHAPTER TWO

An Integrative Model for
Holistic Nurses' Nature Care

The five-step nursing process as discussed in Chapter 1 not only lays a scientific foundation for solving problems and creating care plans with clients, it also provides a platform for the definition of professional therapeutic relationships. The nursing process helps to distinguish social and professional therapeutic relationships. Therapeutic relationships are the central focus of a holistic caring practice that would be fully integrative. I have defined integrative nursing previously as "the creation of evolving, healing relationships with patients in which the nurse observes the patient's need for greater harmony and balance in their life and then addresses those needs by offering care that is a holistic blend of biomedical and caring modalities."[1] This chapter first describes an integrative model of care rooted in a historical tradition of nature cure. It then introduces three paradigms of health and healing that support the integrative process: biomedical, traditional, and holistic nursing, which are fundamental to the practice of nurse-herbalism.

Integration is a quality of heart—a welcoming heart. In health care, people can demonstrate that quality of heart by inviting and applying different health beliefs and practices. A holistic blending or integration

---

1   Martha Libster, *Demonstrating Care: The Art of Integrative Nursing* (Albany, N.Y: Delmar Thomson Learning, 2001), 26.

of cares is an expression of cultural diversity or *pluralism*[2] in health care. Whereas biomedical care may have become the dominant culture in health care and the primary form of care in industrialized societies, other societies continue to invite many ways of knowing, healing, and practicing caregiving. Although the United States is a highly industrialized, biomedically focused health-care culture, it has a strong history of pluralism and integration. For example, Americans, like peoples of other industrialized and developing nations, continue to actively engage in self-care[3] in which they draw upon the services, advice, and insights of many types of health educators and community healers such as herbalists.

In conducting historical research of the early and mid-nineteenth century in America, I found that this period really epitomized the spirit of self-care and integration in health care with a particular emphasis on herbal remedies, which are still an American healing tradition. It is really helpful to understand some of the historical context for herbalism and health care in one's country prior to establishing a practice in nurse-herbalism. That history informs legal, social, cultural, and professional aspects of practice. I focus on American history in this book because that is my country of origin and because my specialty as a historian is American history, but anyone could certainly use the concepts highlighted in this historical overview as a guide for exploring their own country's history of nursing, health care, and herbalism.

During the mid-nineteenth century, the United States underwent numerous social reforms, including health care reform in which the guiding principle for many was to "Be Your Own Doctor." As a result, self-care support groups, advice book and other self-care publications, and home remedy use supported by community healers such as nurses, midwives, bonesetters, herbalists, and physicians were a dominant part of the health care "system" of the day. Herbal remedies, a cornerstone of many self-care practices, were very popular. Herbs were also applied by community healers such as nurse-herbalists and midwives in the care of patients, a practice often referred to as "nature cure."

---

2   Diana Eck, professor and director of The Pluralism Project at Harvard University, defines the concept well as the "energetic engagement with diversity." See: http://pluralism.org/pages/pluralism/meanings.
3   Lowell S. Levin and Ellen L. Idler, *The Hidden Health Care System* (Farmville, NC: Golden Apple Publications, 2010).

THE ROOTS OF NURSES' NATURE CARE

Nature *cure* was a common term used by many nineteenth-century Americans, especially those who were seeking methods for being their own doctor. People learned from physicians, nurses, and healers to apply nature's elements in relieving symptoms and promoting their own health as well as that of their families. The connection with nature was a tradition that has been linked to the healing philosophies of the ancient Greeks.[4] Many thought that rest, a strengthening diet, and/or a mild herbal cathartic were all that was needed to aid nature in most cases of illness. People in America and in Europe "took the waters"[5] by bathing in hot springs and sipping the mineral springs that bubbled out of the earth. Religious communities, such as the Shakers, experimented with diet and lifestyle changes. The Sylvester Graham diet, a nature cure that included lifestyle changes such as sleeping on a hard mattress, horseback riding, removing stimulants from the diet such as coffee, and eating a vegetarian diet with unbolted wheat crackers (today known as Graham crackers), was highly popular. The Botanical Movements of the Thomsonians and Beachites were also popular. Later in the century, these two health and social movements were followed by the Eclectics.

Physicians, both Regulars[6] and Botanics, also endorsed nature cure philosophies, often prescribing trips to the ocean or to sanatoriums in the mountains for curing illnesses from depression to tuberculosis. They, like their patients, valued the healing relationship between people and the natural environment. Physicians defined nature cure when describing their roles in the medical care of the time. In 1835, American "Regular" physician Dr. Jacob Bigelow read his essay on "self-limited diseases" before the Massachusetts Medical Society in which he encouraged physicians to rethink their practice of prescribing medicine for all diseases. He stated that "some diseases are controlled by nature alone"[7] and that the physician was "but the minister and servant of

---

4   Ingunn Elstad and Kirsti Torjuul, "The Issue of Life: Aristotle in Nursing Perspective," *Nursing Philosophy : An International Journal for Healthcare Professionals* 10, no. 4 (2009).

5   Known as "Water Cure"

6   Regulars were defined by the public as university-trained physicians who were orthodox in practice. A Regular was a physician who was not a Botanic or Homeopath.

7   Jacob Bigelow, "Discourse on Self-Limited Disease," in *Medical Communications of the Massachusetts Medical Society* (Boston: The Massachusetts Medical Society, 1836).

nature" who was to endeavor to "aid nature in her salutary intentions, or to remove obstacles out of her path."[8] President Thomas Jefferson had instructed Dr. Casper Wister in 1807 to instruct the "young practitioner, especially, to have deeply impressed on his mind the real limits of his art, and that when the state of the patient gets beyond these, his office is to be a watchful, but quiet spectator of the operations of nature" as it will "re-establish the disordered functions."[9]

Like Bigelow and other physicians, nurses in the early and mid-nineteenth century were also influenced by the notion of nature cure. Lydia Maria Child, a popular authoress of advice books, wrote in *The Family Nurse* (1837): "Both doctors and nurses, as they grow older and wiser, use as little medicine as possible, and simply content themselves with recommending fasting, or such light diet as will best assist the kindly efforts of nature."[10] British nurse Florence Nightingale wrote in 1859: "Nature alone cures ... and what nursing has to do in either case, is to put the patient in the best condition for nature to act upon him."[11] Her understanding of nature cure, like that of her contemporaries on both sides of the Atlantic, was congruent with health beliefs and practices promoting cures that went beyond the common environmental changes typically made by the nurse to the sick room, which was the nineteenth-century nurse's laboratory for the invention and application of herbal remedies and other nature cures.[12]

Nightingale and other nurse-leaders of the time observed and taught about the healing "nature" within each person using their own language of their time. Nightingale identified the healing power of nature as the "vital force" that emanated from the Creator.[13] The Sisters of Charity were commended by their physician colleagues for the creation of a caring environment that supported healing just at the turning point in disease when a cure would manifest. This moment was observed by caregivers

8   Ibid.
9   Thomas Jefferson and others, *The Life and Selected Writings of Thomas Jefferson* (New York: The Modern Library, 1944), 583.
10 Lydia Maria Child, *The Family Nurse* (Bedford, MA: Applewood Books, 1997).
11 Florence Nightingale, *Notes on Nursing: What It Is and What It Is Not* (Edinburgh, Scotland: Churchill Livingstone, 1980, Originally published 1859).
12 Martha Libster, "Elements of Care: Nursing Environmental Theory in Historical Context," *Holistic Nursing Practice* 22, no. 3 (2008): 163.
13 Nightingale, *Notes on Nursing: What It Is and What It Is Not*; Barbara Dossey and others, *Florence Nightingale Today* (Silver Spring, MD: American Nurses Association, 2005), 158.

and referred to as the "curative point"[14] when nature affected her cure.

Putting the patient in "the best condition" for nature to heal him did not mean that the patient was left alone. Nurses and physicians used elements found in the environment, such as water and medicinal herbs, to partner with nature in the comfort, care, and cure of patients. Water cure and herbal therapies were valued therapeutics in the nineteenth century that assisted nature in the healing process. Herbal remedies were so popular in the early and mid-nineteenth century that historians have referred to this period as the "American Botanical Movement."[15] The American Botanical Movement was led in the political domain by men such as Samuel Thomson and Wooster Beach and their followers but often implemented in communities by women[16] nurses and midwives. For example, nurses of the Shaker and Latter-Day Saints communities used herbal remedies extensively in their care of the sick. They routinely prescribed teas and syrups as well as topical remedies such as poultices, liniments, and compresses for their patients.[17]

The Shakers, known for their botanical products enterprise in the nineteenth and early twentieth centuries, are often considered the predecessor of the current pharmaceutical industry. The Shaker nurses officiated over the health care "system" of their communities from their infirmary or "nurses shop." Their infirmary work was the testing ground for the remedies that they and the Shaker men grew and produced. The nurses made their own remedies from the plants growing in their gardens or that they gathered in local fields and forests. Shaker nurses kept infirmary records of their care. Their notes include examples of the clinical decisions made when they employed herbal remedies. For example, on January 14th 1836, Brother Nathan's leg was swollen and so painful that

---

14   Martha Libster and Betty Ann McNeil, *Enlightened Charity: The Holistic Nursing Care, Education and Advices Concerning the Sick of Sister Matilda Coskery, (1799-1870).* (Farmville, NC: Golden Apple Publications, 2009), 172-76.

15   Alex Berman and Michael Flannery, *America's Botanico-Medical Movement: Vox Populi* (New York: Pharmaceutical Products Press, 2001).

16   There is extensive historical evidence that a prevailing belief in antebellum society was that women were experts in nursing. Men who worked in community or institutions as caregivers typically did so as assistants to the women-nurses. This was not the case in colonial America or during and after the Civil War.

17   Martha Libster, *Herbal Diplomats: The Contribution of Early American Nurses (1830-1860) to Nineteenth-Century Health Care Reform and the Botanical Medical Movement* (Thornton, CO: Golden Apple Publications, 2004).

he "could scarcely bear to have it touched with a feather." The Sisters applied a poultice of charcoal and yeast to his leg. On the 15th, Sister Sarah Kendall applied a poultice of stewed pumpkin. The Sisters wrote that, "Both seemed to have a good effect."[18] On the 16th, Sister Sarah "wanted to have applied to Br N's leg a poultice composed of the following articles, Beef brine, Feverfew, Mayweed Flowers, Wormwood, & wheat middlings, it proved to be too harsh for it, caused some irritation & increased the swelling, it was taken off in the P. M. & the pumpkin poultice put on again."[19] This reference documents the science of nature care practiced in early American nursing. There are numerous references in the infirmary and community records and diaries such as this that I have read over the years to the scientific decision making of early nurses—a practice that would be referred to today as "evidence-based practice."

The nurses administered treatments known as emetics, cathartics, injections (enemas), steams, and sweats for mild to moderate illnesses such as stomach pain and influenza. Emetic and cathartic treatments were given orally and were either plant or chemical based. Like many nineteenth-century Americans, Shakers believed that powerful remedies effected powerful cures and the power of a remedy was demonstrated in the "action" of that remedy, such as in the action of vomiting, referred to commonly as "puking." The Shaker nurses most often used plant-based emetics, such as lobelia (*Lobelia inflata*) and cayenne pepper (*Capsicum frutescens*) to encourage puking. These treatments were recorded as daily events in Shaker infirmary records.[20]

The nurses of the Church of Jesus Christ of Latter-day Saints (LDS), referred to in the early nineteenth century as "Mormons," also applied botanical remedies extensively in caregiving. When community members became ill, herbs and mild foods were used as remedies in the care of the ill in keeping with religious belief as demonstrated in the written *Doctrine and Covenants of the Church*.[21] Historical records date

---

18 Harvard Shakers, *Physicians' Journal or an Account of the Sickness at Harvard*, Western Reserve Historical Society, Cleveland, OH, Shaker Manuscripts V:B 41 (1843).
19 Ibid.
20 Ibid.
21 Church of Jesus Christ of Latter-Day Saints, *The Book of Mormon. The Doctrine and Covenants of the Church of Jesus Christ of Latter-Day Saints. The Pearl of Great Price* (Salt Lake City, UT: Church of Jesus Christ of Latter-Day Saints, 1981).

the use of botanicals and a specific connection with the Thomsonian botanical movement back to the founding of the Church in 1830. The Thomsonians, mentioned previously, were a prominent nineteenth-century sect of herbal healers led by Samuel Thomson (1769-1843), whose botanical program was one of the first prescriptive, organized systems of botanical therapies in America. His botanical system of health care was patented and mass-produced for the public. He was an activist against what he perceived as "medical monopoly."[22] The history of LDS nurses includes accounts of a number of nurse-midwife-herbalists including two bonafide Thomsonian nurse healers, Margaret Cooper West (1833-1912) and Patty Bartlett Sessions (1795-1892), who applied Thomsonian philosophy and used the patented formulations in patient care.[23] They made the majority of their herbal remedies, which, as with the Shakers, were most often teas and topical remedies. For example, Patty Sessions recorded in her diary the use of an herbal poultice for a patient with a hand infection:

> Br Filawry came here a week ago with a very bad hand it was poisoned by skinning a cow that died did not know what ailed her he had a small place on his finger where the skin was scrat[c]hed off and it swelled verry [sic] bad & made him sick all over, to day he is better I have took care of his hand polticed [sic] it with catnip & Lobelia mostly put in salt & soap and molasses his finger turned black & the flesh dead when the but it begins to come to its feeling a little now.[24]

Some of the earliest records of hospital nursing in America are represented in the history of the Sisters of Charity (SC) who began their healing mission in 1809 under the leadership of Elizabeth Ann Seton

---

22 Samuel Thomson, *New Guide to Health, or, Botanic Family Physician Containing a Complete System of Practice, Upon a Plan Entirely New: With a Description of the Vegetables Made Use of, and Directions for Preparing and Administering Them to Cure Disease: To Which is Prefixed a Narrative of the Life and Medical Discoveries of the Author* (Boston: Printed for the author by J.Q. Adams, 1835).

23 Libster, *Herbal Diplomats: The Contribution of Early American Nurses (1830-1860) to Nineteenth-Century Health Care Reform and the Botanical Medical Movement.*

24 Patty Bartlett Sessions and Donna Toland Smart, *Mormon Midwife: The 1846-1888 Diaries of Patty Bartlett Sessions* (Logan, UT: Utah State University Press, 1997).

(1774-1821). The first hospital mission of the community was in 1823 at the Baltimore Infirmary in Maryland. Following the healing tradition of the French Daughters of Charity, established in 1633 by Vincent de Paul and Louise de Marillac, the American SC quickly became renowned caregivers of the sick poor, cholera victims, and the insane. One of the roles of a hospital nurse in the Vincentian-Louisian tradition was that of Assistant Infirmarian. According to community records, the duties of the Assistant Infirmarian included sweeping the infirmary, making the beds, and attending the sick by "giving them teas and victuals according to the directions of the Infirmarian."[25]

Teas, known among the French Daughters as "tisanes," were an important part of nurses' nature care. Following French tradition, American Sister Matilda Coskery taught Sister-nurses the importance of simple nursing interventions in the care and cure of patients, such as administering herbal teas. She also defined the influence that the nurse's proper application of teas had on patient care and physician decision making:

> Make them strong, & in a clean vessel, have the water boiling—keep them covered while boiling or steaming. When done, strain & cover it. In warm weather do not make too much at a time, & keep it in a cool place. Nurses are often careless in these things, thinking they are only simple matters, thus, they prepare them negligently, & are irregular in giving them—or give them after they are sour & mouldy, & this makes the stomach sick, or getting them irregular does no good. The Dr thinks it is the fault of the tonic & changes it for something stronger, perhaps brandy or some other thing that does real harm—He loses confidence in that tonic, names it to his students and Medical friends, who likewise discontinue it, in all these cases that fall into their hands, some stronger thing is given, when the thing itself was right, in right hands. How often, these, seemingly small things, are the beginnings of the death-bed & in many, many cases, Life and Death is (in) the hands of the nurses, more than in the Physicians.[26]

---

25 Daughters of Charity, *The Rule of 1812: Regulations for the Society of Sisters of Charity in the United States of America*, Emmitsburg, MD Archives of the Daughters of Charity, St. Joseph's Provincial House, (1812), 1-3-3-5:7(6).

26 Sister Matilda Coskery, *Advices Concerning the Sick* (Emmitsburg, MD: Archives of Daughters of Charity, St. Joseph's Provincial House, n.d. c. 1840).

The Sisters of Charity nurses practiced collaboratively with physicians in the nineteenth century. They developed expertise in nursing care and knew when and how to introduce herbal remedies to patients. For example, Sister Matilda, considered an "oracle"[27] in the care of the insane, suggested a substitute (herbal) treatment for a patient suffering from mania a potu (delirium tremens):

> After the Dr has named the kind, quantity and frequency of the opiates & stimulants, there is still much depending on the attendants, as in many cases these remedies increase excitement & shd therefore be discontinued until the Dr. comes again, & telling why these were not given—Hop tea is a good substitute as opiate & tonic; & often serves better than opiates or spirits.[28]

The Sisters of Charity nurses' work with herbs reflected their values of humility, simplicity, and charity because herbal remedies were considered by early Americans to be, for the most part, gentle, simple, and publicly accessible remedies.[29] Some of the earliest evidence for the roots of nurse-herbalism can be found in the spiritual writings of Louise de Marillac, the founder of the Daughters of Charity with Vincent de Paul, the predecessors of the American Sisters of Charity. Her spiritual writings contain numerous receipts (recipes) for healing with plants. Here is an example of one of Louise's nature care receipts, which she wrote for Monsieur L'Abbé de Vaux in 1641:

> Forgive me, Monsieur, if I take this liberty as well as that of telling you that, if you have not already been purged. I would be pleased to render you this little service by preparing you a potion which I believe should be made up of the weight of three copper coins of senna steeped overnight in a good mixture of refreshing, pleasant-tasting herbs. To this add one-half ounce of cleaned black currants mixed with an ounce of peach syrup (the pharmacist

---

27 Libster and McNeil, *Enlightened Charity: The Holistic Nursing Care, Education and Advices Concerning the Sick of Sister Matilda Coskery, (1799-1870).*

28 Coskery's Advices Concerning the Sick as cited in ibid., 218.

29 Libster, *Herbal Diplomats: The Contribution of Early American Nurses (1830-1860) to Nineteenth-Century Health Care Reform and the Botanical Medical Movement.*

here has given me some that is excellent) or, if this is not available, the same amount of pink rose syrup. However, I believe that you should wait until the pain which is causing the inflammation has subsided completely, or at least for a week, so as not to bring on another attack."[30]

It is not clear from the letter exactly what the man's condition was but it seems plausible that he had some type of inflammatory condition. Black currant berry juice is a diuretic and diaphoretic that has been used traditionally in people with febrile illness, sore throat, and inflammatory conditions.[31] The herb senna (*Cassia spp.*) is still used today with caution as a laxative and purgative for the bowel. Louise demonstrated her holistic approach to nature care in such acts as adding spiritual attention to the patient. For example, she recommended boiling chicory root and a little bayberry as a quick-acting remedy for Sister Claude's intestinal inflammation. These herbs are quite bitter tasting so it is not surprising that Louise offered spiritual advice in keeping with her Christian tradition—that of accompanying the remedy with a "remembrance of the bitter drink offered to Our Lord on the Cross."[32]

The Daughters made excellent herbal syrups that were used as carriers for more bitter herbs such as senna into the body. Many were trained compounding pharmacists who knew how to prepare inexpensive remedies for the sick. More broadly, the French Daughters of Charity were professional nurses renowned for their expertise in the care of the sick poor and insane. They were well versed in many aspects of care with which they often integrated plant remedies. Louise wrote to some of the sister-nurses, for example: "I beg you not to go to visit the sick without rubbing your nose with vinegar and putting some on your temples."[33] Vinegar is a well-known and time-honored, plant-based disinfectant. Their herbal tradition has been documented since the inception of their healing community. The preparation and administration of teas,

30 Louise Sullivan, *Spiritual Writings of Louise de Marillac: Correspondence and Thoughts.* (New York: New City Press, ed. and trans. 1991), 47.
31 Harvey Wickes Felter and John Uri Lloyd, *King's American Dispensatory*, 18th ed., 3d rev ed. (Sandy, OR: Eclectic Medical Publications, 1983), 1675.
32 Sullivan, *Spiritual Writings of Louise de Marillac: Correspondence and Thoughts.*: 615.
33 Ibid., 640.

also referred to as tisanes or infusions, were common in their practice. Their botanical knowledge was so well known that early texts including a little pocket herbal written by a Royal French physician, Arnault de Nobleville (1701 – 1778), reference the extensive knowledge of some, if not all, of the Daughters of Charity.[34] Although the use of herbs was highly condemned during the 550 years of the Inquisition as the favored source of the "witches poison,"[35] the sister-nurses trained by Vincent de Paul and Louise de Marillac carved out a sacred niche for herbs as a spiritual and therefore holistic practice of professional nursing.

Herbal remedies were also part of the caregiving work of indigenous people. Although the term "nurse" was not used, nineteenth-century Native American women typically provided care for their families and for community members when they were sick. Native women were also midwives. Some of the knowledge of healing plants, such as corn, was transmitted along a tribe's matrilineal lines. In the southwestern United States, cornmeal blessings were commonly used to maintain physical, mental, emotional, and spiritual wellbeing. Prayer cornmeal, which at times had turquoise and coral added to it, was used throughout the year in blessings for family members.[36] Elders advised younger people to go outside in the early morning when the spirits were out, offer their cornmeal and "get a fresh wind into themselves."[37] This daily ritual was believed to be the first step toward maintaining balance. Cornmeal also played an important part in the tribal nurses' preparation of the dead for their journey to the spirit world.

Many indigenous peoples' beliefs included the view that plants and animals were their brothers and sisters. American Indians believed that it was respectful to pray to plants and animals and ask for their wisdom and help before using them in healing. The nurses often worked side by side with medicine men. They provided herbal remedies and caring for the ill while the medicine man purified the affected person by removing evil from them.[38]

34   Libster, *Herbal Diplomats: The Contribution of Early American Nurses (1830-1860) to Nineteenth-Century Health Care Reform and the Botanical Medical Movement*: 196.

35   Francesco Maria Guazzo and Montague Summers, *Compendium Maleficarum: The Montague Summers Edition*, Dover ed. (New York: Dover, 1988), 90.

36   Ruth Leah Bunzel, *Zuni Ceremonialism* (Albuquerque: University of New Mexico Press, 1992).

37   Margaret Moss, "Zuni Elders: Ethnography of American Indian Aging" (University of Texas Houston, 2000), 91.

38   Ibid.

In eighteenth- and nineteenth-century African-American slave communities, nurses were recognized female community healers who had nursed family members through serious illness, brought up a large number of children, or had acquired their knowledge regarding health and illness from previous generations in their family.[39] African-American slaves thought that the medicine of whites was less effective and they may have also been aware that white physicians experimented with their medicines on slaves. Slave-nurses, who worked in larger plantations' infirmaries, were often charged with preventing African-American patients from leaving and with compelling them to take unwanted treatments.[40] But these women, labeled "nurse" by their slave masters, also knew where to gather wild medicinal herbal plants for use in their caregiving. Among the most common herbs used were Mullein, Camphor, Chinaberry, Collard leaves, Pine needles, and Sweet Gum.[41] Slave-nurses would often gather their herbs and prepare the remedies for their slave-patients at night when they would not be caught by plantation owners. Enslaved healers such as the midwives and nurses became "agents of transformation, altering the very terms of slaveholder medical attention and creating new claims to healing authority."[42]

Nurse-herbalists in the nineteenth century were agents of change in their communities. They were instrumental in the continuation of their communities' cultural traditions. Nurses demonstrated caring in a way that was creative, scientific, and spiritual, often with herbs and other remedies as their instruments of compassionate nature care. They were often highly respected healers in their communities. Toward the end of the nineteenth and into the mid-twentieth century, nursing care changed its primary focus from community- to hospital-based care. As industrialization boomed, nurses' nature cares gradually became less prominent. While nurses working in hospitals might have offered an herbal tea to a patient, that tea was more often purchased in a teabag

---

39   Glenda Smith, "An Ethnographic Study of Home Remedy Use for African-American Children." (University of Texas Houston, 2001).

40   Emily Abel, *Hearts of Wisdom: American Women Caring for Kin, 1850-1940* (Cambridge, MA: Harvard University Press, 2000).

41   Smith, "An Ethnographic Study of Home Remedy Use for African-American Children.." Botanical genus and species of plants listed not identified.

42   Sharla Fett, *Working Cures: Healing, Health, and Power on Southern Slave Plantations* (Chapel Hill: University of North Carolina Press, 2002).

rather than gathered from the garden or field as the Shakers did. The tea was also presented as a beverage rather than as part of patient care. Part of the reason for this change was that some nurses modeled their profession after physician practice, and in their love of science and a desire to be paid more for their services, distanced themselves from nature as physicians had been doing for some time.

Herbs and other nature cures and cares are likened with Mother Nature herself. In the eighteenth and nineteenth centuries, the "separation of religion or spiritual matters from the practice of medicine was a symptom of a greater cultural change that was occurring, the separation of science and nature and the elimination of nature from medicine."[43] Nature represents chaos, ambiguity, and even death as part of the life cycle. As the industrialization of societies progressed, many thought it possible to apply technology in such a fashion as to ultimately dominate nature. The Greek philosophy of the participatory relationship between healer and patient and nature was gradually overridden. The concept of the *domination* of nature became linked with science, medicine, comfort, social progress, and the conquest of disease.[44] Herbal remedies gradually became equated with self-care, folklore, and domestic medicine and marginalized in American culture as "alternative" medicine rather than indigenous or traditional healing; therefore, it was harder for physicians and nurses to distinguish themselves as an "expert" or professional that deserved to be paid as such[45] if they were applying herbs in cure and care—a system of health care that was also accessible to the lay public.

Nevertheless, curricula until the 1950s included the study of nursing materia medica that incorporated the use of herbs. For example, the popular *Materia Medica for Nurses* by Lavinia Dock originally published in 1890 includes numerous references to herbal tinctures, liniments, syrups, plasters, and poultices made from plants such as hops (*Humulus lupulus*), thyme (*Thymus vulgaris*), mustard (*Brassica nigra*), and

43   Libster, *Herbal Diplomats: The Contribution of Early American Nurses (1830-1860) to Nineteenth-Century Health Care Reform and the Botanical Medical Movement*: 30.
44   Roy Porter, *The Greatest Benefit to Mankind: A Medical History of Humanity*, 1st American ed. (New York: W. W. Norton, 1997), 307.
45   Libster, *Herbal Diplomats: The Contribution of Early American Nurses (1830-1860) to Nineteenth-Century Health Care Reform and the Botanical Medical Movement*.

goldenseal (*Hydrastis canadensis*) along with drugs such as digitalis, Novocain, nitroglycerin, and morphine.

Until the proliferation of pharmaceutical drugs, American nursing texts routinely included the plant medicines of the day. Like Dock, Virginia Henderson included information on plant applications in her theory and practice texts, which have been used worldwide since the mid-1900s. For example, nurses were taught the health benefits of a "counterirritant" action on the skin. Herbs such as mustard (*Brassica spp.*) or cayenne pepper (*Capsicum frutescens*) might be recommended externally for their counterirritant action. The purpose of the counterirritant was to warm and stimulate circulation in a particular area of the body. "Counterirritation relieves the affection of the organ over which it is applied by reflex nerve relation between the skin and the organ, and by producing a change in the blood supply to the organ. The mental effect of substitution of a new and superficial pain also assists in the result."[46]

Since early history, nurse-midwives have routinely applied plant therapies in their work with women. In the Pulitzer Prize-winning book *A Midwife's Tale: The Life of Martha Ballard, Based on her Dairy, 1785-1812*, the American midwife grows, harvests, dries, and applies the medicinal herbs from her garden in her nature care practice. She applied some of the same plant medicines as the physicians in the town, such as rhubarb (*Rheum rhaponticum*) and senna, but did not use the "dramatic therapies" such as the mercurial compound known as calomel that the physicians used.[47] Martha Ballard was held in high esteem in her town and practiced independently. She "summoned a physician twice in twenty-seven years"[48] and she used plant medicines often in practice.

During the 1800s when almost 50 percent of the population of the state of Ohio was using therapies and remedies suggested by practitioners educated in the practices of the Thomsonian Botanico-medico movement,[49] a nurse-herbalist named Mary Ann Bickerdyke from Ohio opened a private practice in physio-botanic medicine. In addition to

---

46 Bertha Harmer and Virginia Henderson, *Textbook of the Principles and Practice of Nursing* (New York: Macmillan Co., 1955), 264.

47 Laurel Ulrich, *A Midwife's Tale: The Life of Martha Ballard, Based on Her Diary, 1785-1812* (New York: Knopf: Distributed by Random House, 1990), 56.

48 Ibid., 180.

49 John Haller, *The People's Doctors: Samuel Thomson and the American Botanical Movement, 1790-1860* (Carbondale, IL: Southern Illinois University Press, 2000).

being in private practice, Bickerdyke was also the staff herbalist at her local hospital. During the Civil War, she served as a noncommissioned nurse of the Union army where she "established over 300 field hospitals and nursed casualties on nineteen battlefields. ... A pragmatic herbalist, she replaced limited medicines with blackberry cordial for diarrhea, jimsonweed for pain, and bloodroot and wild cherry for stimulants."[50] Although she encountered opposition to her use of botanical medicines in the army hospitals, when she was in charge of the hospital, the "patients were bathed, put to bed in clean clothes on clean bedding, dosed with black root and goldenseal, sassafras tea and beet juice, and fed all the milk and fresh vegetables they would take. A surprisingly large number of them recovered."[51] Nurse-herbalist Bickerdyke was known as the "cyclone in calico" and was honored many times for her tremendous service.

History clearly shows the influence plants have had in the development of healing practices of the people, health care systems, and professional nursing. Herbal medicine and the practice of using plants in healing is not a passing fad nor is it simply a complementary or alternative therapy to biomedical care. The use of herbs is a healing tradition that continues to be used and explored by many health practitioners and the public alike. Herbalism, like nursing, is an evolving science and art. Before the advent of modern pharmaceuticals, nurses administered the medicines of the time. For example, in the early 1900s, American nurses administered an "emulsion" of asafoetida (*Ferula foetida*), a pungent gum resin, by mouth to infants and adults with colic or gas pains. They applied flaxseed (*Linum usitatissimum*) poultices to the chest of patients with pneumonia. While many of those herbal remedies may have come to be replaced by pharmaceutical preparations, there is no reason why nurses must totally reject the application of herbal remedies and the centuries of safe use in nature care. The integrative model of nurse-herbalism is a blending of technique, technology, and tradition from three perspectives: the biomedical, traditional, and nursing/self-care paradigms.

---

50 Mary Ellen Snodgrass, *Historical Encyclopedia of Nursing* (Santa Barbara, CA: ABC-CLIO, 1999), 26.

51 Nina Brown Baker, *Cyclone in Calico: The Story of Mary Ann Bickerdyke* (Boston: Little, Brown, 1952), 142.

AN INTEGRATIVE MODEL AS THE
CHALICE FOR NURSE-HERBALISM

A person's interest in healing plants is often sparked by a special, attention-getting experience or interaction with a plant. Personally, I have, for some reason, had many of these experiences with healing plants and have always been surrounded by them. They are part of my life, part of my way of being in the world. One of the earliest pictures of me taken by my parents is of my sister feeding me marigold flowers at 1 year of age. To this day, I have a special connection with marigold (*Calendula officinalis*) and many stories of its place of honor in my life. I have witnessed its many healing properties in the care and comfort of clients' skin, eyes, and digestive systems over the years. I grow the brilliant yellow-orange petals and use them to make tea, eye wash, and salve or ointment. It is a powerful flower, which I have seen soothe and heal corneal abrasion faster than any other remedy. It is also a plant that has deep spiritual meaning for me. In traditional healing, including my Celtic tradition, it is often posited that it is really that connection with the plant that is the source of healing in herbalism. In a spiritual sense, healing flowers and herbs are chalices or cups of healing potential.

It is really our relationship with the plant that provides the opportunity for healing rather than the plant object itself. There are other examples in culture of what I mean here. For example, in the art world, specifically in dance, it is often said that the true *dance* is not the movement itself but that which occurs *between* two movements. Dance is that which is between or in relationship between movements. The individual dancer experiences *dance* in unique ways, often beyond space and time. For example, when dancing to a particular piece of music, the dancer might turn between two movements and on one occasion spin twice to fill that space/time of music and another time spin six times in the same amount of space/time. What was the difference? Many dancers talk about their connection with the movement, the music, and even the change in audience as inspiring the changes manifest in any given performance. In the plant world, the opportunity for healing is much like the dance. The plant provides an opportunity for connection or relationship with a person. The plant matter is a chalice or matrix into which the consciousness, thoughts, feelings, and healing intentions of the persons involved in the application of that plant are stored. The relationship and connection with the plant and the context for its use in healing then become as important, if not more important actually, to the healing outcome. My marigold connection continues today.

In my early twenties I had a connection with a picture in the back of a church in California. It was a photo of an old woman identified as the wise Indian Teacher Ananda Mayi Ma. It was a powerful connection that I would call recognition. I remember feeling completely compelled to speak to that photo and ask her where she was so that I could talk with her. A few months later, she came to me! My husband at that time was a physician and he had a new client visit him in his practice. That person was an American devotee of Ma, whom we learned had made her transition to the spirit world a few years prior. But the woman and her husband had visited Ma in India and had been allowed to take home movies of Ma holding sat sang, a devotional time of song, prayer and teachings. I was invited to watch the movies and afterward the woman gave me a little box. In that box was a marigold flower from Ma's lei that had been around her neck the day that my new acquaintances had taken their movies. The marigold flower was the chalice for my spiritual connection with and memory of a woman whose teachings I came to treasure.[52]

Each time I interact with marigold, I experience what might best be explained scientifically by the theory of morphic resonance. Biologist Dr. Rupert Sheldrake proposes that nature is essentially habitual in that all natural systems or morphic units from plants and crystals to human societies inherit a collective *memory* that influences their form and behavior. Resonance is rhythmic vibration in response to a stimulus. Morphic resonance is the influence of previous activity on subsequent similar activity organized by morphic fields. Morphic fields are defined by Sheldrake as "fields of information."[53] They exert a "region of physical influence" in which matter and energy are "interconnected"; "matter

---

52 The Andover-Harvard Theological Library at Harvard Divinity School houses some of the papers of Ananda Mayi Ma covering the period of 1950–1981: http://www.hds.harvard.edu/library/bms/bms00556.html

53 Rupert Sheldrake, *The Presence of the Past: Morphic Resonance and the Habits of Nature* (Rochester, VT: Park Street Press, 1995), 113.

is energy bound within fields."[54] Morphic resonance occurs between rhythmic structures of activity "on the basis of similarity." The influence of morphic resonance as a "non-energetic transfer of information" is cumulative over time.[55] Memory, conscious or unconscious, is due to morphic resonance. As memory is experienced by one person or many in society as a collective experience known as history, it takes shape or form and carries with it a power to affect human experience such as belief, action, and feeling. Morphic resonance and personal and race memory may account some for how plant remedies work ... or not in any given situation.

People's memories of experiences with plants can be most pleasant, fuzzy, fragrant, tasty, stimulating, and even ecstatic. They also can be unpleasant, thorny, stinging, and bitter. People's experiences of the same plant can also be very different. My sister and I were both on Mount Washington in New Hampshire when mom pulled out her penknife to cut the one tiny checkerberry (*Gaultheria procumbens*) we found into four pieces for us, our brother, and her. I loved the flavor but Sara spit it out. She has never liked the smell, let alone the taste, of wintergreen, aka checkerberry. Pepto-Bismol˚ has the opposite effect for her because she finds that plant unpleasant, to say the least. My favorite ice cream is checkerberry chip, and I am still teaching about the analgesic qualities of the salicylates in the *Gaultheria* leaf and the elegant taste of the berry. "One man's meat is another's poison." That is why an integrative model provides the best chalice for nurse-herbalism that would be practiced to its fullest.

People and practitioners have different relationships with healing plants. They perceive them in different ways. Plants have the power, if you will, to call forth these different relationships because they, like humans, are life forms. They relate to us and us to them. Just as human-to-human relationships vary, so, too, do plant-human relationships. That is how they provide such an excellent chalice for holistic nature care. They hold the potential to work spiritually as did the marigold with me—physically, mentally, and emotionally. People also respond to them in different ways and therefore apply them in different ways.

---

54 Ibid., 367.
55 Ibid., 109.

For example, a group of people might hear of a story about how a man's prostate was "healed" when he took saw palmetto berries. One person who heard the story might think, "Oh my father has prostate problems, maybe the berries would help him feel better." Another person might think, "Oh that's poppycock! How can a little berry heal a prostate?" Another might think, "Well, it helped him, but it probably won't help every man. I want to see some scientific studies that prove it works before I consider it." These reactions represent just a few of the numerous possible responses to any herbal remedy. These thought processes reflect the person's paradigm or philosophy about life. They are perspectives that come from inner belief systems, cultural upbringing, education, and life experiences. A person's paradigm or worldview is important as an expression of their sense of self. Therefore, the paradigm is never judged as "bad" or "good." It just is. Personal paradigms can change, but because they often are rooted deeply in belief patterns that have evolved over time, they rarely change quickly. A person's paradigm or personal philosophy influences both the way they see the world and the way in which they are shaped by the world. The client's and the nurse-herbalist's paradigms are important to understand when discussing plant therapies because the way people view their human world is often what they bring to and project onto the world of plants.

Over the years, the differences in paradigm have contributed to the underlying disagreement between science and healing. I have watched as healers assume that the nurse or medical scientist lacks ability or sensitivity for healing simply because they were educated and work in the biomedical world. The same thing was said in the nineteenth century of medical men who were educated in university settings. Dr. Benjamin Rush had to send his eighteenth-century medical students back to their farms to "get their fingernails dirty" so that the people would trust them and their ability to heal and cure. On the other hand, I have observed indigenous and traditional healers, and myself as well, be the brunt of jokes and jabs, and I have been at the receiving end of accusations and slander from some in the biomedical world suggesting that there is no way that I or my colleagues were rigorous scientists simply because the object of the work we do involves herbs and other healing traditions. A chemist once asked me, "How flakey are you?" and I was told one time in a professional meeting at a hospital to join "the fluff" research group.

Putting aside the blatant prejudices on both sides of the cultural equation, there are some philosophical differences between those who tend to polarize with one or the other paradigm. For example, traditional healers and the public have a tendency to utilize the whole plant and its parts such as the flower or root. Those of the biomedical paradigm tend to value a plant's constituents.

The history of competition and lack of unity between biomedical and traditional worlds is described in social science as being due to the commodification of health care.[56] The competition on the part of some in the biomedical community is exemplified in the gross generalization and marginalization of all non-biomedical healing practices as lesser (i.e. not as "safe and effective") medicine and healing. In the United States, medical, hospital, and pharmaceutical industries vanquished the rival medical sects (that practiced botanical and homeopathic medicine) in the late nineteenth century and destroyed the patent medicine industry, replacing its botanical medicines with synthetic over-the-counter and prescription products while assuring the public that industrialization of medicine making and greater federal controls ensured public safety. It is not clear that this has always been the case.

Nurses historically act as bridges between the people and their traditions and the emerging technologies of the biomedical world. They are trusted professionals who are relied upon in society to fulfill their caregiving role integrating technology and tradition. Nurses' understanding of herbalism as that which is informed by an integrated view of both the biomedical and traditional views of healing plants continues to provide the public a place for discussing plant remedies without judgment and perhaps even a modicum of fun. So often my clients, especially the children, tell me that they did not know that healing can be fun! Plants make the experience and possibility of healing fun especially when a nurse-herbalist provides the opportunity for the inclusion of all knowledge—traditional and biomedical. Plant therapies provide an opportunity for growth in the integration of the understanding that comes from looking at the parts and the whole. Because nurses have

---

56   Ronald Caplan, "The Commodification of American Health Care," *Social Science in Medicine* 28, no. 11 (1989).

a history both with the use of plant medicines and being able to bridge the worlds of biomedicine and tradition, they have much to contribute to furthering the understanding of healing plants from a model in which biomedical, traditional, and holistic nursing paradigms are integrated as holistic practice.

HERBALISM AND THE BIOMEDICAL PARADIGM

Nurses are very familiar with the biomedical paradigm because many nurses work in the culture of the biomedical world every day. Nurses share in the visions and beliefs of biomedical practitioners such as physicians and pharmacists. Some of the strengths of the biomedical worldview include valuing cure, a persistent attempt to find the cause (diagnose) of the disease in need of curing, and the deft use of technology to make discoveries on the cellular level. The cure is highly valued because it is equated with life and health. Research is one means of determining the efficacy of the cure. The biomedical paradigm includes a conviction regarding the benefits of good research in supporting clinical provision of safer and more efficacious health care. The gold standard of research is the randomized, double-blind, placebo-controlled trial because it is a form of inquiry that focuses on a very specific variable and seeks to isolate that variable so that its unique qualities can be recognized. Research questions are often answered through evaluation of quantifiable data. Nurses understand the value of quantifiable data and controls in clinical trials. They, too, perform such studies. How is the biomedical paradigm translated to the field of herbalism? The following are common questions asked by those perceiving herbs from a biomedical paradigm:

1. Are there any clinical trials on the use of this herbal *drug*?
2. How safe is this herbal drug for human consumption?
3. How efficacious is this herbal drug in curing specific disease?
4. What is the dose of the herb used?
5. What are the active ingredients/constituents in the crude herb drug, and can they be synthesized?
6. What are the risks of harmful interactions between herbs and other therapies prescribed such as drug and diet therapies?

I often hear these questions from many nurses, physicians, and pharmacists. These questions stem from the underlying values of the biomedical paradigm. The problem often encountered by patients and traditional healers who use plants in healing when they reveal the use to biomedical practitioners is that if these questions cannot be answered, then the herb is considered suspect, even useless. In industrialized societies where the biomedical view is dominant,[57] there is a sense of ethnocentrism as the biomedical culture raises its values for herbs as the "gold standard" for understanding healing plants. Biomedical dominance can lead to the closing of the heart and mind to inquiry. When this happens, the possibility of integration and consideration diminishes and negotiation ceases. Re-framing the biomedical questions can create a space for dialog. I call this approach "cultural diplomacy."

Cultural Diplomacy

Science and healing are part of culture. The word culture comes from the Latin *cultus* meaning "care" and the French *colere* meaning "cultivate."[58] Cultivation is a term commonly used in the plant world when referring to the nurturance of plant growth. *Ur* in Hebrew means "light." A synthesis of the roots of the word suggests that culture is of major concern in nurse-herbalism because it is in essence "the practice of the cultivation of light in giving care." Culture is also defined in the dictionary as "the integrated pattern of human knowledge, belief, and behavior that depends upon man's capacity for learning and transmitting knowledge."[59] Cultural diplomacy is the *active expression* of the internalized qualities of cultural awareness, sensitivity, and competence so often discussed in nursing as the practice of cultivating light in giving care.

Diplomacy is the highly refined communication skill used in developing and maintaining relationships between different cultures. It is an antidote to the culture clashes between nations and peoples that lead to frustration, power struggle, anger, argument, and violence. While

---

57 Sally Thorne, "Health Belief Systems in Perspective," *Journal of Advanced Nursing* 18 (1993): 1931.

58 Merriam-Webster, *Merriam-Webster's Collegiate Dictionary*, 10th ed. (Springfield, MA: Merriam-Webster, 1999).

59 Ibid.

the term diplomacy is more commonly applied to international, political relationships, *cultural* diplomacy is not unknown. All cultural exchanges often involve diplomacy in developing and maintaining relationships between different peoples. All relations between peoples are cultural in nature. The foundation of cultural diplomacy is education and example.[60] As it is applied to health care, cultural diplomacy suggests acknowledgment of the diversity of health beliefs and practices as represented in the paradigms discussed here and the need to build bridges between diverse groups through education and diplomatic example.

The goal of cultural diplomacy is to build long-term relationships that can lead to an increasingly peaceful global community. The purpose of cultural diplomacy in health care is improving communication and understanding between peoples of the biomedical, traditional, and holistic nursing paradigms or cultures. Because people of all paradigms relate to plants, plants have the potential of bringing people of different health cultures, beliefs, and practices together! This is why I advocate for cultural and herbal diplomacy.

Culture clash is the greatest obstacle to building a global health care community and bridging the gap between the biomedical and traditional worlds. At the center of culture clash is the fear of loss of control and the subsequent need to dominate others and convert them to one's own cultural beliefs and practices. People of every health care culture seek cultural authority. Culture clash occurs when people with different perspectives seek to extend their influence by convincing others of the "rightness" of their views. One example of culture clash in herbalism occurs in discussion about the necessity of formal (textbook-based) education. As I mentioned previously, some traditional healers criticize biomedical and complementary practitioners as being "book" trained about herbs and some suggest that those with formal herbal education are not "real" herbal healers. Biomedically focused practitioners (and some practitioners of complementary therapies as well) criticize traditional healers for not being "scientific" about herb use and suggest that their traditions are outdated and unsafe. Some herbalists, particularly in Europe, started a decade or so ago to refer to their work by the "technical

---

60 Harvey Feigenbaum, "Globalization and Cultural Diplomacy," (Washington, DC: George Washington University Center for the Arts and Culture, 2001).

term—phytotherapy" rather than "herbalism" as a way of distinguishing themselves from herbalism, "which is generally devoted to the folklore and mystical aspects of plant use."[61] After hundreds of years, we find in some of the biomedical and traditional worlds a desire to continue to focus on separating science, art, and spirit rather than bringing them back together as the balanced three-legged stool within the circle of culture. Nursing embodies the integration of science, art, and spirit and therefore nurse-herbalists need not adopt a different title as they continue to contribute to the creation of caring community. Historical tradition does not suggest a need for separation between the technical and the folkloric/mystical.

Psychologist M. Scott Peck wrote that the purpose of community building is peace making. He also stated that as long as people try to "convert and heal" others and attempt to turn them toward their own paradigm of the world, true community is not possible.[62] The diplomat does not seek to convert and heal; s/he uses the skill of tactful negotiation to maintain open communication between parties. This philosophy was very helpful for me when I was invited to create the Integrative Resource Center for Cancer (IRCC) at the University of Colorado Cancer Center a number of years ago when "integrative" centers were not the vogue they are today. The funding for the IRCC came from a very influential family in the community who wanted to provide families with information and resources not only about plant remedies but about all complementary therapies. There was a very influential oncologist who invited me to his clinic to observe him and the team of nurses to learn more about the purpose of the IRCC in patient and family care and support. The physician said to me in the morning, "You know I don't believe in what you are doing down there." My response was simply, "I understand and I want you and the nurses to know that I'm not here to convert you. We do know statistically that at least 75 percent of your patients are using complementary therapies and therefore I would like to find a way to work together to support them." We agreed to interact with an intention

---

61 Dan Kenner and Yves Requeno, "Whole-System Models Commonly Used in European Botanical Therapies, Part 1: The Terrain Concept and the Neuroendocrine Model," *American Journal of Acupuncture* 25, no. 4 (1997): 234.

62 M. Scott Peck, *The Different Drum: Community Making and Peace* (New York: Touchstone, 1987).

to help patients better. After a few hours of demonstrating a sincere interest in their work, the physician asked to see me again. He said, "I think that I have figured it out... how I can refer patients to your program. I was raised a Catholic but am an atheist—but I still refer patients to the chaplain or their priest when they clearly have a spiritual concern. I can refer patients to the IRCC, too, even though I don't agree with complementary therapies in cancer treatment." I received his solution and thanked him. The IRCC is still there for patients and families and that physician and his nurses changed their paradigm of care.

The cultural diplomat in health care and nursing inspires an ideal of a peaceful global health care community working together toward a plan of health care for all that is inclusive of all health beliefs, practices, and systems. Nurse-herbalists, because of their social position and having been educated and experienced in both biomedical and traditional cultures, can act as bridges between a variety of belief systems and practices. Nurse-herbalists can interpret herbal use from different paradigms and therefore can identify the appropriateness of the herbal care plan for a unique patient in a particular situation. Because they have a historical record of inclusion of all paradigms, they are well positioned to act as cultural diplomats for the healing art in general and botanical therapies in particular. They can help clients and caregivers examine plant knowledge from all cultural paradigms and then glean the plant wisdom that will enable them to use plant remedies as safely and effectively as possible. Here is an example of a diplomatic way of re-framing questions that reflect biomedical cultural values about herbal remedies while cultivating light:

1. What type of research questions need to be asked about plant therapies and nursing care, and what methodologies will best answer these questions?
2. How is safe use determined in the use of plant medicines?
3. Do plants "cure disease," or do they act in other ways?
4. How are herbal remedies dosed?
5. What are the healing properties, characteristics, and personality of the plant?
6. Herbs must "interact" with other therapies in some way. How can herbs and biomedical therapies be integrated, and

how can I help the patient understand the benefits and risks associated with choosing a plan of care that includes herbs if they are indicated and the patient wishes to use them?

These are broader, plant-focused questions. Many plant science experts often ask these kinds of questions. Norman Farnsworth, research professor of Pharmacognosy at the University of Illinois, and colleagues raised these kinds of questions in relation to the study of plants used in traditional medicine: "Is it desirable to put in effort to discover pure compounds in the hope of using them as drugs per se or is it preferable to go on using traditional preparations and make no attempt to identify the active principles?"[63] Although they may value understanding the active principles of a plant, they first question the relevance and purpose of the information. In general, those of the biomedical paradigm consider each plant a potential drug. Historically, the plant's constituents have been more highly valued than the plant as a whole. The overarching question of the biomedical paradigm about herbal remedies can be summarized as "What makes this healing plant work?" The following sections discuss four views of the workings of healing plants from the perspective of the biomedical paradigm.

Plants as Potential Drugs

First, plants are viewed as potential drugs. Most pharmaceutical drugs have been developed from plants and their constituents. A primary goal of those of the biomedical paradigm who use healing plants is to discover the plant drug's mechanism of action:

In the developed world, the active constituents of medicinal plants are of major importance; plant extracts are of minor importance as drugs. It is known that ca 119 drugs of known structure are still extracted from higher plants and are used globally in allopathic medicine . . . 10-15% of the 250,000 species of flowering plants on the planet have been used medicinally. However, only a fraction of

---

63 Norman Farnsworth and others, "Medicinal Plants in Therapy," *Bulletin of the World Health Organization* 63, no. 6 (1985): 967.

these are of sufficient importance to be considered as candidates as registration as drugs in developing countries based on widespread and continuous use and with some type of experimental confirmation of their biological activities.[64]

Some of the prescription and over-the-counter drugs for which plants or their derivatives are used include caffeine, opium, tincture of benzoin, oatmeal, chlorophyll, reserpine, scopolamine, vincristine, morphine, ipecac, psyllium, digoxin, ephedrine, and theophylline. These and many more drugs have brought relief to people over the years, and they are the result of the hard work and vision of those with a biomedical worldview. In the United States there is still some effort placed on plant-based drug development (pharmacognosy will be discussed in Chapter 6) but other governments in countries such as South Africa actively support and fund the development of traditional herbal medicines.

The cost of a new prescription drug going through the research and development phases and the formal approval process set forth by the Food and Drug Administration in the United States has been estimated to be between hundreds of thousands and millions of dollars, depending on such things as the number of phases of clinical trials to be undertaken and the drug being tested. This is one of the most expensive drug approval systems in the world today. If drug companies were to put this kind of money into the development of plant drugs, they could only recoup their costs if they held exclusive rights or a patent on the herbal drug to sell it. However, plants are not patentable because they are common, are used by many, and often grow outside our back doors. Drug companies can patent extraction techniques or they can modify some natural compound to make a semi-synthetic from a natural starting material. Although people may prefer a natural drug, the drug companies prefer a synthetic they can legally protect. Although some pharmaceutical companies have begun to take a second look at plant medicines, there are still some very big issues with the approach of searching for the active compounds.

Medicinal plants have very complex chemical structures. Identifying

---

64 Farnsworth in Shigeaki Baba, Olayiwola Akerele, and Yuji Kawaguchi, "Natural Resources and Human Health: Plants of Medicinal and Nutritional Value. Proceedings of the 1st WHO Symposium on Plants and Health for All: Scientific Advancement, Kobe, Japan. August 1991," (Amsterdam: Elsevier, 1992), 87.

one special active constituent that can create a certain health-giving action in the human body is not easy. It would be like saying that "an apple a day keeps the doctor away" solely because of the fructose or the pectin in the fruit. Plant medicines can elude the biomedical mind, which often tries to find the one drug for the particular disease. It may be the ideal, but "the bioavailability of these chemicals in an herbal formula or in an ingested herb is most likely very selective and dependent upon the physiological state of the individual consumer."[65] It is speculated that this may account for why herbs such as ginseng have been used for so many centuries in China for so many different conditions, yet ginseng still has not been proven "effective" by modern science. Herbs deliver a smorgasbord of biochemical constituents to the body and biomedical technology may not be able to identify how they work in multiple pathways at one time. The researcher may pay top money for the research and development of an herb or herbal formula only to end up with more questions about a particular plant's biologic and medicinal activity.

The consumer saves money with herbal remedies, however. One paper on the costs of herbal medicines to Health Maintenance Organizations (HMO) reported that if Saint John's Wort was given to depressed patient subscribers in the HMO instead of Prozac and were effective only in 25 percent of cases, the cost savings estimated to the HMO would be $250,000.[66] The paradox is that although the research and approval of a pharmaceutical drug made from a plant may be valued and desired, the reality is that it is often economically impractical for drug companies to promote the very products those in the biomedical world may want.

Research

The second view of the biomedical paradigm is that plant medicines must be submitted to the same rigorous testing and research controls used for drugs. It is often implied that the potential for harm to a patient taking plant medicines is just as great as if they were using a pharmaceutical

---

65 Albert Leung and Steven Foster, *Encyclopedia of Common Natural Ingredients Used in Food, Drugs, and Cosmetics*, 2nd ed. (New York: John Wiley & Sons, 1996), xii.
66 Lawrence Kincheloe, "Herbal Medicines Can Reduce the Costs in HMO," *Herbalgram* 41(1997).

drug, and therefore, toxicity, dosing, and standardization should be established for all herbal drugs. Some warn that herbs should not be used until such data are thoroughly collected and evaluated.[67] I have heard physicians, nurses, researchers, and even the public say this over the years. Although this concern may arise out of a health practitioner's ethical duty to do no harm, no data support the view that herbs should be considered as potentially harmful as the potent pharmaceutical drugs that scientists have created for diseases that require strong medicines. In sharp contrast, historical data demonstrate the opposite. Although there are herbal remedies that can cause harm if used improperly, such as applying a mustard plaster too long on the skin, community and health care records show that herbs have been considered gentler than pharmaceuticals that are often made of specific chemical compounds. In addition, the cost to support clinical research on every substance used in the healing arts is positively prohibitive.

So often nurses and other health care practitioners suggest that herbs be used only if they can be proven safe and efficacious by randomized clinical trials (RCTs), the gold standard of biomedical science most often used in the testing of pharmaceutical drugs. Some actually dismiss the question of the use of an herb in practice simply because no RCTs justify its use. There are some pros and cons to holding herbs to the same standards as pharmaceutical drugs. First of all, herbs do not have the same history as pharmaceutical drugs. Plant therapies often have been used extensively in one culture or another, sometimes for hundreds of years by humans, whereas drugs have not been used at all. Denying the use of drugs that have not been thoroughly studied is reasonable when they have never been used in humans. But is it reasonable to suggest that herbs that have been safely used by humans for hundreds of years should now be used only based on whether or not RCTs have proved that they are helpful and not just executing a placebo effect?

Secondly, the concept of the standard RCT is not acceptable to all cultures. For example, scientists in some countries do not agree philosophically with the concept of using a placebo. Is it reasonable to believe that all cultures will honor and value the RCT as the gold standard for good

---

67   Carol Newall, Linda Anderson, and J. David Phillipson, *Herbal Medicines: A Guide for Healthcare Professionals.* (London: The Pharmaceutical Press, 1996).

science or good herbal practice? It may seem culturally biased to some that the RCT is the only truly acceptable measure of safety and efficacy of an herb.

Questions have been raised within the biomedical community about the feasibility and the effect of holding the RCT as the gold standard for health science in the first place. RCTs are very expensive and logistically challenging. In fact, RCTs have not been carried out for many of the medical treatments in existence. And even when RCTs are available, it is difficult to extrapolate the findings to the individual patient because the entry criteria into the RCTs are usually very stringent and the clinician may never find an RCT that matches the patient seeking treatment. "The ideal of standardized and rigorous process for evaluating treatments seems at odds with everyday clinical practice, in which small sample sizes, even just one case, are frequently enough to convince clinicians and patients that something works…the treatment of an individual patient in routine clinical practice can be likened to a therapeutic experiment."[68]

Some have suggested that single patient trials (SPTs), or "N-of-1" studies, may be more feasible and more helpful in directing patient care.[69] The SPT provides research that supports the treatment of the *individual* patient. The goal of the SPT is the determination of the most suitable treatment for a given patient. As with all research methods, there are limitations to SPTs. "The limitations of n-of-1 trials arise from the prerequisites for their execution."[70] To perform an SPT, both the clinician and the patient must agree that there is some doubt about the effectiveness of the treatment under consideration. This doubt can be related to one or more of the following circumstances: (1) The client is taking a remedy that the clinician feels is worthless. (2) The client may be experiencing symptoms that may be construed as having adverse effects. (3) The clinician and/or the client are doubtful about the effectiveness of a particular treatment. (4) The clinician and/or the client are uncertain about the quantity of medication or therapy to be used. Although SPTs have been considered in terms of pharmaceutical drug studies, it is

---

68 Eric Larson, Allan Ellsworth, and Janet Oas, "Randomized Clinical Trials in Single Patients During a 2-year Period," *Journal of the American Medical Association* 270, no. 22 (1993): 2708.

69 Roman Jaeschke, Deborah Cook, and David Sackett, "The Potential Role of Single-Patient Randomized Controlled Trials (N-of-1 RCT's) in Clinical Practice," *Journal of the American Board of Family Practice* 5, no. 2 (1992).

70 Ibid., 228.

possible this method may be helpful in working with the individual client using some form of plant therapy, be it an herbal bath, compress, or tea.

The questions regarding the feasibility of any clinical trial involving plant therapies relate primarily to randomization and blindedness. There have been concerns that many herbal therapies as well as other complementary therapies may not best be studied by the clinical trial method. "Alternative medicine therapies may also possess a theoretical basis, may stem from a cultural tradition that is seemingly antithetical to a quantitative, biomedical framework, or may possess little foundation research on which to base a controlled evaluation."[71] Often with herbal remedies, the investigator is seeking to understand the mechanism of action or established therapeutic outcomes. Because the mechanism of action is often unknown, establishing controls for a particular study can be very difficult.

In many cultural traditions, the herbal remedy being studied might preclude the blinding of the practitioner in the study because the relationship between healer, plant, and patient is highly significant and essential to the treatment outcome. For example, if a nurse-investigator wanted to study the effects of *Aloe vera* plasters on second- or third-degree burns, the preparation and application of the plaster (the method) is just as significant as the aloe material itself when considering the therapy as a whole. How the plaster is applied and how the care is demonstrated are as important to nursing practice as the biochemical action of the aloe. These factors also are important in traditional herbalism and, in some cases, are considered more important. This will be discussed more in the section on the traditional paradigm.

If the way in which care is provided did not matter to nurses, we would not spend time teaching students how to communicate or educate patients. Students would not be taught how to manage a sick room as Nightingale[72] and the Sisters of Charity[73] discussed, or how to touch a patient therapeutically, or how to respond when one sees a gross malformation such as a gaping wound on a patient for the first time. None

71 Arthur Margolin, S. Kelly Avants, and Herbert Kleber, "Investigating Alternative Medicine Therapies in Randomized Controlled Trials," *Journal of the American Medical Association* 280, no. 18 (1998): 1626.

72 Nightingale, *Notes on Nursing: What It Is and What It Is Not.*

73 Coskery, *Advices Concerning the Sick.* As cited in Libster and McNeil, *Enlightened Charity: The Holistic Nursing Care, Education and Advices Concerning the Sick of Sister Matilda Coskery, (1799-1870).*

of this would matter. But it does matter to nurses, and to patients. "How nurses creatively demonstrate caring is the art of nursing. It is the beauty of nursing. It is also the science of nursing."[74] How an herb is prepared and applied matters, too. Herb research in nursing should complement and inform nursing science and professional values and lend itself to ready application in meaningful evidence-based practice.

Evidence-Based Practice

In 1990, I was moonlighting on a medical-surgical ward in rural Montana. As I was performing my rounds as charge nurse and assessing my patients, I entered the room of a 50- year-old woman who had been admitted for a cholecystectomy. She was receiving intravenous antibiotics for an inflamed gall bladder and resting for a few days in preparation for surgery. She asked me quietly if I had ever heard of a "gall bladder bursting." I told her that I had not but after looking at her face I knew that I had to ask, "What makes you ask?" She said that she thought that her "gall bladder had burst" that morning. She had asked the day nurse the same question she had asked me and been told "no," the nurse knew of no such thing. She had tried unsuccessfully to go back to sleep. Over the years I had learned through interaction with many pediatric patients to always trust what children and their parents tell me. Based on those experiences I said to her, "If you think that your gall bladder burst this morning then we can call the doctor to get an order for an ultrasound to check it out." Sure enough, the woman's gall bladder had indeed ruptured. I had taken care of patients whose appendices had ruptured but never had I heard of nor seen a ruptured gall bladder. And while it did not seem to me to be out of the realm of possibility, I had not read about it in a text or in a medical or nursing journal.

This experience I had is just one of many examples of how nurses gather "evidence" from their experiences with patients. I remember this event not only for what I learned about the gall bladder. I also remember the process of how I came to know more about the gall bladder. From this one experience, I remember the important lessons I learned about patients' intuitions, body awareness, and ways of communication. This

---

74 Libster, *Demonstrating Care: The Art of Integrative Nursing*: 3.

patient taught me well that the "evidence" upon which nurses and health care practitioners make decisions is not always concrete, reasonable, or supported given our professional experience, paradigm or framework in that particular moment of interaction. Knowledge and evidence in health care and nursing are not only gained through research in laboratories and clinical trials. They are created by patients and nurses within the context of the healing relationship. My experience with this patient's burst gall bladder taught me that a nurse's evidence-based practice is a professional construct founded upon an ongoing scientific process that includes keen observation, listening, and interaction.

Evidence-based practice (EBP) is best used to support the nurse-herbalist focus on integrative care. It is part of the problem-solving approach in which the practitioner consciously includes knowledge, ideas, insights, feelings, and intuitions from such sources as randomized clinical trials, descriptive and qualitative studies, theories, client preferences and experiences, client health patterns, nurse and client dreams and interactions, and plant knowledge, memories, and experiences. The concept of EBP originated in the United Kingdom with an epidemiologist named Dr. Archie Cochrane and was also developed in Canada. It is a reflection of those cultures' health beliefs, values, and practices. How nurses of other countries translate and implement the concept of EBP into practice is also a reflection of their own professional culture. For example, while British nurses might link evidence from a clinical trial to a hospital policy and procedure, a nurse using that policy is not required, in Britain, to use that policy or the evidence in the care of the patient. Each patient is treated as a unique person and the "evidence" from a study is applied only if the nurse, through his or her assessment, deems it rational and pertinent to do so.

One British colleague once told me that to *require* nurses to use the evidence as policy and procedure without allowing for critical examination of how that evidence should or should not be used in the care of the client would be considered by British nurses an act of the "thought policing." David Sackett of the National Health Service in the UK and his colleagues clarify that, "Evidence-based medicine is not 'cook-book' medicine."[75] Hence it seems that in the United Kingdom,

---

75   David Sackett and others, *Evidence-Based Medicine.* (London: Churchill Livingstone, 1998), 3.

EBP is used as a conceptual framework for a practice that is patient-focused and promoting of the practitioner as critical thinker. The British approach to EBP also resonates with "fourth-generation evaluation" in nursing, a framework for critical evaluation of nursing care that includes the patient experience and is transactional as opposed to the first three generations of evaluation of care that focused on measurement, objectives, and judgment.[76]

In light of the cultural shift to EBP, the nurse of the twenty-first century is challenged to find ways to examine not only the evidence of its more conventional technology-based inventions but to include in that examination process the historical healing traditions and complementary therapies used by nurses for centuries. Some have questioned whether or not the concept of EBP can be applied to complementary therapies and ancient healing traditional practices. I would argue that healing traditions and complementary therapies can indeed be included in EBP as long as the construct of EBP being used is one that is inclusive of all ways of knowing, such as that which is stated in the definition above. For example, the historical evidence of centuries of use of a modality, such as a particular botanical therapy, is best considered equally with the evidence provided by the randomized clinical trial. Over the years, I have heard health practitioners, community leaders, scientists, the media, and members of the public question the legitimacy of the "evidence" around traditional healing, called "complementary therapies" in industrialized countries. The argument most often used is that there are "no clinical trials supporting the use of these healing methods." This is simply not the case. The Cochrane Library reports that they housed, as of 2002, more than 80 complementary therapies-related, full-text systematic and comprehensive reviews and approximately 5,000 reports of complementary therapies-related clinical trials.[77]

What is a significant challenge, however, in the application of EBP to healing traditions/complementary therapies is the ability to directly apply the randomized clinical trial, a highly valued research method in

---

76 Tomasz Koch, "Beyond Measurement: Fourth-Generation Evaluation in Nursing," *Journal of Advanced Nursing* 20, no. 6 (1994): 1148-9.

77 Jeanette Ezzo and others, "Use of the Cochrane Electronic Library in Complementary and Alternative Medicine Courses in Medical Schools: Is the Giant Lost in Cyberspace?" *Journal of Alternative and Complementary Medicine* 8, no. 5 (2002).

the biomedical culture, to the investigation of the efficacy and safety of these therapies. Many research questions scientists and practitioners of healing traditions have are not best answered by the clinical trial. Historical evidence, such as the hundreds of years of human use of a specific botanical therapy, is a significant source of evidence of the safety and efficacy of that plant when used within its historical cultural context. There are also ethical as well as philosophical and clinical issues related to the study of certain healing modalities that preclude the use of research techniques such as the use of the double blind technique and the administration of placebos.

Therefore, the inquiring nurse who seeks to apply an evidence-based approach to healing traditions and complementary therapies must keep in mind the most inclusive definition of evidence possible so as not to lose sight of valuable resources, information, and data supplied by historical traditional evidence, patient experience, and practitioner expertise. Just as some nurses need to be encouraged to move beyond their traditional patterns of practice and explore clinical trial and laboratory evidence, some need to be challenged to integrate historical and traditional evidence into their expression of EBP. Nurses who are able to rationally inquire into numerous ways of knowing about healing traditions and complementary therapies as well as conventional nursing interventions add to their talent for reflective practice. This integrative, inclusive approach to the evidence builds potential for finding new ways of moving nursing research into new arenas of creative, scientific exploration. By applying different paradigms, nurses can experience the integrative insights that allow even the smallest piece of the puzzle of healing evidence, such as a burst gall bladder, a rightful place in the development of a twenty-first century nursing science.

Outcomes measurement, evidence-based practice, and research in general are an ongoing concern for nurse-scholars. The concern about developing quality research in nursing that informs holistic caring practice is very similar to the concerns about researching complementary therapies such as herbal medicine. Although clinical trials have been done with herbal medicines, especially with standardized extract preparations, there are questions as to whether or not these studies actually promote understanding of the herbal *therapy*. Many studies that help in identifying plant constituents that are possibly responsible for the action of a medicinal plant are done as *in vitro* studies in a laboratory. Can understanding the mechanism of action of a plant or its constituents give a clinician a reasonably good understanding of the safety and efficacy of the plant as a remedy or healing modality?

Studies using *in vitro* and other scientific methods can be helpful in adding to the body of healing plant knowledge. Nursing practice benefits from quantitative studies, such as *in vitro* and the RCT, and also from qualitative studies. For example, ethnographic and narrative inquiries could be helpful in understanding traditional uses of herbal remedies that are highly valued by communities. Studies that lead to a greater understanding of the relationship of the plant in the healing rituals of an individual may be just as insightful as the studies that lead to greater understanding of the inner workings of the plant itself. Integration of understanding gained from biomedical and traditional research may be the most reasonable approach when the nurse-herbalist seeks to meet individual client needs for healing and greater well-being.

Reporting the Outcome and the Evidence

Because nurses have a history of supporting and promoting self-care, they often encounter patients who are using plant remedies in self-treatment or treatment of their family members. Nurses are often in a position, as in the consumer model of care, to provide research and information to patients about the herbal remedies they are using or considering using. The public, although interested in scientific research, is often uninformed regarding the variation of methodologies used to study herbs. It is the ethical responsibility of health practitioners and researchers to clearly report findings and include any limitations of the study to the consumer. This means that if a large clinical trial on an herb shows favorable, generalizable responses, consumers must not be led to believe that *they* are assured benefit. This also means that if an RCT shows no benefit for an herb that traditional herbalists or a community has used for hundreds of years, then there is *no* health benefit. RCTs are very specific, and the results must be reported regarding the study's inclusion criteria, the herb(s) included in the study, and how they were applied. For example, if the RCT involved the use of standardized extract of a particular constituent from an herb such as alliin from garlic (*Allium sativum*), it should not be reported in a way that would leave the consumer with the impression that whole garlic or other garlic products would have the same results.

One example of ethically flawed reporting occurred with the release of results of an *in vitro* study of four herbs' effect on penetration of *hamster* oocytes and the integrity of donor (presumably human) sperm deoxyribonucleic acid.[78] The results of the *in vitro* study were that flooding the oocytes with a "concentrated herbal solution" of each of the four herbs resulted in reduced or zero penetration of oocytes. Exposure of sperm cells to some of the herbs resulted in denaturation of DNA. One well-known American physician appeared on a major national news program and reported to the public that anyone trying to conceive should not take any of the herbs evaluated in the study. He mentioned that many herbs are not "studied" and therefore are potentially unsafe. It was never mentioned that the study was on hamster instead of human cells. The physician did mention in passing that the study was an *in vitro* study, but he did not clarify for the listener what that meant. The essence of the report was that the four herbs have not been studied, they are unsafe, and pose a danger to those trying to conceive. The report was made without consideration of the need for clear, unbiased representation of research findings.

In reporting orally or in written form any research findings or evidence about herbal remedies it is important to include the following plant science perspective:

1. Include the Plant Perspective
   a. Botanical names should include scientific name if known.
   b. Format for botanical name: Common name (Scientific name)
   c. Include relevant information on the historical and traditional applications of the plant or plants discussed.

---

78 Richard Ondrizek and others, "An Alternative Medicine Study of Herbal Effects on the Penetration of Zona-Free Hamster Oocytes and the Integrity of Sperm Deoxyribonucleic Acid," *Fertility and Sterility* 71, no. 3 (1999).

    d. Be sure to distinguish whole plant from plant constituents and their applications when discussing botanical therapies. Examples:

        i. Identify the Botanical Application: Ex. In citing an article on St. John's Wort (*Hypericum perforatum*) for mitigating episiotomy, state that the infused oil of St. John's Wort was massaged on the perineum.

        ii. Plant Constituent: If discussing risks of oral doses of St. John's Wort for mild depression, quote the article and be sure to state if risk is related to *Hypericum* whole plant or a constituent such as hypericin.

2. Control Bias –Health sciences literature in which plants are discussed should follow guidelines for professional scientific reporting and writing.

    a. Discuss the data and avoid gross generalizations from unsupported data, which imply or state a risk from using botanical therapies

    b. Call for further research as is customary in scientific writing rather than debunk a plant, its use in health care or herbalism in general.

    c. Be fair to plants and cultural traditions and rituals that include them. Just as scientific writing calls for sensitivity to marginalized humans, respect should be shown to plants and associated cultural traditions. Slurring of any plant, botanical therapy or cultural tradition is not appropriate.

3. Include a Literature Review from a Plant Perspective

    a. Demonstrate that botanical literature has been reviewed. See publications in phytopharmacy, ethnobotany, botany, folklore, etc.

    b. Consider including international research publications, particularly if a plant is indigenous and well known outside the USA.

c. Use botanical databases such as NAPRALERT and HERBCLIPS (American Botanical Council).

d. Include book publications – Some of the plant expertise, such as on medicinal mushrooms, for example, is well documented in experts' book publications.

Here is an example of reporting research information to a client: "The randomized, double-blind, placebo-controlled study involved 30 men taking whole garlic *(Allium sativum)* in capsules (amount if known) for 3 months. The study of these men showed that taking the garlic capsules did lower total cholesterol levels in all of the men by _____ (number) points." If speaking to a woman, it might be emphasized that the study only included men. If someone were taking whole garlic in their diet, it might be emphasized that the results of the study were related to the use of capsulated whole garlic. Nurses have a responsibility not only to perform reasonable research but also to reasonably report research findings in a manner that clearly informs the public and does not mislead them to believe strongly in benefits or risks that do not necessarily exist.

Standardization

The third biomedical view is that controlling the quality and quantity of plant constituents in a standardization process (such as European phyto-pharmaceuticals) provides for safer and more effective use of herbal remedies. In the biomedical paradigm, it is believed that standardization to a specific plant constituent makes the remedy more potent, more effective, and easier to use, at least for those who are more familiar with dosing pharmaceutical drugs than with traditional or clinical herbalist dosing strategies for a particular herb. Standardized herbal products have become "drugs of choice" in some countries. It is important to know that in plant science, standardization based on one particular chemical constituent is not considered representative of the total activity of a medicinal plant. The selected components are meant to be biologic markers of product quality of total plant extractions rather than medicinal effectiveness.

Standardization of chemical constituents may appear to be easier to study in clinical trials and often is touted by biomedical practitioners as an "evolution" in herbal medicine. Along with standardization comes a cleaner, smaller package. Processed standardized herbs are usually sold in capsule or tablet form, similar to pharmaceuticals. The consumer is spared the fuss of dealing with whole herb products and knowing how to prepare them for their healing applications. Some consumers and nurses may believe that taking a pill is easier and more enjoyable (i.e., no odd taste). Even though biomedical practitioners may feel they are providing a service to patients, some may question the so-called evolution in the use of herbal medicines just as they might other technologic advances.

Clinical science in botanical medicine was well developed among nineteenth-century physicians in America and England. Doctors knew how to choose plant medicines for clients and knew their common dosages, which were individualized for the client. The use of standardized plant extracts is now being promoted as "a professionalization of botanical medicine, an enhancement of nature by laboratory science creating a quasi-pharmaceutical for 'scientific' professional use."[79] The role of technology in general is being questioned among members adhering to the biomedical paradigm. "It is apparent that technology has indeed come between the patient and the doctor and that although scientific devices disgorge much information, knowledge as to how to treat the patient properly may still be lacking."[80] Nurses must seriously consider any unstudied biomedical belief that a standardized herbal preparation is inherently better or safer for use than a remedy that is not standardized.

Herbal Revolution

A revolution is defined as a "change in paradigm."[81] If the change in paradigm were for biomedical practitioners to once again consider using herbs and also to work together with traditional healers and clinical

79 Dan Kenner and Yves Requena, "Whole-System Models Commonly Used in European Botanical Therapies, Part II: The Five Phases Model," *American Journal of Acupuncture* 26, no. 1 (1998): 55.
80 Franz Ingelfinger, "Medicine: Meritorious or Meretricious," *Science* 200, no. 4344 (1978): 945.
81 Merriam-Webster, *Merriam-Webster's Collegiate Dictionary.*

herbalists, some would want to change and others would not. The fourth view of the biomedical paradigm has to do with the two perceptions of what would happen if there were to be an herbal revolution or change in paradigm. The first, perhaps stemming from the historical issues between the scientists and the people, is that there needs to be a revolution on herbal medicines to expose what biomedical practitioners consider to be "dangerous" practitioners and practices with plant therapies. Some believe that those who heal with herbs are pretending to have medical skills—that they are "quacks." "Orthodox medicine does not reject medicines derived from herbs but it does reject quackery,"[82] possibly implying that biomedical practice with herbs is not subject to quackery. Others of the biomedical paradigm understand that "herbal medicine differs from orthodox medicine not only in the form in which plants are administered but also in its underlying philosophy"[83] and the way herbal practitioners provide their service. They understand that quackery can exist in any group of professionals and that philosophical differences must be respected.

Secondly, some biomedical practitioners are revolutionary in that they realize that there are valid viewpoints other than those often held in biomedical and research domains regarding the best means of studying the efficacy and safety of herbal medicines. Some biomedical practitioners suggest that "long and widespread use together with closely-detailed records of individual case histories"[84] be considered when examining an herb's safety and efficacy. Others recommend including experimental case studies as a way of studying efficacy of herbs. It also is thought to be important that biomedical practitioners broaden the scope of literature searches associated with herbal research to go beyond the available literature in Western publications or a MEDLINE database as I suggested above. For example, I have been involved in any number of circumstances in which journals with published, peer-reviewed studies, even RCTs from countries outside the United States are excluded simply because they were not done in this country. These are just a few of the potential responses to an herbal revolution.

---

82 R Penn, "Adverse Reactions to Herbal and Other Unorthodox Medicines," in *Iatrogenic Diseases*, eds. Patrick D'Arcy and John Griffin (Oxford: Oxford University Press, 1986), 898.

83 Peter Houghton, "The Role of Plants in Traditional Medicine and Current Therapy," *Journal of Alternative and Complementary Medicine* 1, no. 2 (1995): 137.

84 Ibid.

At the same time that herbs and the philosophy regarding their use are being questioned in the biomedical world, some beliefs regarding some of the oldest biomedical drugs are even being questioned. Aspirin, first introduced to the American public in 1899, is considered the most popular drug of all time. Aspirin, acetylsalicylic acid, was developed from the plant, *Filipendula ulmaria,* also known as *Spiraea ulmaria* or meadowsweet. It is among the top ten drugs prescribed in the United States.[85] A pioneer in biotechnology who has developed drug delivery systems for cancer and heart patients questions the recommendation of other biomedical colleagues who prescribe an aspirin a day. He writes that:

> Taking an aspirin for the rest of your life can, in proper doses knock out bad eicosanoids [a family of biological substances including thromboxanes and prostaglandins] at a slightly faster rate than it knocks out good eicosanoids. But taking aspirin is a tricky game to play, sort of like lighting a cigarette with a stick of dynamite. . . . No one knows what the 'proper' dose of aspirin is, especially over a long period of time. . . . Long-term aspirin may be the biological equivalent of a loose cannon.[86]

Changes are happening in the biomedical paradigm in relationship to drugs and especially with plant therapies. As interaction among disciplines increases, new questions about herbs and new ways of answering those questions emerge.

Nurses must not rely completely upon the values and standards of the biomedical paradigm, which work well for the biomedical world but do not seem best fitted to the use of plant therapies. There is a call for a new worldview even among those who may have held the biomedical paradigm for some time. Nurse-herbalists will note that as changes occur, they will be able to observe which aspects of their own biomedical paradigm inform their work with medicinal plants and which do not. This examination of one's own paradigm is part of reflective practice and also part of developing skills in integrative nursing.

---

85   Carol Lewis, "Medical Milestones of the Last Millennium," *FDA Consumer* 34, no. 2 (2000).
86   Barry Sears, *The Zone.* (New York: Regan Books Harper Collins, 1995), 161.

HERBALISM AND THE TRADITIONAL PARADIGM

History demonstrates some of the vast differences between traditional healers' and biomedical views of healing, health care, and medicinal use of plants. "In keeping with scientific tradition modern biomedicine has striven to separate itself from broader cultural concerns and influences (and has considered itself largely successful in the attempt)."[87] Biomedical science continues to separate itself from the people and traditions in an attempt to increase the objectivity and therefore the rigor of the inquiry. Striving for objectivity does not always work in medicinal plant science because, as those who partner with plants know well, plants are living beings with which people have relationships. Those relationships sometimes include memories of years of application in numerous health conditions, healing rituals, and practices. Plant knowledge in the traditional paradigm is most often embedded in story.

There is an old story in Chinese herbal medicine that helps illustrate a traditional paradigm of the use of herbs. It goes like this. ... A group of herbal students was ready for their final exam. Their teacher told them to search eight miles out on all sides of the town and bring back samples of all the plants they could find that had absolutely no medicinal value. Within a few days all but one of the students had returned, each with a few plants. Finally on the fifth day, the last student returned looking very sad indeed, for he was empty handed. "Why so sad?" asked the teacher. "You are the only one qualified to pursue the herbal path."

This story illustrates the plant values of the traditional sphere. The traditional paradigm represents the "people's" cultural beliefs about plants and their rituals and habits of use over time. One dictionary definition of tradition is the "continuity of culture."[88] Because cultures and plant populations differ geographically, the specifics of a particular traditional plant paradigm also differs from country to country. It is beyond the scope of this book to examine each individual culture's traditional uses of herbs; however, the traditional use of herbs and herb use in the biomedical world, which is also a culture in its own right, will be compared and contrasted.

---

87 Bonnie O'Connor, *Healing Traditions: Alternative Medicine and the Health Professions* (Philadelphia: University of Pennsylvania Press, 1995), 22.

88 Merriam-Webster, *Merriam-Webster's Collegiate Dictionary*.

Traditional medicine is defined by the World Health Organization (WHO) as "the ways of protecting and restoring health that existed before the arrival of modern medicine . . . approaches to health that belong to the traditions of a country and have been handed down from generation to generation."[89] Some traditional healing with plants has been passed by word of mouth as part of the folklore of a country. The oral tradition of passing on information about herbs includes a belief system and a philosophy as well as the details of the actual use of the healing plants. Some traditional systems such as Traditional Chinese Medicine (TCM), Kampo medicine in Japan, and Ayurveda in India are highly documented, theoretically based, and researched. In addition to herbalists, WHO classifies acupuncturists, traditional birth attendants, and mental healers as traditional healers. Many countries have traditional healers who are indigenous peoples who use herbs as part of their healing practices.

Balick and Cox define indigenous people as those "who follow traditional, non-industrialized lifestyles in areas that they have occupied for generations."[90] So a TCM practitioner in the United Kingdom, for example, although a practitioner of a traditional form of medicine, would not be considered an indigenous healer in Britain the way a Celtic person might. Indigenous healers serve as great resources about the plants growing in their regions. Their relationships with plants are strong and direct. Indigenous healers wildcraft or cultivate their own herbs, and use the plants directly. They retain their knowledge of use of plants. Many indigenous cultures "perceive the earth as existing not in the realm of the profane, but in the realm of the sacred, a worldview that distinguishes them from many Western traditions. Indigenous legends emphasize the need to protect the earth not because it is useful to humans but because it is sacred."[91] Traditional healing practices emphasize balance and harmony between the elements, person, all living creatures, Earth, and the universe. Holistic nursing also has a history with the same values.

---

89 World Health Organization, "Fact Sheet No. 134 Traditional Medicine," (Geneva, Switzerland: WHO, 2003), 1.

90 Michael Balick and Paul Alan Cox, *Plants, People, and Culture: The Science of Ethnobotany* (New York: Scientific American Library, 1996), 5.

91 Ibid., 182.

North American Indian or First Nation indigenous medicine is connected with the history of nursing in North America. Midwives and caregivers, often the women of the households of the European settlers, learned early on from Native American healers how to apply plant remedies when caring for themselves and their families.[92] Early North American medical dispensatories included plant medicines commonly used by various Native American tribes. Yet the Native American contributions to the medical practices of North Americans are often devalued if not grossly under-recognized.

North American Indian medicine includes the use of plant remedies for wounds, fractures, and numerous illnesses. Some illnesses are not only treated with plant remedies. For example, "persistent internal disease" is thought to be caused by supernatural forces; therefore, other methods of healing besides plant remedies, such as chant, dance, and drumming, also are used in healing. North American Indian herbalists, called "Mashki-kike-winini" by one tribe, receive a calling to know the various mysterious properties of medicinal plants. "Although these herbalists are aware that certain plants or roots will produce a specified effect upon the human system, they attribute the benefit to the fact that such remedies are distasteful and injurious to the demons who are present in the system and whom the disease is attributed."[93]

The term "medicine" to a North American Indian has meaning that extends well beyond the remedy or treatment. Medicine is equated with the "mysterious, inexplicable, and unaccountable."[94] This book does not even begin to account for the rituals and mystical understanding held by the American indigenous healers regarding plants. Much of this plant wisdom and understanding is protected as a valuable treasure and is not shared even by tribal members without the express permission and spiritual guidance of the tribal elders and healers. Ethnobotanical studies have revealed the richness of the healing traditions of various American Indian tribes such as the Zuni and Cheyenne, and that knowledge of traditional beliefs and customs in regard to medicinal plant healing is diminishing. But there are some tribal wisdom keepers and medicine

---

92   Libster, *Herbal Diplomats: The Contribution of Early American Nurses (1830-1860) to Nineteenth-Century Health Care Reform and the Botanical Medical Movement.*

93   Virgil Vogel, *American Indian Medicine* (Norman: University of Oklahoma Press, 1970), 23.

94   Ibid., 25.

people, such as Cecilia Mitchell known as Zezi, an elder from Akwesasne Mohawk Country,[95] whom I have worked with, who teach, heal, and tell stories that help root their people's knowledge of healing plants deeply within the community so that the understanding of the plants is preserved. Zezi also fights to preserve her herbal "apothecaries" from political and corporate land claim and other potential public developments.

I have lodged with Zezi. Being with her at the nexus of five rivers in a land that my cell phone told me was Canada and the map said was New York State, USA, is always a peaceful experience. Zezi carries the legends of the people of Six Nations (Iroquois). We talk plant, take medicine walks, pray, and share medicine stories. Zezi also gave me the gift of the story of the Peace Maker and history of the White Roots of Peace that is one of the most important stories of the Six Nations people and therefore fundamental for understanding their medicine traditions. To begin to understand medicine as fully as is possible from traditional and indigenous healers, one must experience the stories and legends of the people.

In traditional ways of knowing and being, the way life is viewed is quite different from views of the biomedical culture. Whereas the main question of those of the biomedical culture might be "What makes this plant work?" the main question of those of the traditional paradigm might simply be "How can this plant be used for healing?" The need for understanding the components that make up the plant before deciding whether or not it can be used is not necessarily part of the traditional paradigm. "Typically, practitioners of traditional medicine view the biomedical search for a single, so-called active ingredient as an inappropriate application of their empirically and culturally grounded health knowledge."[96] In traditional practice, herbs are most often used synergistically in combination as opposed to the biomedical approach of targeting a single constituent.

In folkloric healing or domestic medicine—types of traditional practice—herbs often have been used historically as single-plant remedies, called "simples." In the twelfth century, European apothecaries

---

95 Steve Wall, *Wisdom's Daughters: Conversations With Women Elders of Native America* (New York: Harper Perennial, 1993).

96 Gerard Bodeker, "Traditional Health Systems: Policy, Biodiversity, and Global Interdependence," *Journal of Alternative and Complementary Medicine* 1, no. 3 (1995): 235.

or pharmacists were busy developing all sorts of new complex drugs from animals, vegetables, and minerals because they could not have "made the barest living by selling the simples that grew in their customers' gardens or flourished in the nearest patch of waste land."[97] Today, many pharmacies are selling large amounts of herbal preparations to people who have no knowledge of the plant, let alone the ability to grow it themselves. A simple today might be considered a capsule of a single herb. This is very different from the approach of those practicing from the domestic or folkloric view in which a single fresh or dried herb might be used as a tea, topical application or solution such as a syrup or alcohol extract.

Traditional practitioners also have their own language for describing illness. The paradigm does not include seeking to control nature, destroy pathogens, or eradicate diseases. Although the explanations about cause for illness and rationale for use of a particular herb may be very different from that of the biomedical paradigm, they are similarly scientifically based. Indigenous knowledge systems (IKS) include ways of knowing about medicines, healing, communication, art, agriculture, education, and all other cultural arenas from the views of indigenous peoples. Indigenous knowledge is local knowledge that is unique to a given culture or society. It is the foundation for decision making within a culture.

Traditional and indigenous practitioners use logic and some form of pattern recognition when describing illness. They match the pattern of illness or discomfort with an herb or herbs that bring about greater balance and health. Traditional medical knowledge is typically coded into household cooking practices, home remedies, and health prevention/maintenance beliefs and routines.[98] It is not uncommon for people who use traditional and folk medicines to also use biomedical treatments and medicines. Traditional health care alternatives abound in areas well served by conventional medical care, as a survey in any major metropolitan area in the United States would demonstrate.

There has been an enduring awareness of the ability to integrate the values and practices of biomedicine and tradition in the use of

---

97   Barbara Griggs, *Green Pharmacy* (Rochester, VT: Healing Arts Press, 1991), 29.
98   Bodeker, "Traditional Health Systems: Policy, Biodiversity, and Global Interdependence," 232.

plant medicines for centuries.[99] It has also been demonstrated in many countries that people often choose to combine the use of herbs and conventional biomedical practices in some way. One American study showed that, "Among the 44% of adults who said that they regularly take prescription medications, nearly 1 in 5 (18.4%) reported the concurrent use of at least 1 herbal product, a high-dose vitamin, or both."[100]

People choose to use traditional healing methods for many reasons. Their decisions can be quite logical and are often based on trust. People who have seen the effectiveness of plant remedies used by their families may suspect the newest treatment introduced by the biomedical practitioner. That is human nature, and it is also very logical. People also know from experience and from long historical use that plant medicines are gentler medicines and have not had the same adverse effects that pharmaceutical drugs do. Because many of the day-to-day health concerns are not life threatening, many people logically turn to lifestyle issues such as diet and home remedies (e.g., plant medicines) to effect changes that result in greater comfort and health. People have a sense of timing in their healing process. Although they often prefer to provide self-care and not rely on someone else for care, they also ask for help when it is needed. Ethnographic fieldwork has "repeatedly revealed that vernacular health belief systems have among their central values concerns for the appropriate and timely intervention and for seeking the proper specialist."[101] These concerns are shared by those with a biomedical paradigm. The differences lie in the treatment that is deemed necessary and where the search for relief ought to begin.

In my experience, culture clashes frequently occur in private, public, hospital or community-based health care facilities. I have seen how cultural gaps, such as how folk remedies from one culture can be misinterpreted by those who work in the biomedical culture, cause great tension in the healing relationship and environment. For example, when I was a school nurse in Minnesota where many Hmong refugees had

---

99 Libster, *Herbal Diplomats: The Contribution of Early American Nurses (1830-1860) to Nineteenth-Century Health Care Reform and the Botanical Medical Movement*; Levin and Idler, *The Hidden Health Care System*

100 David Eisenberg and others, "Trends in Alternative Medicine Use in the United States, 1990-1997: Results of a Follow-up National Survey," *JAMA* 280, no. 18 (1998): 1572.

101 O'Connor, *Healing Traditions: Alternative Medicine and the Health Professions*: 21.

immigrated, I had been given some education as to their cultural beliefs. One day a child came to school with small, circular burn marks along his spine. The teachers thought that the parents were abusing the small child by burning him with what looked like might have been a cigarette, but the child had been burned on certain acupuncture meridian points to heal the cold sore on his lip. I realized the burn pattern because of my background in Asian medicine, not because of the cultural training I had been given by the county. Although other treatments for cold sores are less physically harmful, the Hmong parents' intent was not to harm their child with the moxibustion treatment, but to heal him. It is important that the traditional paradigm and practice be understood before making any kind of assumption about healing practices, including the use of herbs. Had child protective services been called in on this case, the family who spoke little English could have been devastated by the enactment of a law that did not apply to them.

The tension between the herbal practices of those of the traditional paradigm and those of the biomedical paradigm is often fanned by the clashes of the two paradigms. In my experience, people respect and use their own herbal traditions and like to learn from other traditions, too. People often like to learn about the herbal science of the biomedical world as well. They seek information about all options from both paradigms, especially for chronic conditions, health promotion, and day-to-day discomfort. Biomedical practitioners who understand as much as possible about their patients' belief systems and what their traditional use of plants is like can better develop a healing and helping relationship with their clients when they seek help from the biomedical world.

Because of their extensive history of use and their prevalence in contemporary societies, herbal remedies continue to be an ever-present part of the traditional health care practices of people. As countries continue to address the struggle to provide health care for all, traditional/indigenous healers are becoming more valuable each day. In some countries, they are part of a community's primary health care network.

Primary Health Care and the Promotion of Diplomacy and Integration

Integration has been initiated by the World Health Organization's Traditional Medicine Programme. The Alma-Ata Declaration of 1978 marked the beginning of a health policy with a goal of health for all in the spirit of social justice. Alma-Ata accepted the primary health care (PHC) approach defined as "essential health care based on practical, scientifically sound, and socially acceptable methods and technology made universally accessible to individuals and families in the community through their full participation and at a cost that the community and country can afford to maintain at every stage of their development in the spirit of self-reliance and self-determination."[102] PHC is not to be confused with the concept of primary care, which is a health care delivery system stressing first contact and maintenance care. Primary care is also a costly system of care stressing the importance of 1:1 care and physician leadership and specialty care rather than promoting the growth of a network of community healers. PHC has been implemented with the intent of increasing accessibility of affordable health care. Alma-Ata specifically recognized "traditional medical practitioners and birth attendants as important allies in organizing efforts to improve health of the community and recommend that proven traditional remedies should be incorporated in national programmes for the provision of essential drugs for primary health care."[103] In addition, Resolution WHA44.34 of the 44th World Health Assembly urged member states (i.e., countries participating in WHO) to "identify activities leading to cooperation between those providing traditional medicine and modern health care, respectively, especially in regards to the use of scientifically proven safe and effective traditional remedies to reduce national drug costs."[104]

For years, WHO and its Traditional Medicine Programme have been pursuing the goal of cooperation between traditional and biomedical

---

102 Donelle Barnes and others, "Primary Health Care and Primary Care: A Confusion of Philosophies," *Nursing Outlook* 43, no. 1 (1995): 8.

103 Baba, Akerele, and Kawaguchi, "Natural Resources and Human Health: Plants of Medicinal and Nutritional Value. Proceedings of the 1st WHO Symposium on Plants and Health for All: Scientific Advancement, Kobe, Japan. August 1991.," 64.

104 Ibid., 65.

practitioners primarily in developing countries. Primary health care is the foundation for this cooperation. There is an important role for nurses in achieving this vision, which has not come to fruition yet. In 1985, the WHO executive board, concluded that the role of nurses "would move from the hospital to everyday life in the community, that nurses would become resources to people, rather than to physicians, and that nurses would become leaders and managers of PHC teams, including supervising nonprofessional community health workers."[105] I would settle for nurses simply being more active participants in the global health community than maintaining alliances strictly within the biomedical culture. Nurses have an important role to play in the furthering of the plan of primary health care and health care for all. Whenever I hear people talking about global plans for health care for all I ask the question, "What health care?" I find that many clinicians trained in biomedically dominant university programs will assume that the health care-for-all programs are supported by biomedical values. This would include medical care and surgeries. These are very important but to many peoples so is access to their indigenous healers, practices, and traditional remedies. Dr. Margaret Moss, a nurse ethnographer who has studied Zuni elders, reports that the elders place such great importance on their spiritual rituals that they will not seek care that would preclude them from in any way being able to attend to their spiritual practice.[106] In reflection, who would criticize or question this? But, in practice, the Zuni elders are questioned. "Why won't they comply with care," asks the nurse? The answer is quite simple. They cannot break with tradition because their belief is that interrupting their prayer ritual will be spiritually harmful to the extent that the risk far outweighs the benefit of the offered biomedical care. Their decision, from the standpoint of their culture, is sound.

Dr. Sally Thorne, a Canadian nurse-scientist, has written extensively on health belief and the social context of health and illness.[107] She identifies Western biomedicine as a belief system rather than a "standard against which all other healing traditions should be evaluated."[108] She

---

105 Barnes and others, "Primary Health Care and Primary Care: A Confusion of Philosophies," 8.

106 Moss, "Zuni Elders: Ethnography of American Indian Aging."

107 Thorne, "Health Belief Systems in Perspective"; ———, *Negotiating Health Care: The Social Context of Chronic Illness* (Newbury Park, CA: Sage Publications, 1993).

108 ———, "Health Belief Systems in Perspective," 1938.

calls for nurses to "fix their gaze beyond cultural sensitivity and begin to appreciate the degree to which the western biomedical tradition has influenced all aspects of their practice and the organizational structures within which that practice occurs."[109] She wrote this 18 years ago and yet the focus on cultural competency without study of biomedically based nursing as a professional culture remains. Only three years ago, I was part of a team that received federal funding for creating a curriculum that addressed raising awareness of nurses in graduate education regarding their identification with biomedical culture. I often find that even suggesting the notion of nursing as a professional culture raises the tension in a room, suggesting that the status quo has been challenged. This was never my intention. It is just that my experience has propelled me forward as an advocate for health care pluralism. A few years ago, for example, I was informed by a global health official that indigenous healers in many developing nations in particular perceive that nurses and physicians trained in the biomedical culture (particularly in the USA) possess an "arrogance" toward community healers.

I realize that many nurse educators have worked diligently to increase awareness of the diverse needs of clients when they enter the biomedical culture's hospitals and public clinics. More work is needed to prepare nurses and students to participate in the global health care community. I agree with Thorne and others in their assessment that nursing is in an ideal position to distance itself from the biomedical status quo and pursue re-alignment with what my historical data show is its sociocultural position of strength—alliance with community and the balance created within a profession that embodies cultural diplomacy, and provides and promotes integrative care from the heart that understands the value of pluralism. What is needed now is student education in cultural diplomacy that exemplifies highly sensitive communication and negotiation skills, and increased exposure to health beliefs and models of care outside the biomedical paradigm.

Discussion of plant remedies and herbalism can be a natural entrée into the study of cultural diplomacy. Students are familiar with the negative effects of plants such as that which they hear about in tobacco cessation and alcohol addiction programs. But they are learning less and

109 Ibid., 1939.

less about the positive effects of plant remedies, some of which their patients use based upon extensive evidence of safe and effective use. Nurse-herbalists are the teachers that students and practicing nurses need to become better informed. They can bring comfort to nurses when they experience the culture clashes that occur when patients reveal that they are using herbs. For example, I once had a student in a class who knew that I was a clinical herbalist. She told me that she had an elderly Asian patient in the hospital who was chewing an herb that made her mouth red. The woman spoke little English but conveyed that she would not give up the herb as the nurses wanted her to do because it helped her digestion.

My student acknowledged her own frustration and that of the other nurses who told her that they only knew that the herb was a "nut" (Authors note: Most likely Betel nut – *Areca catechu*) with "mind altering and appetite suppressant effects." As a Chinese herbalist, my assessment of the Asian woman's herbal treatment was much different than that of the student and other nurses. After listening to the story, I gave the student information about the herb and a possible rationale for its use by the patient based upon the use of betel nut in the traditional paradigm of Chinese herbal medicine. Although I do not know the outcome with the patient, I did observe that the student was relieved to know that there was someone she could talk to about the difficult culture clash experience.

Nurses, who work so closely with people, potentially hold an important position in creating opportunities for diplomatic cultural exchange between traditional healers and the biomedical world, and in integrating plant therapies with biomedical services as deemed appropriate for the unique needs of their communities. The WHO report identifies the advantages of integration of biomedical and traditional healing systems as the following:

- Improving general health care knowledge for the greater welfare of mankind

- Providing wider and more efficient population coverage

- Enhancing the quality and numbers of practitioners

- Promoting dissemination of Primary Health Care (PHC) knowledge

- Providing a means of achieving the goal of health care for all

Some of the obstacles to integration include lack of interest, fear of harmful effects of traditional medicines, doubting the results of integrated trainings, resistance to change by advocates of biomedical or traditional systems, and fear of litigation.[110] There have been obstacles to the approach, which ultimately leads to some type of greater recognition of the importance of traditional healing systems, including herbal medicines. In the 1970s, "some medical circles sarcastically denigrated WHO with lead headlines in their journals announcing that the Organization had sold its soul to the 'witch doctors.' "[111] However, there was tremendous growth in the acceptance of herbal and other traditional health practices after the early 1970s.[112] And the governments of countries such as South Africa have increased their support of IKS and traditional medicine exponentially.

Some nurses are already involved in the integration process in community centers. In the United States for example, Native American healers in the Southwest and indigenous healers in Hawaii participate in the programs of their community health centers led by nurses. In South Africa, historical research distinguishes the evolving role of the nurse as a "culture broker . . . whose work was at the intersection of two health care worlds. Digby and Sweet write that the nurses "acted as a bridge between the 'modern' western medical model of their training and the African 'traditional' medicine of their patients."[113] What actually happens with integration can differ from place to place and nurse to nurse. Bodeker suggests that there are four possible relationships between biomedical and traditional medicine.

---

110 World Health Organization, "The Promotion and Development of Traditional Medicine: WHO Technical Report Series 622," (Geneva: World Health Organization, 1978).

111 Baba, Akerele, and Kawaguchi, "Natural Resources and Human Health: Plants of Medicinal and Nutritional Value. Proceedings of the 1st WHO Symposium on Plants and Health for All: Scientific Advancement, Kobe, Japan. August 1991," 73.

112 Ibid.

113 Anne Digby and Helen Sweet, "Nurses as Culture Brokers in Twentieth-Century South Africa" in Plural Medicine, Tradition and Modernity, 1800-2000, ed. Waltraud Ernst (London and New York: Routledge, 2001).

1. The health care system can be "monopolistic" where physicians have the sole right to practice medicine.
2. Relationships can be "tolerant" where traditional practitioners freely practice without official recognition and agree not to claim to be medical doctors.
3. There can be a "parallel" relationship, such as exists in India, in which both systems are officially recognized and provide services to patients through equal but separate systems.
4. There can be an "integrated" relationship such as in China where traditional and biomedical systems merge in educational and practice settings.[114]

The question still remains whether or not full integration of traditional and biomedical systems is truly the ultimate answer in health care. For example, one patient who trusts their community elder healer implicitly might not be as comfortable going to that practitioner if the healer had been trained in primary health care and had become part of a government-sponsored facility that allowed the practitioner to only use herbs that had been scientifically proven by biomedical standards as set forth in WHO guidelines. Alternatively, patients used to being given medications for their asthma might think it odd if their practitioner started recommending acupuncture and herbs.

Does the full integration of traditional and biomedical health practices mean that health will become increasingly medicalized? For instance, because the biomedical paradigm is primarily focused on the eradication of disease, will the only herbal applications used in a clinic be those that are approved and proven to treat *disease*? What would happen to the practice of using herbs for promoting health and longevity? Biomedicine does have a history of "establishing claims to expertise and authority over many areas of life not viewed as medical in other cultures or at other times."[115] The question might be raised about the ability of traditional healers to maintain their individuality within the sphere of conventional medicine if chiropractors and nurses have

---

114 Bodeker, "Traditional Health Systems: Policy, Biodiversity, and Global Interdependence," 232.
115 David Hufford, "Integrating Complementary and Alternative Medicine Into Conventional Medical Practice," *Alternative Therapies in Health and Medicine* 3, no. 3 (1997): 81.

difficulty maintaining their individuality. I had this very discussion with the Aunties in Hawaii with whom I taught. They were Kahuna from the island of Molokai and they told me that there was talk of legislation to require all indigenous healers to take certain courses in the university before they could be given permission to care for people. One of the Aunties was in her 70s and would never submit to such a ruling.

Having worked in a clinic with many complementary therapies practitioners, it is my experience that the biomedical practices and practitioners are often viewed by some team members, including the nurses, as superior. The belief was that biomedical practices were to be offered first before traditional practices such as herbal medicine. Some practitioners with a strict biomedical paradigm that focuses on safety and efficacy may erroneously believe that they must be the gatekeepers to complementary therapies such as herbal medicine. Although they may be well intended, the gatekeeping approach couched in an expressed desire for integration serves only to alienate patients, traditional practitioners, and biomedical practitioners who are seeking integration without a belief in the superiority of one paradigm over another. Biomedical practitioners can best serve the consumers of health care when they recognize their own paradigm for what it is—a set of cultural beliefs— and diplomatically consider and discuss what approaches may be best for an individual client. Ethnocentrism undermines the healing relationship and, therefore, the ultimate goal of integrative health care for all.

According to WHO, 80 percent of the world's population continues to use their traditional methods of healing, including the use of medicinal plants.[116] This is important information for nurses. As both plant and biomedical therapies evolve in the twenty-first century, nurses will be called upon more than ever to explore ways of helping people integrate their traditional healing methods and the gifts of biomedicine into their lives. For years, WHO and its Traditional Medicine Programme have been pursuing the goal of cooperation between traditional and biomedical practitioners primarily in developing countries. WHO provides training to traditional and indigenous healers who work alongside nurses. Nurses who specialize in holistic care are well positioned to fine-tune their practice to incorporate skills in cultural diplomacy, integration,

116 Farnsworth and others, "Medicinal Plants in Therapy."

and indigenous knowledge systems necessary to not only partner with plants but also to partner with those community healers who specialize in partnering with plants.

In 1985, the WHO executive board concluded that the role of nurses "would move from the hospital to everyday life in the community that nurses would become resources to people, rather than to physicians, and that nurses would become leaders and managers of primary health care teams."[117] Boards of Nursing and federal and state agencies must expect that nurses will work closely with practitioners of complementary therapies and traditional healers and perhaps use traditional modalities such as herbs in practice themselves for the good of community. Accepting the concept of health care pluralism—that there are many healing paths used by patients and practitioners alike—is recognized as one of the foundations of ethical health care practice.[118] The use of herbal remedies in the care of patients is a healing tradition in which nurses and midwives in many countries around the world, including the USA, participate.

THREE KEYS TO CREATING AN ENDURING INTEGRATIVE PRACTICE

While many nurses may realize the importance of integrating their biomedical knowledge of health care with healing traditions, how they should actually integrate the two, such as integrating herbal remedies and conventional nursing care, is often difficult to accomplish. I have defined *integrative nursing* as "the creation of evolving, healing relationships with patients, in which the nurse observes the patient's needs for greater harmony and balance in their life and then addresses those needs by offering care that is a holistic blend of biomedical and caring skills."[119] Integrative care is collaborative and respectful of personal and societal cultural differences. It includes the concepts of unity and equal membership.[120] Integration does not mean, nor does it imply, *cooptation*

---

117 Barnes and others, "Primary Health Care and Primary Care: A Confusion of Philosophies."

118 Committee on the Use of Complementary and Alternative Medicine by the American Public, Board on Health Promotion and Disease Prevention, Institute of Medicine of the National Academies, Complementary and Alternative Medicine in the United States. Washington, DC: The National Academies Press: 2005.

119 Libster, *Demonstrating Care: The Art of Integrative Nursing*.

120 Merriam-Webster, *Merriam-Webster's Collegiate Dictionary*.

of one group and their beliefs and practices by another. Unfortunately, some biomedical practitioners of integrative care have adopted and operationalized the title to mean the use of evidence-based (i.e. clinical research supported) complementary therapies within the established, orthodox model of providing biomedical services.

Practice within the biomedical paradigm includes the curing or removal of disease. The traditional paradigm is focused on the balancing of symptoms. The focus of the holistic nursing paradigm is discovering, in relationship with clients, a healing blend of caring and comfort while supporting the biomedical and traditional paradigms of curing and balancing. Integrative care is a creative process. The ability of the holistic nurse-herbalist to express integration in which all aspects of care are respected as contributing to the greater whole of health care comes as a result of a quality of heart that seeks to serve in the caring spirit of diplomacy and peacemaking. The practice of nurse-herbalism, working with beautiful plant life forms to help people, can inspire a quest for the deepest meaning of integrative care as peacemaking.

Herbs are recognized historically as gentler remedies.[121] The history of nursing holds within it three important keys for exemplifying a holistic paradigm of integrative nurse-herbalism that will promote a gentler system of healing and comfort that contributes to an enduring, peaceful life regardless of which way the winds of change blow in health care reform. These three keys are discernment, pattern recognition, and self-care support. These keys answer one of the main questions of the holistic nursing paradigm: "How can plants be integrated in the support, care, and comfort of people?"

Discernment

When I was conducting research on the history of the Sisters of Charity's use of herbs in nursing care over the centuries, I learned a lot about community of women back to their formation in seventeenth-century France. I came to appreciate, although I was not raised a Catholic, the spirituality of the community founders, Vincent de Paul and Louise

---

121 Libster, *Herbal Diplomats: The Contribution of Early American Nurses (1830-1860) to Nineteenth-Century Health Care Reform and the Botanical Medical Movement.*

de Marillac. One of the talks Vincent gave the early nurses was a teaching on discernment. They needed some guidance of this nature as their task of serving the sick poor in Paris at that time was nothing short of monumental. They often were faced with decisions in the care and comfort of people for which they needed discernment. Those decisions covered the full range of professional practice. They had to decide whom they could treat so that the local surgeons would not feel as if their practice and livelihood were being threatened by knowledgeable nurse-caregivers. They also had to decide which herbs to use in the care and comfort of patients. The early nurses' decisions could be life-saving and therefore they—as did Sister Matilda Coskery—placed great emphasis on the attention to detail even in the simplest of tasks, such as preparing tisanes. Vincent de Paul was a religious man. He was also very practical. In reading the history of the formation of the early nursing community in Paris, women nurses were faced with helping thousands of sick poor people. When I read Vincent's teaching to the early Daughters of Charity on "discernment,"[122] I realized that he had given them and perhaps us today a key for professional practice, a process for holistic decision making.

Vincent taught the women that discernment was a three-part process: unrestricted readiness, weighing the evidence, and taking counsel.[123] By unrestricted readiness, Vincent meant that the sisters would be open to God's will and listening in a way that was detached from any personal agenda. Readiness, like centering practice in holistic nursing today, involved prayer, meditation, and reflection on life events. Vincent was very mindful of the role that life events played. He believed that life events were signs sent by Divine Providence to reveal God's plan. It is in the state of readiness that Vincent instructed the sisters to weigh the evidence and examine the pros and cons of an action—a process that bears a striking resemblance to today's nursing instruction in ethical practice and critical thinking. Lastly, Vincent encouraged the Sisters to seek the counsel of a wise person, which in the case of a sister-nurse

---

122 Libster and McNeil, *Enlightened Charity: The Holistic Nursing Care, Education and Advices Concerning the Sick of Sister Matilda Coskery, (1799-1870).*

123 Hugh O'Donnell, *Vincent de Paul: His Life and Way.* In Francis Ryan and John Rybolt, *Vincent de Paul and Louise de Marillac: Rules, Conferences, and Writings* (Mahwah, NJ: Paulist Press, 1995), 34.

would have been the Sister Servant or head nurse. He taught that God's will was revealed in the process of taking counsel or mentoring with an elder. In essence, the praxis of early holistic nurses—readiness, weighing the evidence, and seeking counsel —is much like holistic nursing practice today, which encourages centering, ethical decision making, and mentoring with an elder. Active, conscious practice in discernment is an enduring healing tradition in nursing that is one of the keys of the holistic nursing paradigm.

Pattern Recognition

The second key of the holistic nursing paradigm emerges out of intervention and experience in providing care, comfort, and support. When one works with hundreds of people over the months and years of one's life, it becomes quite apparent that not only are there patterns of disease that can be observed in people, nurses also recognize health, healing, lifestyle, emotional, and thought patterns as well. Healing traditions throughout the world all acknowledge pattern as important in the work of healing disease and health promotion. TCM, Celtic healing, Ayurveda, Unani, Native American medicine, and homeopathy are whole systems of "medicine" in which pattern recognition is fundamental. Pattern recognition is also a key to the practices of herbalism and nursing.

Pattern recognition is the grouping of symptom-sign observations. Holistic pattern recognition requires an assessment of the spiritual, emotional, mental or psychological and physiological aspect of the person, family or group. There are some philosophical similarities between herbalism and nursing practice in terms of symptom-sign observation. An herbal assessment is done with the intent to identify the symptom-sign pattern so that the proper herbal remedies can be suggested for the client. Pattern recognition is also a key feature of nursing science and theory. The writings of Martha Rogers and Margaret Newman, for example, provide clear descriptions of the importance of understanding pattern when engaging in a healing relationship with a patient. Pattern is described by Rogers as "the distinguishing characteristic of an energy field . . . it is an abstraction. . . . Pattern is not directly observable. However, manifestations of field patterning are observable events in the real world. The implications of this for increased individualization of nursing services are explicit."[124] Newman defines pattern as "information that depicts the whole, understanding of the meaning of all the relationships at once. An understanding of pattern is basic to an understanding of health. . . . Pattern recognition comes from within the observer."[125]

My first understanding of the science of pattern recognition in nursing came from studying the Roy Adaptation Model of nursing while working on my BSN at Mount St. Mary's College in Los Angeles in the mid-1980s. A decade later, I studied Traditional Chinese Herbal Medicine[126] with Dr. Roger Wicke at the Rocky Mountain Herbal Institute during which time I learned about symptom-sign assessment. The TCM assessment includes the observation of behaviors that are also assessed in nursing, such as energy level, nutritional and fluid intake, elimination, skin, sleep and rest, and emotions to name a few. Practitioners of herbal medicine use a clinically based system of assessment that includes such methods as pulse, tongue, and face diagnosis along with extensive history taking, symptom-sign patterns, and discussion of concerns with patients. The assessment is then matched with the personality or unique qualities of plants. The clinical assessment allows the practitioner to match the unique picture of a patient with the herbs necessary to create balance in that picture. This type of clinical assessment and pattern recognition represents "biological individuality rather than a standardized nosology. In clinical science, systems of correspondence, that is, whole system models are used as a foundation for practice. Using a whole system model as a foundation for clinical practice makes mastery of botanical

---

124 Martha Rogers, "Nursing Science and the Space Age," *Nursing Science Quarterly* 5, no. 1 (1992).

125 Margaret Newman, *Health as Expanding Consciousness* (New York: National League for Nursing Press, 1994), 71,73.

126 For ease of reading, this book will refer to Traditional Chinese Herbal Medicine (TCHM) as Traditional Chinese Medicine (TCM). The TCHM program I studied included over 660 hours of study of herbal medicine in the traditional paradigm of theories such as 8 Principle Patterns and Fundamental Processes. While I learned tongue and pulse diagnosis, I did not study acupuncture, moxibustion and cupping interventions that are typically part of TCM training. In TCM philosophy, healing patterns are best affected in the following order: Lifestyle Changes, Dietary Changes, Introduction of Herbal Remedies, and then other modalities such as acupuncture and moxibustion. The foci of assessment and intervention in my TCHM studies were lifestyle/environmental patterns, the energetics of foods, and herbal formulation (teas).

medicine, or any therapeutic modality possible."[127] The nursing models mentioned here emphasize wholeness. Nursing process and theories can be used as a foundation for the study of plant therapies. Learning herbal medicine theory, such as is part of TCM, is often a smooth transition for nurses who have studied nursing theory based on wholeness models.

TCM

Herbs have been used in traditional medicine practices throughout Asia for centuries. There are highly developed systems of medicine in China, Japan, and Korea, for example, that include the use of plants. TCM was the system I learned, though I only studied herbalism not acupuncture. I recommend TCM herbalism in the creation of a holistic nurse-herbalist practice. The use of herbs in TCM is based on the principle of balance, a major concept in Taoist philosophy, and on the recognition of patterns of symptoms and signs unique to a given patient. Like nursing, the Chinese system of herbalism recognizes that no two of the same symptom such as a headache are alike when the whole picture, or symptom-sign pattern, is assessed. The Chinese system of herbal medicine has been very successful because of the way the herbs are used.

The herbs in a Chinese *Materia Medica* are not necessarily native to or cultivated in China per se. The Chinese have historically collected the best medicinal plants from around the globe to add to their *Materia Medica*. Yet some species of "Chinese" herbs are found primarily, if not exclusively, in Asia. The successful treatment of a patient with Chinese herbs stems from the understanding of the patient's unique *response* to illness, disease, or discomfort. This is similar to the nursing process of understanding and intervening in actual and potential responses to illness.

Response to illness often occurs incrementally. I have noticed this, for example, when working with patients with back pain. When a thorough history and assessment of the signs and symptoms are taken without discounting any data reported by the patient, a pattern of acute episodes is often easily recognized. Patients might discover that every time they eat a specific food they get slightly constipated and then their

---

127 Kenner and Requena, "Whole-System Models Commonly Used in European Botanical Therapies, Part II: The Five Phases Model," 54.

back begins to go into spasm, leading to another acute episode. "It is commonly observed by TCM doctors that clearly detectable imbalances in a patient's health and their corresponding symptoms manifest long before they are usually detected as an abnormality in blood chemistry, x-rays, electrical activity, etc. . . . The success of TCM health care is partly due to its ability to detect imbalances in health in their early stages."[128] The assessment process includes history; determination of symptom-sign patterns (a grouping of symptoms), such as whether the person likes cold or hot drinks; the consistency of the patient's stool; the tone of their voice; their skin color; and a diagnosis of the tongue and pulse. Once the pattern or patterns are identified, an herbal tea is formulated specifically for the patient. The formula is designed to promote balance. One example of designing a balancing formula is giving a formula with herbs that warm the interior to the patient who has interior cold.

TCM has its own language related to symptom-sign patterns and classification of herbs that is learned by practitioners and the public. An herb in China might be sold for "yin deficiency" condition. Westerners who use Chinese herbs, those herbs in a Chinese *Materia Medica*, can easily learn the language and underlying philosophy of the system so as to be able to effectively apply the principles and methods of the system. I always use TCM language with clients so that they not only learn the system of health care but also tap into the success of the healing tradition, which is "stored" or embedded energetically in the culture of that tradition. I typically recommend that my clients read *The Tao of Healthy Eating* by Bob Flaws on TCM diet therapy[129] since people can readily recognize the energetic pattern of a common food, such as a chili pepper (energetics – hot and spicy), that they have eaten many times as opposed to an herb that may only grow in China.

The Chinese have had hundreds of years of trial and error and scientific observation that has laid the foundation of a highly effective system of herbal medicine. Herbal tea formulations are one of the primary foci in the TCM treatment system. Formulations typically include more than three herbs, sometimes many more. The herbs are

128 Roger Wicke, *Clinical Handbook of Herbal Medicine Vol. I* (Hot Springs, MT: Rocky Mountain Herbal Institute Publications, 1992), 14.
129 Bob Flaws, *The Tao of Healthy Eating : Dietary Wisdom According to Traditional Chinese Medicine* (Boulder, CO: Blue Poppy Press, 1998).

used not only for their individual properties but for the ways in which they have been observed over many centuries of use to interact with other herbs with which they have a synergistic effect. This synergistic effect is a phenomenon that may not be able to be fully explained from a conventional pharmaceutical paradigm. I and others who "formulate" know the unique energetic properties of individual plants, synergistic effects of plants used in formulation together, and how to create formulations or recipes that specifically meet the energetic needs of a client for greater physical, mental, emotional, and spiritual balance.

A TCM herbal practitioner begins treatment with suggesting lifestyle and dietary changes. If the imbalance is not affected by the changes, then herbs and other modalities are introduced. Herbs are used to treat acute and chronic patterns in China. They are also used to treat disease. For example, since the cultural revolution (until 1975), as many as 20,000 cases of appendicitis have been treated with herbal formulas (different in various hospitals) with a 90 percent overall cure rate.[130] Many herb gardens are situated in traditional medical colleges for students to see as they are studying. Although studies of the herbs are always being done (usually human not animal studies), some Chinese have opposed the placebo-controlled trial over the years because of ethical issues. They believe that placebo use is deceptive.[131] Because of the many years of traditional use of herbs in humans, the studies on Chinese herbs are often performed to understand why and how the herbs have worked rather than to discover *if* they work. Chinese researchers believe that safety is not an issue in human trials because the herbs have already been shown to be safe for human consumption, and therefore they may not feel that animal trials are necessary.

In China, nurses may be educated to work in TCM hospitals. Nurses in conventional hospitals also may administer herbal therapies in practice. There are numerous oral, topical, and intravenous applications of herbs. Many of the herbs and prepared herbal products are exported to other countries. Analgesic salves with names like "tiger balm" (does not contain tiger)[132] are common in Western use. Western practitioners

---

130 National Academy of Sciences, "Herbal Pharmacology in the People's Republic of China," (Washington, DC: National Academy of Sciences, 1975).
131 Ibid., 67.
132 One way I use tiger balm is for blood stagnation muscle or joint pain – that is pain aggravated by rubbing or massage. Some of the herbs in the salve "move" blood.

often voice concerns about the quality of some of the Chinese products. Chinese whole dried herbs must be washed thoroughly because fertilizers are used liberally in China. When using whole herbs, care must be taken to clearly identify herbs and sources of product. This is a good practice regardless of where the herb comes from. There is also a concern about patent formulations—prepared remedies, often in tablet form, in which unwanted ingredients might be included. Examples of substances that have been known to be included in patent formulas include steroids and heavy metals such as lead. For this reason, it is recommended that a TCM practitioner be consulted for use of patent formulas.

When nurses partner with plants and herbal tea formulations in practice and then observe for responses and changes in behavior, they enter into a consciousness of pattern recognition. They encounter the moment when they, as Newman says, may begin to understand the meaning of relationships: the client and their environment, the herb or formulation and the client, and the herbs in formulation. Understanding of pattern can lead to insight. How the parts of the pattern fit together is "*Integrative Insight.*" Integrative insight is awareness of the relationships between objects and patterns that emerges in the consciousness of the nurse during the process of considering two or more perspectives, concepts, objects that may even seem to be in opposition. For example, insight can demonstrate the meaning of care and comfort delivered to people from an integration of TCM herbal and nursing sciences. The opportunity for integrative insight begins with assessment.

Pattern recognition takes place in all phases of the nursing process, most particularly during assessment and diagnosis. Assessment is observation of symptom-signs and diagnosis represents the period for grouping those symptom-sign patterns. In the Roy Adaptation Model[133] of nursing, physiological patterns are assessed using the following language:

Oxygenation – Nutrition – Elimination – Activity/Rest – Protection

Senses- Fluids and Electrolytes – Neurological function – Endocrine function

---

133 Sister Callista Roy, *The Roy Adaptation Model*, 3rd ed. (Upper Saddle River, NJ: Pearson, 2009).

In TCM the following are assessed:

Systemic characteristics – Respiration – Intake/Outflow – Pain – Sensation – Sleep – Motion – Speech – Behavior – Tongue Tissue/Coat – Pulse

Having performed numerous assessments in both systems, I have experienced the similarities and complementariness of the two systems. They equally inform the understanding of clients' patterns without separation or distinction.

TCM and nursing are complementary whereas other health systems may not be. Chinese nurses seem to agree. Nursing schools in China often have included in their three-year curriculum the subject of "native medicine," TCM, and acupuncture. The nurses in the intensive care units in China are familiar with a "unique aspect of care . . . the use of a Chinese herbal medicine called don-sen for intravenous infusion."[134] Don-sen is used in cases of myocardial infarction and is reported to have a positive effect on dilation of coronary arteries. Chinese nurses, or any others whose education includes the use of traditional medicines such as herbal remedies, are socialized professionally to regard plants and other remedies as part of their practice. Therefore, I think it important in the preparation of nurse-herbalists and the creation of a nurse-herbalist practice to ground intuitive, integrative insights in specific cognitive links between pattern recognition in nursing science and traditional healing such as TCM. This is best done through selection of the assessment models from a specific nursing theory and healing tradition. As I mentioned, I recommend Roy Adaptation Model for nursing assessment and TCM for herbal assessment as a highly complementary blending of the science of East and West that can lead to accurate levels of pattern recognition and profound integrative insight. The way in which I employ these two assessment models in my practice of nurse-herbalism will be further outlined in Chapter 3.

---

134 Margaret Chang, "Nursing in China: Three Perspectives," *The American Journal of Nursing* 83, no. 3 (1983): 391.

Self–Care Support

The third key of the holistic nursing paradigm has to do with supporting and promoting the client's relationship with their own Self (with a capital "S"). This is to say, that Self that has been referred to in so many ways: the still small voice, the inner healer, or the inner wisdom. I refer to this Self as "the Gentle Healer Within" whose voice, vision, and instruction is always caring, comforting, soothing, joyful, illuminating, loving, and meaningful. Nurses are the witness to this Self or Gentle Healer in their own being and in that of their clients. Much the way the physicians and nurses of the nineteenth century referred to their work as supporting nature in her healing work, I let clients know that I support self-care and the work of their inner nature—their Gentle Healer Within.

Nursing has a long history of supporting self-care. This work was discussed previously in the section on the consumer model of herbalism where the focus of care and comfort was providing resources, information, and education when needed. In the integrative model of nurse-herbalism, nurses discern what kind of care would be most appropriate for a given situation. When clients choose to take care of themselves with herbs, the nurse can provide support. If and when clients have no knowledge of herbs, the nurse may decide that providing more directed or dependent care is important for a period of time.

Dorothea Orem's nursing theory guides nurses in their support of self-care and dependent-care nursing.[135] Nurses acknowledge that even when a client is dependent in their need for care, they are striving for the ability to ultimately care for Self. I often test this idea with people and ask them if and how they take care of themselves. Then I ask if they enjoy being able to care for themselves and solve their own health concerns or problems. I have never had anyone say that they do not like to solve their own health concerns. The consistent pattern in the responses, however, is that many people believe, feel, and think that they do not have the resources or knowledge to care for themselves in a way that will solve the problem. They may not have the knowledge of the body anatomy and physiology, disease process, or options for care and comfort. Self-care

---

135 Dorothea Orem, *Nursing Concepts of Practice*, 6 ed. (St. Louis, MO: Mosby, 2001).

supported by knowledgeable practitioners is oftentimes helpful. It is also a healing tradition in nursing with roots in the elements of nature care.[136]

The elements of nature care—ether, fire, air, water, and earth—are the elements of Self and the same elements from which all matter in the universe is and has been created. The creation and re-creation of Self is an ongoing process of healing. Viewing self-care from the perspective of consumer model is one level of care. In the integrative model, self-care is viewed as a calling that moves beyond the focus on solving a health concern and repairing the body. Self-care support, comfort, and care repairs the body and solves health concerns with a greater purpose in mind; the integration and alignment of the four "bodies" or elements of Self —fire, air, water, earth—and the fifth element, ether or vital energy, which the Greeks called "pneuma." These five have been considered the elements of creation and were clearly defined in hermetic texts, the oldest spiritual tradition in the West. Hermeticism is known to have inspired Judaism, Christianity, Islam, Paganism, and Gnosticism. Buddhism, Taoism, and Hinduism also share similar concepts.[137] The Greeks described the qualities of the four fundamental archetypes in their system of humoral medicine as: fire – hot and dry; water – cold and moist; earth – cold and dry; and air – hot and moist. The Greeks believed that health was most affected by changing the natural elements. For example, one could turn excess water in the body into steam by applying heat, creating a change in the environment, in the elements of care that promoted heat. Representatives from the diet or herbs, as well as rest and lifestyle, could all affect the heat in the body and thereby help relieve excess water.

In many healing traditions, from the Greek humoral to Indian Ayurveda to African medicine, the proper balance of the spiritual, mental, emotional, and physical bodies and their associated elements are thought of as being the platform for health. Health is also believed in many traditions to occur when all elements align and become congruent and harmonious with the vital energy (pneuma), which is expressed as the divine purpose of the person. Dr. Edward Bach (pronounced

---

136 Martha Libster, "Perspectives on the History of Self-Care," *Self-Care, Dependent-Care & Nursing* 16, no. 2 (2008).

137 Dennis Hauck, *The Emerald Tablet: Alchemy for Personal Transformation* (New York: Penguin Putnam Inc., 1999).

"batch"), a British physician who created a system of remedies called the Bach Flower Remedies, wrote eloquently of his research in the support of self-care and the importance of engagement in divine purpose:

> Thus we see that our conquest of disease will mainly depend on the following: Firstly, the realization of the Divinity within our nature and our consequent power to overcome all that is wrong; secondly, the knowledge that the basic cause of disease is due to the disharmony between the personality and the Soul; thirdly, our willingness and ability to discover the fault which is causing such a conflict; and fourthly, the removal of any such fault by developing the opposing virtue. The duty of the healing art will be to assist us to the necessary knowledge and means by which we may overcome our maladies, and in addition to this to administer such remedies as will strengthen our mental and physical bodies.[138]

He goes on to say that it is in the process of "harmonizing body, mind, and soul" that disease is cured and even averted all together if addressed early on. The remedies that assist in the harmonizing of the body, mind, and soul are from the "most beautiful plants and herbs to be found in the pharmacy of Nature."[139] Striving for harmony of the body, mind, and soul (which I identify as four bodies—spiritual, emotional, mental and physiological) is the spiritual practice of healing and integrative care from the heart. Bach writes:

> For our own part we must practise[sic] peace, harmony, individuality and firmness of purpose and increasingly develop the knowledge that in essence we are of the Divine origin, children of the Creator, and thus have within us, if we will but develop it, as in time we ultimately surely must, the power to attain perfection. . . .We must steadfastly practise peace, imagining our minds as a lake ever to be kept calm, without waves, or even ripples, to disturb its tranquility, and gradually develop this state of peace until no event of life, no

---

138 Edward Bach, *Heal Thyself: An Explanation of the Real Cause and Cure of Disease* (Mount Vernon, England: Bach Centre, 1996 (Originally published 1931), 52.
139 Ibid., 53.

circumstance, no other personality is able under any condition to ruffle the surface of that lake or raise within us any feelings of irritability, depression, or doubt. . . .We are not all asked to be saints or martyrs or men of renown; to most of us less conspicuous offices are allotted. But we are all expected to understand the joy and adventures of life and fulfil[sic] with cheerfulness the particular piece of work which has been ordained for us by our Divinity.[140]

Bach, like all other healers I have worked with, reverences the Divinity within as that connection with God, The Creator, or many other names. That Divinity within is also the gentle healing power within. Bach was challenged with life-threatening illness at one point in his life. He seems to have fully understood what he was asking us to consider. His focus was the uplifting of the spirit through the engagement with the *beauty* of flowers and herbs; hence the Bach Flower Remedies, a self-care system, came into being. I have used these remedies in practice for decades and find them most helpful in moving people through tough emotions that cloud the ability to recognize the client's health patterns. I include in my initial assessment a scan of the remedies and help the client select their remedies. I use psychological and body-mind techniques of free-association and mindfulness meditation as well as herbal assessment in the process of matching the remedies with the client at a specific time. Continuing education is also available through the Bach Centre in England for those who wish to study the remedies.[141]

The Bach Flower Remedies, like herbs, are easily applied in nursing care and comfort. Nurses are well positioned to help people implement self-care systems such as the Bach Remedies. The effects of gentler, subtle remedies such as flower essences and herbs are not always readily experienced by the public. I have found that teaching clients about pattern recognition as I work with them helps them be more attuned to the harmonization effects of gentle remedies. The nurse-herbalist is the calm clear lake for the client while they sort out their health concerns and move into a state of readiness to contact and learn from the Gentle Healer Within. The ultimate purpose of nursing care is to support the

---

140 Ibid., 53-54.
141 See www.Bachcentre.com for information.

person, who is becoming whole and fully tethered to their true nature, their Gentle Healer Within, and their true Self. Flower essences and herbs help catalyze this process of harmonization, transformation, and healing. This is why they are used historically in self-care and why nurse-herbalists can apply them in their holistic practice of support, comfort, and care.

REFERENCES

Abel, Emily. *Hearts of Wisdom: American Women Caring for Kin, 1850-1940*. Cambridge, MA: Harvard University Press, 2000.

Baba, Shigeaki, Olayiwola Akerele, and Yuji Kawaguchi. "Natural Resources and Human Health: Plants of Medicinal and Nutritional Value. Proceedings of the 1st WHO Symposium on Plants and Health for All: Scientific Advancement, Kobe, Japan. August 1991."Amsterdam: Elsevier, 1992.

Bach, Edward. *Heal Thyself: An Explanation of the Real Cause and Cure of Disease*. Mount Vernon, England: Bach Centre, 1996 (Originally published 1931).

Baker, Nina Brown. *Cyclone in Calico: The Story of Mary Ann Bickerdyke*. Boston: Little, Brown, 1952.

Balick, Michael and Paul Alan Cox. *Plants, People, and Culture: The Science of Ethnobotany*. New York: Scientific American Library, 1996.

Barnes, Donelle, Carmen Eribes, Teresa Juarbe, Martha Nelson, Susan Proctor, Linda Sawyer, Muriel Shaul, and Afaf Meleis. "Primary Health Care and Primary Care: A Confusion of Philosophies." *Nursing Outlook* 43, no. 1 (1995): 7-16.

Berman, Alex and Michael Flannery. *America's Botanico-Medical Movement: Vox Populi*. New York: Pharmaceutical Products Press, 2001.

Bigelow, Jacob. "Discourse on Self-Limited Disease." In *Medical Communications of the Massachusetts Medical Society*. Boston: The Massachusetts Medical Society, 1836.

Bodeker, Gerard. "Traditional Health Systems: Policy, Biodiversity, and Global Interdependence." *Journal of Alternative and Complementary Medicine* 1, no. 3 (1995): 231-43.

Bunzel, Ruth Leah. *Zuni Ceremonialism*. Albuquerque: University of New Mexico Press, 1992.

Caplan, Ronald. "The Commodification of American Health Care." *Social Science in Medicine* 28, no. 11 (1989): 1139-48.

Chang, Margaret. "Nursing in China: Three Perspectives " *The American Journal of Nursing* 83, no. 3 (1983): 389-91.

Child, Lydia Maria. *The Family Nurse*. Bedford, Massachusetts: Applewood Books, 1997.

Church of Jesus Christ of Latter-Day Saints. *The Book of Mormon. The Doctrine and Covenants of the Church of Jesus Christ of Latter-Day Saints. The Pearl of Great Price.* Salt Lake City, UT: Church of Jesus Christ of Latter-Day Saints, 1981.

Coskery, Sister Matilda. *Advices Concerning the Sick*. Emmitsburg, MD: Archives of Daughters of Charity, St. Joseph's Provincial House, n.d. c. 1840.

Daughters of Charity. *The Rule of 1812: Regulations for the Society of Sisters of Charity in the United States of America*, Emmitsburg, MD: Archives of the Daughters of Charity, St. Joseph's Provincial House, 1812.

Digby, Anne and Helen Sweet. "Nurses as Culture Brokers in Twentieth-Century South Africa" in *Plural Medicine, Tradition and Modernity, 1800-2000*, edited by Waltraud Ernst, 113-29. London and New York: Routledge, 2001.

Dossey, Barbara, Louise Selanders, Deva Beck, and Alex Attewell. *Florence Nightingale Today*. Silver Spring, MD: American Nurses Association, 2005.

Eisenberg, David, Roger Davis, Susan Ettner, Scott Appel, Sonja Wilkey, Maria Van Rompay, and Ronald Kessler. "Trends in Alternative Medicine Use in the United States, 1990-1997: Results of a Follow-up National Survey." *JAMA* 280, no. 18 (1998): 1569-75.

Elstad, Ingunn and Kirsti Torjuul. "The Issue of Life: Aristotle in Nursing Perspective." *Nursing Philosophy : An International Journal for Healthcare Professionals* 10, no. 4 (2009): 275-86.

Ezzo, Jeanette, Katherine Wright, Victoria Hadhazy, Mary Bahr-Robertson, William Mac Beckner, Maggie Covington, and Brian Berman. "Use of the Cochrane Electronic Library in Complementary and Alternative Medicine Courses in Medical Schools: Is the Giant Lost in Cyberspace?" *Journal of Alternative and Complementary Medicine* 8, no. 5 (2002): 681-6.

Farnsworth, Norman, Olayiwola Akerele, Audrey Bingel, Djaja Soejarto, and Zhengang Guo. "Medicinal Plants in Therapy." *Bulletin of the World Health Organization* 63, no. 6 (1985): 965-81.

Feigenbaum, Harvey. "Globalization and Cultural Diplomacy." Washington, DC: George Washington University Center for the Arts and Culture, 2001.

Felter, Harvey Wickes and John Uri Lloyd. *King's American Dispensatory*. 18th ed., 3d rev ed. Sandy, OR: Eclectic Medical Publications, 1983.

Fett, Sharla. *Working Cures: Healing, Health, and Power on Southern Slave Plantations*. Chapel Hill: University of North Carolina Press, 2002.

Flaws, Bob. *The Tao of Healthy Eating : Dietary Wisdom According to Traditional Chinese Medicine*. Boulder, CO: Blue Poppy Press, 1998.

Griggs, Barbara. *Green Pharmacy*. Rochester, VT: Healing Arts Press, 1991.

Guazzo, Francesco Maria and Montague Summers. *Compendium Maleficarum: The Montague Summers Edition*. Dover ed. New York: Dover, 1988.

Haller, John. *The People's Doctors: Samuel Thomson and the American Botanical Movement, 1790-1860*. Carbondale IL: Southern Illinois University Press, 2000.

Harmer, Bertha and Virginia Henderson. *Textbook of the Principles and Practice of Nursing*. New York: Macmillan Co., 1955.

Hauck, Dennis. *The Emerald Tablet: Alchemy for Personal Transformation*. New York: Penguin Putnam Inc., 1999.

Houghton, Peter. "The Role of Plants in Traditional Medicine and Current Therapy." *Journal of Alternative and Complementary Medicine* 1, no. 2 (1995): 131-43.

Hufford, David. "Integrating Complementary and Alternative Medicine Into Conventional Medical Practice." *Alternative Therapies in Health and Medicine* 3, no. 3 (1997): 81-3.

Ingelfinger, Franz. "Medicine: Meritorious or Meretricious." *Science* 200, no. 4344 (1978): 942-6.

Jaeschke, Roman, Deborah Cook, and David Sackett. "The Potential Role of Single-Patient Randomized Controlled Trials (N-of-1 Rct's) in Clinical Practice." *Journal of the American Board of Family Practice* 5, no. 2 (1992): 227-29.

Jefferson, Thomas, Adrienne Koch, William Harwood Peden, and Thomas Jefferson. *The Life and Selected Writings of Thomas Jefferson*. New York: The Modern Library, 1944.

Kenner, Dan and Yves Requeno. "Whole-System Models Commonly Used in European Botanical Therapies, Part 1: The Terrain Concept and the Neuroendocrine Model." *American Journal of Acupuncture* 25, no. 4 (1997): 233-40.

Kenner, Dan and Yves Requena. "Whole-System Models Commonly Used in European Botanical Therapies, Part II: The Five Phases Model." *American Journal of Acupuncture* 26, no. 1 (1998): 5-18.

Kincheloe, Lawrence. "Herbal Medicines Can Reduce the Costs in HMO." *Herbalgram* 41 (1997): 49.

Koch, Tomasz. "Beyond Measurement: Fourth-Generation Evaluation in Nursing." *Journal of Advanced Nursing* 20, no. 6 (1994): 1148-55.

Larson, Eric, Allan Ellsworth, and Janet Oas. "Randomized Clinical Trials in Single Patients During a 2-Year Period." *Journal of the American Medical Association* 270, no. 22 (1993): 2708-12.

Leung, Albert and Steven Foster. *Encyclopedia of Common Natural Ingredients Used in Food, Drugs, and Cosmetics*. 2nd ed. New York: John Wiley & Sons, 1996.

Levin, Lowell S. and Ellen L. Idler. *The Hidden Health Care System*. Farmville, NC: Golden Apple Publications, 2010.

Lewis, Carol. "Medical Milestones of the Last Millennium." *FDA Consumer* 34, no. 2 (2000): 8-13.

Libster, Martha. *Demonstrating Care: The Art of Integrative Nursing*. Albany, N.Y: Delmar Thomson Learning, 2001.

———. "Elements of Care: Nursing Environmental Theory in Historical Context." *Holistic Nursing Practice* 22, no. 3 (2008): 160-70.

———. *Herbal Diplomats: The Contribution of Early American Nurses (1830-1860) to Nineteenth-Century Health Care Reform and the Botanical Medical Movement*. Thornton, CO: Golden Apple Publications, 2004.

———. "Perspectives on the History of Self-Care." *Self-Care, Dependent-Care & Nursing* 16, no. 2 (2008): 8-17.

Libster, Martha, and Betty Ann McNeil. *Enlightened Charity: The Holistic Nursing Care, Education and Advices Concerning the Sick of Sister Matilda Coskery, (1799-1870)*. Farmville, NC: Golden Apple Publications, 2009.

Margolin, Arthur, S. Kelly Avants, and Herbert Kleber. "Investigating Alternative Medicine Therapies in Randomized Controlled Trials." *Journal of the American Medical Association* 280, no. 18 (1998): 1626-28.

Merriam-Webster. *Merriam-Webster's Collegiate Dictionary*. 10th ed. Springfield, MA: Merriam-Webster, 1999.

Moss, Margaret. "Zuni Elders: Ethnography of American Indian Aging." University of Texas Houston, 2000.

National Academy of Sciences. "Herbal Pharmacology in the People's Republic of China." Washington, DC: National Academy of Sciences, 1975.

Newall, Carol, Linda Anderson, and J. David Phillipson. *Herbal Medicines: A Guide for Healthcare Professionals.* London: The Pharmaceutical Press, 1996.

Newman, Margaret. *Health as Expanding Consciousness.* New York: National League for Nursing Press, 1994.

Nightingale, Florence. *Notes on Nursing: What It Is and What It Is Not.* Edinburgh, Scotland: Churchill Livingstone, 1980, Originally published 1859.

O'Connor, Bonnie *Healing Traditions: Alternative Medicine and the Health Professions.* Philadelphia: University of Pennsylvania Press, 1995.

Ondrizek, Richard, Philip Chan, William Patton, and Alan King. "An Alternative Medicine Study of Herbal Effects on the Penetration of Zona-Free Hamster Oocytes and the Integrity of Sperm Deoxyribonucleic Acid." *Fertility and Sterility* 71, no. 3 (1999): 517-22.

Orem, Dorothea. *Nursing Concepts of Practice.* 6 ed. St. Louis, MO: Mosby, 2001.

Peck, M. Scott. *The Different Drum: Community Making and Peace.* New York: Touchstone, 1987.

Penn, R. "Adverse Reactions to Herbal and Other Unorthodox Medicines" in *Iatrogenic Diseases,* edited by Patrick D'Arcy and John Griffin. Oxford: Oxford University Press, 1986.

Porter, Roy. *The Greatest Benefit to Mankind: A Medical History of Humanity.* 1st American ed. New York: W. W. Norton, 1997.

Rogers, Martha. "Nursing Science and the Space Age." *Nursing Science Quarterly* 5, no. 1 (1992): 27-34.

Roy, Sister Callista. *The Roy Adaptation Model.* 3rd ed. Upper Saddle River, NJ: Pearson, 2009.

Ryan, Francis, and John Rybolt. *Vincent De Paul and Louise De Marillac: Rules, Conferences, and Writings.* Mahwah, New Jersey: Paulist Press, 1995.

Sackett, David, W. Scott Richardson, William Rosenberg, and R. Brian Haynes. *Evidence-Based Medicine.* London: Churchill Livingstone, 1998.

Sears, Barry. *The Zone.* New York: Regan Books Harper Collins, 1995.

Sessions, Patty Bartlett, and Donna Toland Smart. *Mormon Midwife: The 1846-1888 Diaries of Patty Bartlett Sessions.* Logan, UT: Utah State University Press, 1997.

Shakers, Harvard. *Physicians' Journal or an Account of the Sickness at Harvard,* Western Reserve Historical Society, Cleveland, OH, Shaker Manuscripts V:B 41, 1843.

Sheldrake, Rupert. *The Presence of the Past: Morphic Resonance and the Habits of Nature.* Rochester, VT: Park Street Press, 1995.

Smith, Glenda. "An Ethnographic Study of Home Remedy Use for African-American Children." University of Texas Houston, 2001.

Snodgrass, Mary Ellen. *Historical Encyclopedia of Nursing.* Santa Barbara, CA: ABC-CLIO, 1999.

Sullivan, Louise. *Spiritual Writings of Louise De Marillac: Correspondence and Thoughts*. New York: New City Press, ed. and trans. 1991.

Thomson, Samuel. *New Guide to Health, or, Botanic Family Physician Containing a Complete System of Practice, Upon a Plan Entirely New: With a Description of the Vegetables Made Use of, and Directions for Preparing and Administering Them to Cure Disease: To Which Is Prefixed a Narrative of the Life and Medical Discoveries of the Author* Boston: Printed for the author by J.Q. Adams, 1835.

Thorne, Sally. "Health Belief Systems in Perspective." *Journal of Advanced Nursing* 18 (1993): 1931-41.

———. *Negotiating Health Care: The Social Context of Chronic Illness*. Newbury Park, CA: Sage Publications, 1993.

Ulrich, Laurel. *A Midwife's Tale: The Life of Martha Ballard, Based on Her Diary, 1785-1812*. New York: Knopf : Distributed by Random House, 1990.

Vogel, Virgil. *American Indian Medicine*. Norman: University of Oklahoma Press, 1970.

Wall, Steve. *Wisdom's Daughters: Conversations With Women Elders of Native America*. New York: Harper Perennial, 1993.

Wicke, Roger. *Clinical Handbook of Herbal Medicine Vol. I*. Hot Springs, MT: Rocky Mountain Herbal Institute Publications, 1992.

World Health Organization. "Fact Sheet No. 134 Traditional Medicine." Geneva, Switzerland: WHO, 2003.

———. "The Promotion and Development of Traditional Medicine: WHO Technical Report Series 622." Geneva: World Health Organization, 1978.

the Earth Element

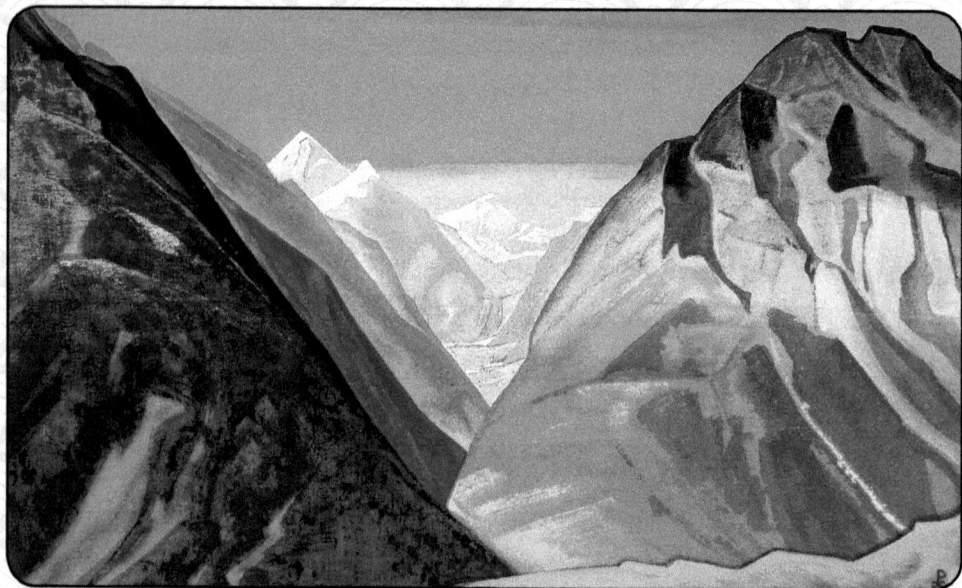

Lahul
Nicholas Roerich, 1932

CHAPTER THREE

Entering the Earth Element

Integration is a quality of heart. How one integrates herbal and nursing science and art is a process that unfolds within the being of the nurse-herbalist. The outcome of this process is as unique as the personality of each and every nurse. There is no specific recipe for the creation of *the* practice in nurse-herbalism, but I will share what I have learned from my experiences and opportunities. These next four chapters are some of my insights and reflections on the elements of nurses' nature care that continue to provide a strong foundation for my evolving nurse-herbalist practice. Chapters 3-7 are the manifestation of some of the integrative insights I have had over the years with plants as partners. They are a detailed account of what I believe to be the best approaches and techniques for creating and sustaining a practice in nurse-herbalism. The chapters follow the holistic nursing process from centering to assessment and diagnosis, to planning and implementation and then evaluation. The chapters, with their corresponding phase of the nursing process, are also organized according to the five elements of Self: earth, air, water, fire, and ether.

In Chapter 3, we begin with the first part of the holistic nurse-herbalist's process: a centering preparation I call "Entering the Earth Element." The earth element is associated with the physical self. The content of the chapter focuses on the physical connection with the environment, specifically healing plants. There are opportunities to engage earth through physical, sense-stimulating experiments with plants. Chapter 4—Awakening the Air Element—expands upon the content on integrative assessment and diagnosis found in Chapter 2. The air element is associated with the mental self and how we *think* about the application of healing plants in comfort and care. Chapter 4 focuses on educational preparation for nurse-herbalism, nursing theories that support nurse-herbalist assessment and diagnosis of symptom-sign patterns in clients, decoding the scientific data on herbs, and the mindful integration of nursing theory and herbal practice. Chapter 5—Welcoming the Water Element—presents nature care solutions and how to plan and implement them. The water element is associated with the emotional self. The content of this chapter focuses on techniques for strengthening the healing relationship that is the "cup" for the solutions or remedies for change and healing that are chosen and then implemented in a plan of care as a result of integrative insight. Chapter 5 addresses the importance of negotiating goals, solution-focused counseling tips, and the power of herbal simples. Chapter 6—Fanning the Fire Element—is the chapter in which we reflect upon and evaluate client transformation that occurs during nurse-herbalist care. The fire element is associated with the spiritual self that I equate with the laws of man and Creator. The content of this chapter focuses on evaluation of client outcomes within the social context of legal, ethical, and the personal-professional standards of practice and care related to nurse-herbalism as well as issues of safety for people and plants. The seventh and final chapter—Effecting the Ether Element—concerns the fifth element of Self, which is associated with the essence of Self or what I will refer to as the "Higher Self." The content of this chapter focuses on bringing about a living ethic for nurse-herbalism to guide peace-making and planet healing based upon the wisdom of elders and ancient tradition.

The ways in which nurse-herbalists provide care and comfort for their client or clients is a manifestation of the elements of their Self: body, mind, emotions, spirit, and essence. The nurse-herbalist creates a healing formula for the nurturance of the healing relationship. That formula is a unique representation of the five elements of Self of nurse and client in a particular moment in time and space. The presence of all five elements of Self, in formula or harmonious pattern, is essential to the fullest expression of holistic nurse-herbalist comfort and care. It is the nurse-herbalist's conscious commitment to connection with the natural world, plants in particular, and with the pattern of the elements of Self that ultimately determines the quality of holistic comfort and care and the opportunities for healing provided. For example, if the nurse-herbalist focuses only on the air element or mental self in practice, s/he might only focus on the scientific or traditional data on the application of a healing plant. Some might think this integrative care because the nurse-herbalist's approach is integrative, but commitment to holistic, integrative nurse-herbalism is demonstrated by the inclusion of all five elements in a practice plan.

STARTING A PRACTICE PLAN

As you read the next chapters, experiment with herbs and reflect upon integrative insights, I recommend that you begin to write down your aspirations and plans for your own nurse-herbalist practice. This chapter is about the earth element of Self. It is a good place to start to root your love of herbalism and your creative ideas for nurse-herbalism care into the garden of design. This is your garden plan that you will use as a guide and organizing framework for ideas and inspirations. There is no right or wrong way to create your plan. But there is one "rule" I like to suggest for any creative endeavor. Do not edit or critique your ideas or work. Turn off the critical thinker mode so highly cultivated in nursing and turn on the free thinker and dreamer modes! Give yourself the luxury of time to dream your dream while you read this book. Know that your practice plan for meaningful work can be inspired and aided by the most beautiful plants, flowers, and trees.

As you start your practice plan, begin to observe what plants come into your world— waking and dreaming. Be sure to enter them also into your practice plan though you may not know immediately what role they will play. Just let the images, ideas, impressions, and dreams come into being. Open the gate to the flow of creativity. This book suggests a professional structure, the line drawings, if you will, that lend definition to the work;

but only you can provide the color and meaning for your design within that definition. Begin by picking a medium for your practice plan. It might be a journal, a canvas, or a sketch pad. Then pick your instrument for documenting your notes: a pencil, pen, or paintbrush. You may find that you prefer to document in words or pictures. The professional structure provided throughout this book for the development of your practice plan is the five elements of nature care. Decide how you will organize each of the five elements within the confines of the medium you have chosen. For example, will you use a section of a journal for each element and how will that section be identified? You are already beginning the process of manifesting your vision for nurse-herbalism.

In this chapter, you have an opportunity to first consider the physical space—the earth element—and the decisions that you make as to the appropriate positioning of location and services provided. How to establish natural pharmacies for wildcrafting is addressed along with the nurse-herbalist tradition of keeping a kitchen laboratory with medicinal gardens. As you enter the earth element, you mindfully establish connection with the healing plants that represent the earth element and begin to learn their qualities, constituents, and history of application in comfort and care.

HALLOWING SPACE

Assessment is typically identified in nursing as the first step in the process of providing comfort and care. There is, however, a time of preparation that occurs prior to assessment that is really vital to the accuracy, efficacy, safety, and perfection or beauty of the care and comfort provided within the healing relationship. In the practice of holistic care, nurses practice centering prior to client interaction. Centering is a time for personal spiritual practices such as meditation (receiving), prayer (requesting), reflection (observation), and body scanning for tensions that could impede the work. I also suggest that creating or *hallowing space* be added to the preparatory repertoire of the nurse-herbalist as the active expression in the material plane for the light and energy garnered through spiritual centering. Hallowing space—connecting with nature and the creation of a healing environment—starts the flow of energy from the spirit world into the earth. This is, in essence, the process of bringing "heaven to earth," an important part of the healing process that I will explain throughout this book. This process is symbolized as a descending triangle.

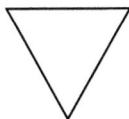

$$\triangledown$$

I learned a lot about hallowing space from my upbringing as a dancer. Dancers are taught how to enter into and participate in a space in such ways as engaging the objects and persons in a space, finding the energetic hotspots, standing in the light, and filling a void. One of my favorite things is sharing and hallowing space with plants. I have "danced" with plants in a wide variety of spaces, including the New York Botanic Garden, the star-shaped Fort Hipo on the lush island of Kauai, a greenhouse filled with loofa hanging from the vines climbing the walls and ceilings, and a field of red clover.

I also learned so much about hallowing space as the creation of a healing environment for clients when I worked with a German healer named Oma in the 1980s in her foot reflexology clinic in Glendale, California. Oma was very connected with nature, plants, and the nature spirits. She told me many stories and allowed me to work beside her for two years while I continued with the pre-licensure phase of my nursing education. Because of the opportunity with Oma, my integrative nursing experience really started as soon as I entered nursing school! Oma and I always spent a good amount of time before opening the clinic each morning preparing for receiving our clients. We cleaned carpets, organized treatment rooms, freshened oils, prepared teas, and even hosed down the outside of the building with cold water. We "demagnetized" the space with our visualizations of the brilliant white light of purity and the gentle violet fires of transmutation. Oma taught me that it was the caregiver's responsibility to manage the energies in a space and she was right.

I use those same techniques that I was taught more than twenty-five years ago and more to establish a space that is settled and energetically clear. Why is this important? Because the nurse-herbalist will first assess what the client needs and what their health patterns are. Clear vision begins with a clear space. Every person's energy field—clients' and nurses'—can be cleared. Before receiving a new client, the nurse-herbalist clears the space so that the new client's pattern can be understood without interference. To dissipate a previous client's energies, I use various herbal solutions in the environment along with visualizations. One of my favorites is eucalyptus essential oil, which I place on my hands before stripping the residual energy from the treatment table in between clients. Some people burn incense, but I find that the action of partnering with plants in stripping the energy from a client's feet or demagnetizing the treatment table with my hands in what I have come to know as the ancient ritual of ablution is the best. I measure the experience by the weight I feel in my body. Energy is felt as weight. After a eucalyptus or other herbal ablution, I feel, as do my clients, lighter. Ablution with herbal foot baths will be discussed in Chapter 5.

Placement of objects in a space is also important to how the energy flows through a space. Furniture can assist or impede the flow of energy and therefore have an effect on the outcome of the session. If nurse-herbalists have their own offices, they can place the furniture where it works the best for client care and comfort as well as where it will facilitate their own well-being as they work throughout the day. When nurse-herbalists work in hospitals, clinics or facilities that they do not own, it is important to first identify if the space is really going to be conducive for the work —that is, provide the proper energetic platform for the nurse-herbalist to have clear vision, assessment, diagnosis, planning, and intervention.

When I first started as a nurse-herbalist, I was fortunate to have a mentor in Oma and a private space in which to work and learn. From that experience, I would suggest that a nurse-herbalist have a room at home or an office space reserved and consecrated as a healing space. Nurses are trained in hospitals that rarely (unless they are Planetree Model hospitals) attend to the level of detail in preparation of the healing environment that I am referring to here. Hospital units and rooms also rarely have any connection with nature. Welcoming "representatives" from the plant, animal, and mineral worlds into a healing space in some form is an amazing experience in the healing art for clients and nurse-herbalists alike. There are hospitals that do include the other kingdoms in their facilities. For example, the Anthroposophical[1] Medicine Hospitals of Germany and Switzerland are large trauma centers that fully integrate nature into the space. In one hospital I visited, I was greeted walking in the door by a four-foot amethyst geode. Each unit is painted in a certain pattern that is considered harmonious with nature. All buildings are constructed with rounded angles, reflecting the knowledge that there are no right angles in nature. Like biodynamic gardening, also founded on Anthroposophical teachings, the hospitals are built to harmonize with patterns and rhythms that occur naturally in the environment. While these hospitals still deal with similar economic, practice, and legal issues found anywhere, the healing environment is a strength of that healing tradition and culture that is palpable.

Herbal Experiment: Entering the Green World

Make a list of the five elements of nature care. Go outside and find a representative in nature of each of the five elements that you can legally and ethically take home. Create a healing space in your home and position your elements in that space. You can integrate the representatives into an existing space or create a new space. Record your reflections. What drew you to the objects you chose? What do the elements mean to you?

---

1   Anthroposophical medicine is part of the culture of Germany and Switzerland. Rudolf Steiner (1861–1925), philosopher, writer, and scientist, whose work was inspired by Goethe's teachings on nature, emphasized that every person has the potential to know the spiritual world. He opened a college in Switzerland specifically for the study of the "sciences of the spirit." He used his research with the assistance of a Dutch physician named Ita Wegman to develop a spiritual medical doctrine that was connected to nature. Plants and plant therapies are a very important part of Anthroposophical healing practices. Anthroposophical practitioners, including nurses, not only use plants in their interventions with clients, they also value interaction with and observation of the live plants they use in practice. The nursing students who receive their education at Anthroposophical hospitals (I have visited hospitals with as many as 450 beds) in Germany and Switzerland tend the plants in the medicinal herb gardens. Pharmacists at these hospitals prepare herbal remedies for client care on site. Nurses' clean utility and medication rooms are stocked with herbal oils and other plant-based remedies. Nurses can receive instruction on Anthroposophical herbal applications, such as rhythmical embrocation with herbal oils, in addition to conventional nursing curriculum. Anthroposophical nurses have a system of practice and education that has integrated the use of herbs, primarily topicals, into client care. Nurses who work in Anthroposophical hospitals do not have to be formal students of the Steiner teachings to learn and apply the wisdom and techniques of plant use that have been developed in Anthroposophical healing practices.

Green Medicine Begins at Home

Over the years after graduating from nursing school and moving away from Glendale, I have had the opportunity to practice in a number of different environments. I have practiced nursing in medical clinics, hospitals, infirmaries, schools, locked psychiatric care units, community clinics, my own office space, and in my home. I have practiced nurse-herbalism in group practice settings where I had my own office and acres of cultivated herb gardens as my laboratory. I have practiced herbalism in hospitals, in home health care, and in private practice offices without gardens. For the past ten years, however, I have chosen to practice in and from the privacy and beauty of my and my husband's home and gardens. I say "in" and "from" because clients can either visit our medicine house for help or I talk with them on the phone. For face-to-face appointments, the lower floor of the house and the gardens is dedicated to receiving and helping people. We have a lending library where clients can read and rest before or after an appointment and where they can borrow recommended resources for continuing their healing work. Throughout the years, I have found that some of the most powerful medicine is that which people pick and make themselves. In addition to serving clients herbal teas and special snacks in the foyer and counseling them in my office, I use the gardens and the kitchen for teaching clients how to make their own medicine, their own herbal remedies.

I have a hypothesis that when people make their own medicine, they actually heal more easily, more thoroughly, and often more gently. Gentle herbal simples, such as a cup of tea or soup, take on more meaning for the client and therefore more power. Participation in making medicine and the direct relationship with medicinal plants is also a part of the creation of the healing environment in which the nurse and client work together to form a chalice to hold the healing energy of the chosen plants. I have found little evidence of research or papers published on this subject of making medicine in the nursing science literature. There was one publication on folk remedies a number of years ago. That phenomenological study by Ruth Davis titled "Understanding Ethnic Women's Experiences with Pharmacopeia" found that among women who used folk remedies such as herbs, foods, and over-the-counter medicines, the actual remedies were not as critical to the care of the person who was ill as the "meaning of the cultural memories inherent in acts of caring."[2] Davis, unfortunately, did not continue her line of research.

My evidence for supporting the promotion of helping clients make their own medicine is historical, anecdotal, and experiential. As discussed earlier, my historical research shows that self-care and being one's own doctor is an American tradition. Prior to the emergence and expansion of the influence of the pharmaceutical industry in the late nineteenth and early twentieth centuries, making one's own medicine, especially from plants from the garden and natural environment, was common and highly valued. With the industrialization of society comes a separation not only from nature but also from the medicines from the earth. When others make our medicines for us, we are not only faced with issues of physical quality and safety. The energy infusing the medicine or even the prepared herbal remedy is critical to the healing of the client.

When a client and their herbalist make their own remedies, they can saturate any remedy with exactly the right energy that will channel the remedy to the specific part of the body needing the medicine. Through visualization, the remedy is infused with the hearts' healing intention and purpose. Not unlike the research on the power of prayer, this hypothesis and experience are based on spiritual as well as natural and behavioral sciences that inform nurse-herbalism and the creation of the healing environment.

Nurse-herbalists and clients are the healing environment. Their energy is a vital element in the making of the herbal remedies and the healing environment in which those remedies are designed and created. The way in which those remedies are made and how they are applied are as important to the healing outcome as the remedy itself. The demonstration of caring that imbues the way in which the herbs are prepared and applied may be of vital importance to the overall effectiveness of the remedy, and perhaps be even more important than the biochemical constituents in the plant.

Nurse-herbalists, in their integration of biomedical and traditional evidence, are well positioned to mobilize a new dimension in caring science that is distinctly inclusive of all elements of care, including

---

2   Ruth Davis, "Understanding Ethnic Women's Experiences with Pharmacopeia," *Health Care for Women International* 18 (1997): 425.

spiritual connection with plant remedies and the environment from which they are grown. Nursing scientist Afaf Meleis wrote of nursing's connection with the greater sociocultural environment in 1996 that, "Over the past three decades, there has been a gradual conceptual shift from nursing as a biomedically driven discipline to a more socioculturally informed discipline. ... Human beings, as defined in nursing, are integrated wholes and are not distinct from their culture, sociopolitical values, family, biology, genetics, physiology, and societal attributions."[3] I would add that nurses and clients are not distinct from their gardens or the natural world, either. This is why I have found a home- and garden-based practice to be the most supportive of holistic nurse-herbalism.

Nurse-Herbalism and Community Health

Practicing in one's own home office and garden is not always a possibility. While perhaps not optimum, it is possible to practice effectively in a variety of settings from hospitals to the World-Wide Web. I know because I have practiced in many of them. From an herbal standpoint, nurse-herbalism can really be applied in any client care situation and in any environment. It is typically the policy of a facility or a state statute that regulates whether or not a nurse-herbalist would practice in a particular setting or not. The statutes I have read typically state that the nurse seeking to implement a particular holistic intervention such as herbs follow the institution's policy. So if one is working from home, there is no institutional policy that would preclude the use of herbs in practice. Other legal and ethical aspects of nurse-herbalism that must be considered are discussed in Chapter 6 on the fire element. But if a nurse-herbalist is working in a hospital where applying herbal simples such as witch hazel distillate compresses to a woman's perineum post-partum, providing chamomile tea at bedtime or serving cranberry juice are common because they are in the pantry and clean utility rooms, then the nurse can really capitalize on the opportunity to not only practice with a simples approach, but educate about herbs and perhaps even conduct research on the herbal applications readily available.

---

3   Afaf I. Meleis, "Culturally Competent Scholarship: Substance and Rigor," ANS: Advances in Nursing Science 19, no. 2 (1996): 4.

One of the nurse-herbalists I met at one of the Anthroposophical medicine hospitals I visited in Germany told me about the extensive research she and a team of practitioners including a physician had done on the application of a lemon compress in fever reduction. She said that they had two file drawers of data that they had collected and that the simple was highly effective in fever reduction. (See Appendix A for the recipe for lemon compress.) Nurse-herbalists can be quite effective in hospitals, particularly when they pick one plant to partner with in the care and comfort of clients. There are many simples that can be developed and researched in the hospital. Community nurses, however, have even greater opportunity to teach, learn, and apply herbal remedies and create healing environments that recognize the environment, nature, and plants in particular. Community health nurses, who are often immersed in the culture of the community in which they work, often see the traditional uses of plant remedies first hand and are ideally positioned for integrative nurse-herbalism. As history demonstrates, nurses' expertise with herbal remedies was developed in community. The Shaker nurses applied the herbal remedies created by their communities in their infirmaries. They were, in essence, the product testers for the Shaker herb industry. They also implemented and tested popular plant-based dietary and herbal programs such as the Graham diet and Thomsonian medicines.[4] They, like nurses in earlier centuries and nurses today, had the opportunity to also influence a community's relationship with certain plants. Because the nature of their work includes a close connection with culture and environment, I encourage community health nurses, in particular, to consider the role nurse-herbalism can play in care planning and their ability to promote trust and relationships with clients and communities. Opportunities for further learning, research, and implementation abound in community practices, including home health, hospice care, and occupational/environmental health. Qualitative studies such as histories and ethnographies are helpful in understanding different communities' herbal healing traditions. There are some ethnographic studies that have been published in nursing on different cultures'

---

4   Martha Libster, *Herbal Diplomats: The Contribution of Early American Nurses (1830-1860) to Nineteenth-Century Health Care Reform and the Botanical Medical Movement* (Thornton, CO: Golden Apple Publications, 2004).

botanical home remedies use. One example is a study that looked at herbal remedies applied in common ailments of rural African-Americans living in Virginia. Remedies identified were onion syrup, lemon, catnip, cabbage leaf compress, and flaxseed poultices.[5] Being able to listen to and include local, traditional remedies in care and comfort is important to building and sustaining community health. The community nurse is well positioned for the role of Herbal Diplomat™—the cultural diplomat who partners with plants in a community building, particularly around health care issues.

Think about the role you currently play in your community's knowledge and understanding of medicinal plants. Start with tobacco or marijuana use for example. How do you talk about these plants? As a nurse-herbalist and nursing faculty member, I am often asked about medical marijuana use and legalization. I remember first being asked my opinion about the subject in 1998, when I served on an ethics board for a hospital in Denver. I decided at that time, which was about the same period I encountered the St. John's Wort that I would respond from a plant perspective. To this day I say that marijuana is a "loud plant," meaning that it gets a lot of attention. In some cultures, such as in India, it has a very sacred use by the rishis or holy men. Hallucinogens are revered in many cultures as part of sacred ritual. In the United States, however, the plant may be used repetitively but is not exactly used ceremonially. I am always concerned about the choices to use any plant routinely—particularly the smoking of it—because of its potential harm to the lungs from the heat of the smoke. I also have questions about the use of any substance to obtain an elevated or out-of-body state that can be achieved through spiritual practice when a person's energy centers are prepared and they have the attainment to be able to apply the experience for service to humanity.

As for tobacco, I was introduced to the plant by my mother, who smoked the leaf every day for many years. I learned at age 17 that I was dangerously allergic to the smoke that comes from cigarettes but, interestingly, I do not react to the smoke of whole dried leaf that an Indian elder burned as a ritual smudge or purification ritual. Tobacco is

---

5   Mildred H. Roberson, "Home Remedies: A Cultural Study," *Home Healthcare Nurse* 5, no. 1 (1987).

considered a sacred plant by indigenous peoples in America. I was taught to use it ceremonially by, Cecilia (Zezi), with whom I have worked. As I mentioned before, Cecilia is a wisdom keeper[6] for all of Turtle Island and the Iroquois People, in particular. When I moved to North Carolina, she gave me some tobacco (*Nicotiana tabacum*) seeds and a vision. I have yet to plant the seeds, but I have worked with a number of tobacco growers in North Carolina who wished to switch from tobacco to herb growing. It is not an easy choice to make as the growers' livelihood and the state economy are entwined with the tobacco industry. From a plant perspective, the mass production and marketing of the tobacco plant might suggest that the plant is actually still enslaved to the tobacco industry while the human slaves who used to cultivate and harvest it were liberated decades ago.

Nurses have a tradition not only in cautioning the public about the safe use of herbs. More often, nurses have historically been able to introduce communities to certain plants that are helpful in health and healing, such as when the Mormon and Shaker women started using lobelia (*Lobelia inflata*) in the nineteenth century. Nurses have also promoted topical applications of plants, such as the Shaker nurses' use of rose (*Rosa gallica*) water in the comfort of those with pain related to migraine headache[7] and the Sisters of Charity's use of hops (*Humulus lupulus*) poultices for allaying the pain of battle wounds. [8] It is a healing tradition for community-based nurse-herbalists to educate and inform the public about healing plants and plant applications and demonstrate their use in comfort and care. The expansion of the community's knowledge base about herbal remedies is important to the health care of the community. The use of herbal remedies can lead to an increase in the connection between people and nature, which some are now considering to be a significant part of health care reform.

---

6   Steve Wall, *Wisdom's Daughters: Conversations with Women Elders of Native America* (New York: Harper Perennial, 1993).

7   Libster, *Herbal Diplomats: The Contribution of Early American Nurses (1830-1860) to Nineteenth-Century Health Care Reform and the Botanical Medical Movement.*

8   Martha Libster and Betty Ann McNeil, *Enlightened Charity: The Holistic Nursing Care, Education and Advices Concerning the Sick of Sister Matilda Coskery*, (1799-1870). (Farmville, NC: Golden Apple Publications, 2009).

BECOMING THE GREEN MAN
AND GREEN WOMAN

Some scientists and historians have suggested that there is a growing disconnect between people and the natural world, particularly the plants that provide the oxygen we breathe and the food that sustains our bodies. This disconnect is often identified as an all-too-common phenomenon of those living in highly industrialized communities where humans have sought dominance over nature.[9] In 2005, news columnist Richard Louv coined a new informal psychiatric diagnosis, "nature-deficit disorder," in his book *Last Child in the Woods* in which nature is revealed as the "antidote" that brings greater health, stress reduction, a "deeper sense of spirit," increased creativity, play, and a safer life[10] to families, in particular children. Children need to connect with nature on a daily basis. Some have speculated that the obesity epidemic along with the significant rise in environmental allergies and depression are just some of the health concerns that arise from a population physiologically, psychologically, and spiritually/energetically starved for their connection with the natural environment.

It seems like it should be common sense that we are meant to interact with the natural world that surrounds us. And yet so many people seem to fear it. I remember meeting people when I moved to New York City who never left the pavements of the city. I asked them if they wanted to go to the "country" where they could sleep in the dark, be surrounded by plants, and experience quiet on a daily basis, some things that I considered "natural." They told me something I would never forget. They said that they did not want to leave the Big Apple because when they went to the country, they "got sick." They said that they experienced headaches, stomach pain, and were often just plain terrified of the dark and quiet! Nature was not for them.

While some people love the comforts of the space of their home and its four walls, others prefer the comfort of the vast open spaces of the outdoors.

---

9   Edward Osborne Wilson, *Biophilia: The Human Bond with Other Species* (Cambridge, MA: Harvard University Press, 1984); Carolyn Merchant, The Death of Nature: Women, Ecology, and the Scientific Revolution (New York: Harper & Row, 1989).

10   Richard Louv, *Last Child in the Woods : Saving Our Children from Nature-Deficit Disorder* (Chapel Hill: Algonquin Books of Chapel Hill, 2005), 161.

As is the case in the broader community, there is also a range of relationships nurses have with nature and the plant world. While some nurses may have no interest in the connection between themselves or their practice and the plant world and the elements of nature care, nurse leaders, educators, and scholars often value nature and the environment. In the 1990s, for example, Dorothy Kleffel encouraged nurses to adopt a more "ecocentric" worldview or philosophy in which all life forms, including human beings, were understood to be essentially interrelated and that the health of Earth affected the health of all.[11] This consciousness that Earth and its plant and animal life forms are interrelated and harmonious rather than animals and plants as separate servants of the human race is not new. In the ancient healing traditions, animals, plants, Earth, and the stars and sky are all considered vital to health and life itself; therefore, they are often fully integrated into creation stories, life events, health beliefs, and healing practices. For example, Cecilia talks about nature, such as the trees, plant medicines, and animals, as if they are family. Her connection with nature is profound. Steve Wall recorded her as saying:

> The amazing thing is our environment. As I get older, I tend to listen to the world, listen to our mother, like our mother the earth and the planets and the trees and the bugs and animals and everything all round me. I pay attention to what our environment says. The moon and the sun and even the wind affects us. ... Like us, us Indian people, our land is like a mother, because she gives us everything, like medicine. Anything we hold dear is sacred to us, like our land because that's where our medicine comes from. You take care of the land, it takes care of you. That's why we call it Mother Earth.[12]

When I have lodged with Zezi in her home where the five rivers come together, I have had one of the best night's sleeps of my life. She and I have gone on medicine walks and we have talked about many things. She has taught me about the Peacemaker who unified Six Nations. We

---

11 Dorothy Kleffel, "Environmental Paradigms: Moving Toward an Ecocentric Perspective," ANS: Advances in Nursing Science *18, no. 4 (1996).*

12 Wall, *Wisdom's Daughters: Conversations with Women Elders of Native America*: 261.

thanked the Creator for many things. Truly, my favorite Zezi saying is, "Thank you Creator – No wonder I love you!" Her love of the Creator and nature is what brought us together. Zezi exudes a reverence for earth mother and her herbal medicines that I cannot, nor do I really want to, describe in words. I can attest that I am always comfortable when we talk and walk medicine. Our love of plants brought us together in Akwasasne where Mother Earth's hair, the sweet grass, is really fragrant and beautiful.

I am also comfortable in my own Celtic tradition in which the connection with seasons, the cycles of the animals and birds, and the herbs of forests, fields, mountains, and waters are also rooted in the deepest reverence for God, the Creator. This spiritual connection was passed to me by my mother, whose people are Cornish Celtic. Perhaps the strongest connection with nature in Celtic tradition is with the sacred spirit of the trees that provide not only fuel and material with which to build houses and furniture, but also are precious sources of food and medicine. Celtic peoples believe that the real healer is the spirit of the tree itself. In some places in Britain the "oak tree was considered so powerful that healing could occur simply by walking around the tree and wishing the ailment to be carried off by the first bird alighting on its branches."[13]

In Celtic tradition the Druids, or learned people in society, often led the rituals celebrating different aspects of nature's beauty and bounty. For example, the early Druids, like the Mohawk, held water, particularly rivers, in such high esteem that they referred to the rivers as "mother goddess." One Celtic historian writes that, "The Celts had developed a concept of water veneration so ingrained in their folk-consciousness that Christianity could not overturn it but had to adapt it for its own uses; hence the preponderance of Holy Wells in the Celtic countries."[14] One of the most famous of healing rituals in Celtic tradition is the cutting or sickling of the mistletoe (*Viscum album*) from its host tree, the sacred oak, on the sixth day of the moon. Mistletoe was called a name that meant "all healing." In modern Cornish, mistletoe is called *ughelvar*, meaning high

---

13 Mara Freeman, *Kindling the Celtic Spirit : Ancient Traditions to Illumine Your Life Throughout the Seasons* (San Francisco: HarperSan Francisco, 2001).
14 Peter Berresford Ellis, *The Druids* (Grand Rapids, MI: W.B. Eerdmans Pub. Co., 1995), 133.

branch. Mistletoe grows high in the trees. I have found it everywhere in eastern North Carolina. It is a succulent evergreen parasite that is strong medicine used as an "antidote to all poisons."[15] Peter Berresford Ellis writes that in Celtic perception, "Mistletoe is neither this nor that; it is neither shrub nor tree. As a plant it neither grows from the ground nor falls to it ... thus mistletoe might be seen as a means whereby one is freed from the restrictions of convention."[16] It is such an interesting and yet small part of our natural world. There are so many plants with which we can associate. Nurse-herbalists specialize in the exploration of that association.

The association between humans and the green world is preserved in a curious part of Celtic tradition known as "The Green Man." This motif, while found throughout the world, is a part of Celtic nature tradition that is preserved in British culture such as in the carvings found in the decorative architectural ornamentation of cathedrals. The Green Man motif is a human face surrounded by and often emerging from the leaves, vines or branches of plants or trees. Peoples who are close to Earth Mother often see faces emerging from the plant world. The Green Man, described as the "archetype of our oneness with the Earth,"[17] symbolizes the plant-person connection.

Biology reveals the nature of our special physiological connection with green plants. On a molecular level, plants and humans are very similar. The chlorophyll found in green plants and the oxygen-carrying molecule, hemoglobin, found in human red blood cells is nearly identical in atomic design.

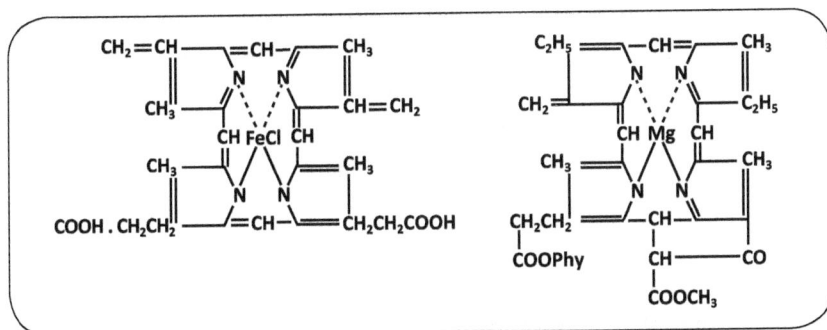

Figure 3.1: The Chlorophyll Connection

15 Ibid., 139.
16 Ibid.
17 William Anderson, *Green Man: The Archetype of Our Oneness with the Earth* (London: HarperCollins, 1990).

The most striking difference between the two is that the porphyrin ring of heme is built around iron (Fe), and the porphyrin ring of chlorophyll is built around magnesium (Mg). Although science has found that heme and chlorophyll are not interchangeable, their similarity in structure and respective functions still captures our interest. Though we are deeply interconnected, plants do not depend upon us for their existence. We, however, depend upon the green world for the very oxygen we breathe. We are partners and yet so often humans forget the reciprocal nature of green arrangement that is also encoded on our genetic experience. Charles Lewis, renowned horticulturalist, researcher, and author of *Green Nature/Human Nature*, wrote:

> A green world was our teacher at a time when the species' survival was a continuous challenge. The sight of living vegetation stimulates the neural pathways established then, so we are biologically prepared to feel a sense of connection with green environments. ... Plants possess life-enhancing qualities that encourage people to respond to them. In a judgmental world, plants are non-threatening and non-discriminating. They are living entities that respond directly to the care that is given them, not to the intellectual or physical capacities of the gardener. In short, they provide a benevolent setting in which a person can take the first steps toward confidence.[18]

The Green Man image suggests an intermingling of plant and human life forces that is mutual rather than human-dominant. As Kleffel suggested an emphasis on a more ecocentric worldview in nursing, physician Larry Dossey has written about "green" awareness as an archetype of consciousness about the plant-human connection. He suggests that a "counterproductive approach would be to regard green medicine in a purely pragmatic, utilitarian way, to consider herbs as merely the latest tricks in our black bag."[19] The ethic of plant-infused health care he proposes incorporates awareness of the inherent goodness and contribution of plants to all life. The nurse-herbalist practice must

---

18 Charles A Lewis, *Green Nature/Human Nature: The Meaning of Plants in Our Lives* (Urbana, IL: University of Illinois Press, 1996), 116.

19 Larry Dossey, "Being Green: On the Relationships Between People and Plants," *Alternative Therapies in Health and Medicine* 7, no. 3 (2001): 139.

exemplify the importance of this ethic. As will be discussed throughout the remainder of this book, it is from the position of being the Green Man or Woman, being in direct relationship with the world of healing plants, that the nurse-herbalist can best understand the safety and efficacy of that plant. As the nurse-herbalist becomes the Green Woman/Man, s/he becomes more attuned to the personality of plants, their unique characters and characteristics. This green attunement invites the emergence of greater awareness and insight into the applications of a specific plant for a specific client.

Like sleeping at the nexus of five rivers in Akwasasne, I find the path of integrative insight with herbs to lead to a nexus as well. The person who actively seeks the Green Man or Green Woman adds a dimension to the practice of nurse-herbalism that I consider fundamental to true holistic care. While standing at the crossroad of herbal tradition and nursing history with their biomedical education and experience intact, *the green nurse* stretches in two more dimensions like the tree, up with branches and leaves toward the sun and deeply into the earth with roots. In Celtic tradition, this image is referred to as *axis mundi*, or the world tree. The three realms of being are represented in the apple or oak tree. The trunk of the tree represents middle Earth or this dimension of daily existence and consciousness where we learn nature's cycles and the patterns of all living things, including health patterns. It is in the dimension of the roots that we connect with the unconscious. Carl Jung defined the unconscious or root world in terms of dreams:

> Even though dreams refer to a definite attitude of consciousness and a definite psychic situation, their roots lie deep in the unfathomably dark recesses of the conscious mind. For want of a more descriptive term we call this unknown background the unconscious. We do not know its nature in and for itself, but we observe certain effects from whose qualities we venture certain conclusions in regard to the nature of the unconscious psyche. Because dreams are the most common and most normal expression of the unconscious psyche, they provide the bulk of the material for its investigation.[20]

---

20   Carl G. Jung, *Dreams*, Bollingen Series, (Princeton, NJ: Princeton University Press, 1974).

The great tree is the place where the strengths of the spirit and dream worlds are drawn for earthly manifestation that is mater-ialization. When the nurse-herbalist connects with the green world, becoming the Green Man or Woman, they enter into the understanding of the ancient teaching of many cultures, "As Above … So Below." Partnership in the application of healing plants is then informed by many ways of knowing which come together at the center, the nexus of the rivers or world tree axis mundi that is represented in the human body as the heart. The green nurse has access to plant knowledge that comes from the dimension of the heart with all of its power, wisdom, and love. It is from this place that the nurse-herbalist can most ethically, respectfully, and safely create a holistic practice and a healing repertoire of green pharmacy.

Green Pharmacy

People rarely have knowledge of what goes into the making of the medicines they receive from hospitals, medical offices or local pharmacies. Nurses are taught the basics of pharmaceutical science with the goal that they safely administer medications under the direction of practitioners with prescriptive privileges. However, nurses and prescribing practitioners are not expected to know about the production, source, and chemical composition of the drugs they prescribe, administer or discuss with clients. Historically, physicians have often prepared, prescribed, and administered their own medications. Now there is a more collaborative system where pharmacists, physicians, and nurses all have varying responsibilities for the use of pharmaceutical drugs. Each practitioner and client trusts the health care system and the education of the practitioners to support the development and application of medicines of excellent quality.

In herbal medicine, however, there is a similar desire for remedies that are of excellent quality. Therefore, the standard of care is often higher in terms of providing herbal remedies, especially in the care of traditional healers and herbalists who utilize whole herbs in care rather than supplements. While the practitioner using herbal supplements in care might not know any more about the growing or production of the herbal remedy than they would know of a pharmaceutical drug, traditional healers and herbalists often grow or wildcraft (harvest from the wild) the medicinal plants themselves. If they do not, the practitioner cultivates a practice in which they are highly mindful of the quality of their sources for herbs and herbal products. Herbalists often make the medicine themselves that they apply in care or teach clients how to make the medicine for themselves from available plant sources. There is no unit dose system in herbalism because the dosages are traditionally individualized.

People who work with medicinal plants are expected to understand the plant in much the same way, and perhaps even in more ways, than nurses are expected to understand pharmaceutical drugs. Nurses who work with plant medicines find that they often have more of a relationship with the medicine they administer or discuss with a client than they do with pharmaceuticals, simply because they may grow the plant, harvest it, and prepare the medicine. But it is still possible for nurses to use herbs in practice much the way they do pharmaceuticals. For example, in the early 1900s, American nurses administered an "emulsion" of asafoetida (*Ferula foetida*), a pungent gum resin, by mouth to infants and adults with colic or gas pains.[21] Asafoetida is indigenous to Persia and Tibet, which means that the nurses most likely bought their herb from an importer rather than growing the plant themselves. They may have had to purchase the emulsion also. In another example, nurses used to apply flaxseed (*Linum usitatissimum*) poultices to the chest of clients with pneumonia.[22] It is probable that nurses living and working in more rural areas had access to flax fields. But what has also occurred historically in nursing is that nurses have maintained their own herb gardens, their own green "pharmacies." Nurse-herbalist midwives such as Martha Ballard[23] of the eighteenth century and nineteenth-century Mormons Patty Bartlett Sessions[24] and Anne Carling[25] kept their own gardens as sources

21 Margaret Tracy, *Nursing: An Art and a Science* (St. Louis, MO: C.V. Mosby, 1938), 367.
22 Bertha Harmer, *Text-Book of the Principles and Practice of Nursing* (New York: Macmillan Co., 1924), 206.
23 Laurel Ulrich, *A Midwife's Tale: The Life of Martha Ballard, Based on Her Diary, 1785-1812* (New York: Knopf, Distributed by Random House, 1990).
24 Patty Bartlett Sessions and Donna Toland Smart, *Mormon Midwife: The 1846-1888 Diaries of Patty Bartlett Sessions* (Logan., UT: Utah State University Press, 1997).
25 Libster, *Herbal Diplomats: The Contribution of Early American Nurses (1830-1860) to Nineteenth-Century Health Care Reform and the Botanical Medical Movement.*

for such healing plants as Joe Pye weed (*Eupatorium purpureum*)[26], onion (*Allium cepa*), and sage (*Salvia officinalis*).

Nurses in rural areas who collect the herbs they use in practice must also be aware of legal and ethical wildcrafting practices for their areas. In general, plants are considered by the public as a product of nature, which may be freely collected by anyone. It is not hard to imagine what can happen if a locally grown plant is discovered to be highly medicinal and the market price skyrockets. People have been known to trespass on private properties and to gouge the earth of the plants. Countries in which the culture of respecting medicinal plants has been taught from generation to generation have protected the right to collect what is needed for personal use, not economic gain. For example, in Bavaria in Germany, the right to gather wild plants anywhere is "enshrined in the Constitution."[27] In some countries, such as Austria and Switzerland, the uprooting of plants is prohibited and the amount of the aerial parts that can be wildcrafted is limited to five to twenty flowering stems or branches, depending on the area, and in some cases, the maximum amount that can be harvested is that which can be held in the palm of one hand.

Because nurse-herbalists are not just using that which they would normally use in their own self-care or family care, they must be aware of the impact that wildcrafting the herbs they use in practice will have on plant populations. If wildcrafting is to be done, the nurse-herbalist may want to consider teaming with a local botanist, who is often highly informed about local plant populations. When I was coordinating the herb program in Montana, I regularly checked in with the lead botanist associated with the Lewis and Clark National Forest. We went out on herb walks together to identify the plants in my area. It was fun and educational!

---

26 The root of Joe Pye Weed, also known as gravel root, has been applied orally as a tea or alcohol extract (drops) for health patterns related to chronic urinary concerns, uterine irritability, atonia, and prolapse, gout, rheumatism, chronic cough and asthma, and impotence. Harvey Wickes Felter and John Uri Lloyd, *King's American Dispensatory*, 18th ed., 3d rev ed. (Sandy, OR: Eclectic Medical Publications, 1983). However, because of the presence of toxic pyrrolizidine alkaloids (PA), the plant is not recommended today for long-term use. Some PAs are known to cause liver toxicity with extensive exposure.

27 Cyril De Klemm, "Medicinal Plants and the Law," in *The Conservation of Medicinal Plants*, eds. Olayiwola Akerele, Vernon Heywood, and Hugh Synge. (Cambridge: Cambridge University Press, 1991).

Conservation of medicinal plants is not a simple matter. Legislation protecting endangered species, although necessary, is considered inadequate. Plant habitats also must be protected to sustain the growth of medicinal plant populations. In the 1991 *Proceedings of an International Consultation* on the conservation of medicinal plants organized by WHO and others, seven points related to legislation regarding the management of medicinal plants were raised: Prevention of over collection, Use permits as management instruments, Use of a management plan, Implementation of controls on the trade of medicinal plants, Collection of license fees, Habitat protection, and Incentives for artificial propagation. [28] Nurses who use herbs in practice may want to consider cultivating and propagating their own plants as much as possible. It is also good practice to send samples of the plants to laboratories for analysis each year when growing plants for use in nursing care and comfort. The analysis of plant constituents provides an additional understanding of the quality of the plants.

When purchasing herbs for practice, it is best to order organically grown plants. Pesticides and herbicides are chemical compounds that when ingested orally or topically also have effects, as would any drug. It is counterproductive, if after performing an energetic clearance to enhance the ability to assess the client's health patterns, a nurse-herbalist were to introduce herbs that include chemical residues from pesticides and herbicides rather than simply providing the herb to the client. Pesticides and herbicides can cause changes in health patterns that "muddy the water" for the nursing process. When purchasing aerial parts of plants, such as leaf and flower, it is best to buy *whole* plant versus cut and sift. Leaves and flower petals can always be chopped before use. Purchasing whole plant helps to prolong the shelf life of volatile oils, in particular. Roots are cut prior to drying so as to increase surface exposure to air drying. They can be decocted or pulverized for oral or topical use when needed.

Create a special pharmacy space or spaces in your home and/or office. In our medicine house, I have an air-conditioned room in the attic with a sink where I can process and dry herbs and also keep them dry in the muggy summer/fall heat of North Carolina. I also have herb cabinets and an antique apothecary chest in my home office that I inherited from my paternal grandmother. It was my grandmother's relatives who

---

28 Ibid.

were medical missionaries to Canton, China. I enjoy having our family tradition—East meets West—represented in my herb practice! I keep my TCM herbs and Western herbs organized in separate closets because I typically (though not always) access the Western herbs for simples and the TCM herbs for formulations. I regularly open packages and test crispness and dryness of the herbs. I keep bay leaf (which I grow here in abundance) in my herb closets to repel any potential insects or moths. The herbs in the kitchen, pantry, and apothecary chest are used more frequently, so I keep those herbs in jars with lids that I remove whenever I use them. My herbs for long-term storage are kept in bags with an opening so that any residual moisture can escape. When I was the director of herb programs in Montana, I oversaw the processing of hundreds of pounds of herbs. I learned the best techniques for drying herbs. More information about herb processing and herbal applications is in Chapter 5.

In most states and practices I have worked in, I have given out the herbs that I recommend. However, in Colorado, I always sent TCM clients to a TCM pharmacy to pick up their herb formulations. In Colorado, there is a history of restricting herbalists from dispensing herbs directly to clients. I learned this through my connections with other herbalists in the state and also by researching state guidelines. It is important to explore this issue prior to setting up your practice if you plan to dispense from your green pharmacy. To buy or order TCM herbs or prescriptions at most reputable places, you have to demonstrate completion of a recognized TCM herb education program. As a TCM herbalist, I am able to buy herbs from Spring Wind Herb Company at retail prices and then create formulations for my clients as needed. I do not mark up the price of the herbs but I do charge clients what we paid for the herbs. Providing the herbs is a service to my clients. I produce as many of the Western herbs as I can from my gardens or from local growers and then purchase organic bulk herbs, such as red raspberry leaf, red clover, chamomile, and calendula flowers from Frontier Coop. My company, Golden Apple Healing Arts, has a wholesale agreement with Frontier and we provide starter supplies from our stock to clients. My clients do not take any one herb or formula for more than three months at the most. I am typically able to provide them with what their body needs.

A Few More Words on Wildcrafting

It is important to always have the safe and judicious use as well as the protection of medicinal plant populations on your heart when you partner with plants. Conservation of natural resources consists of any act that follows the belief that the resource is valuable and must be used prudently in the present so that the resource is not depleted for future generations. Plant medicines are valuable and must be conserved, which is why the WHO Traditional Medicine Programme, clinical herbalists, and herb associations focus on the importance of conservation.

To protect medicinal plants, the environment in which they are nourished must be cared for as well. Because plants obviously do not speak out, it is up to humans to understand and provide for their needs. Plants thrive in healthy environments just as people do. The plant itself produces its medicinal constituents in relationship to its environment. For example, Indian studies on the *Ephedra sp.* plant have shown that the amount of rainfall in a particular area has a relationship with the ephedrine content of the plant. The greater the annual rainfall, the smaller the ephedrine content, and occasional heavy showers also lower the ephedrine content.[29] Altitude affects plants. It also has a great bearing on which plants grow in a particular area. High altitudes have different plant life than those found at sea level. People who live at different altitudes have traditionally learned to use the plants that grow in their areas for healing.

Indigenous people use the plants for medicine as directed by what grows in their environment; hence, they have a strong connection with Earth and specifically the environment in which they live. More recently, increasing agricultural, mining, and lumber industries pose threats to the habitats of medicinal plants. Pollution is also a serious threat to plant life and their environments. In 1950, 30 percent of the globe was forested, and in 1975 only 12 percent of the surface of Earth was covered by forest. In 1995, it has been reported that the tree populations in the 1990s shrank by 10,000 per minute.[30] "Transformation of local ecosystems

29 Krishnarao Mangeshrao Nadkarni, *Indian Materia Medica*, 2 vols. (Bombay: Popular Prakashan, 1976), 501.
30 Charles Anyinam, "Ecology and Ethnomedicine: Exploring Links Between Current Environmental Crisis and Indigenous Medical Practices," *Social Science & Medicine* 40, no. 3 (1995).

wrought through human economic activities has been exercising severe constraints on the availability and accessibility of specific types of plants and animal species used for medicinal purposes."[31] Along with the disappearance of the forests is the disappearance of indigenous people, who not only have the expertise in the use of the medicinal plants in a particular location but who also protect and respect the environment. With the numbers of these people who are national treasures dwindling, the habitats of many medicinal plants, the plants themselves, and the knowledge of the use of these plants are at serious risk.

It is up to those who value medicinal plant life to speak up and protect the environments of these plants. People such as Rosita Arvigo, an American herbalist who apprenticed with Don Elijio Panti, one of the last surviving Maya traditional healers in the rainforest in Belize, help preserve the traditional healing methods and the plants of the areas in which they live. Arvigo has been an advocate for conserving the medicinal plants of the rainforest, and *Sastun,*[32] her story of her relationship with a Mayan healer, can be very inspiring to those who work with healing plants.

WHO has produced numerous documents and guidelines regarding the importance of protecting medicinal plants in their native habitats.[33] In addition, many countries have botanical gardens, even in the inner cities, where plants are preserved for the public so that they can have a place to go to connect with the plants and gain a greater awareness of how the plants that are responsible for many of the medications used in healing grow. Interacting with the plants that provide medicine or the inspiration for medicine is one way that nurses also can move into a more ecocentric paradigm and reconnect with the essence of Earth as the source of the natural beauty and abundance of unique healing plants. Kleffel states that "moving to the ecocentric paradigm will encourage nurses to address worldwide environmental problems that affect the health of everything that exists."[34]

Other nurse scientists also stress the inherent value of environment

---

31 Ibid., 323.
32 Rosita Arvigo, *Sastun* (New York: Harper San Francisco, 1994).
33 World Health Organization, *The Conservation of Medicinal Plants: Proceedings of the International Consultation, 1988, Chiang Mai, Thailand.* (Cambridge: Cambridge University Press, 1991); ———, *Guidelines on the Conservation of Medicinal Plants* (Geneva: World Health Organization, 1993).
34 Kleffel, "Environmental Paradigms: Moving Toward an Ecocentric Perspective," 5.

and its importance to the practice of nursing.[35] Nursing care exists in relationship with clients and the environment. The environment, comprised of thousands of plants that are potential medicine for people, is one of the major foci of nursing practice. Unfortunately, spiritual connections between people and nature are often marginalized in nurses' practice as diseases and biomedical treatments become "louder" and the lure of technology-based care and its demands on nurses increases.[36] Plant remedies that have provided the blueprints for human drug creations are gradually equated with synthetic drugs. But not all plant medicines lend themselves to constituent isolation and drug production. Creating plant-based medicines is not as lucrative for pharmaceutical companies that seek protection of investments through the patent process. Nurses who nurture attunement and connection with medicinal plants and develop a basic understanding of plant science are better prepared to advise clients about the use of herbal remedies. Nurturing plant connections begins with awareness and attention to the environment, to nature. As nurse-herbalists connect with the natural world, hallowing healing spaces that include plants, they open new "doorways into an infinite universe"[37] that the Celtic people have said occurs with the natural elements, those elements of care and of Self represented in powerful momentums in nurses' herbal traditions.

---

35 Margaret Burkhardt, "Healing Relationships with Nature," *Complementary Therapies in Nurisng and Midwifery* 6, no. 1 (2000).

36 Eric Cassell, "The Sorcerer's Broom: Medicine's Rampant Technology," *Hastings Center Report* 23, no. 6 (1993); Judith Erlen, "Technology's Seductive Power," *Orthopaedic Nursing* 13, no. 6 (1994).

37 John Matthews, *Drinking from the Sacred Well* (New York: Harper Collins, 1998), 267.

EARTH – INTEGRATIVE INSIGHT – REVERENCE FOR LIFE

One of the most important integrative insights I have had in partnering with plants over the years has been the healing power of reverence for life—nature, plants, and the Creator. The indigenous healers with whom I have worked continually exude this reverence. It is palpable in the healing space. One of the most precious moments of insight occurred in 2004, when I was invited to teach herbs and healing in Honolulu, Hawaii. I accepted the invitation with one condition: that the first evening would include three other native teachers who would introduce attendees to Hawaiian plants and culture. A nurse-geographer friend and colleague of mine, Dr. Nanette Judd, was invited and two indigenous healers, Auntie Marie and Auntie Anita, graciously flew from Molokai with their plants in arms to Honolulu. The memory of the insight is attached to the Hawaiian ritual of placing a lei of flowers around the neck of another as a gesture of the aloha spirit. The Aunties presented me with a stunning white lei of thin ginger flowers with stems woven together into a delicate breastplate. I had never seen nor smelled anything so vibrant. But they did not simply give me the box with the lei. They took it out of the box and Auntie Marie, the elder of the three, placed the circlet of cream-colored buds over my head and around my shoulders with such reverence. It was the person and the manner in which the plant was presented in the moment that conveyed reverence. I wore and absorbed the healing energy of the lei all week long as we cruised the islands. I learned a beautiful lesson in that simple act of reverence. Earth matter, plant matter, imbued with the power, wisdom, and love of the heart, and the peaceful spirit of aloha is powerful, simple green medicine. I have kept the dried flowers of the ginger flower lei as a reminder of the insight that occurred while in the presence of three Hawaiian women who embody aloha. I try to mindfully demonstrate the reverence I feel for the life in the person I am serving with every herbal remedy I make and each cup of tea I give. Simple demonstrations of reverence create the hallowed space for the herbs to be infused with aloha and the spirit of caring to rise.

REFERENCES

Akerele, Olayiwola, Vernon Heywood, and Hugh Synge, eds. *The Conservation of Medicinal Plants.* Cambridge: Cambridge University Press, 1991.

Anderson, William. *Green Man: The Archetype of Our Oneness with the Earth.* London: HarperCollins, 1990.

Anyinam, Charles. "Ecology and Ethnomedicine: Exploring Links Between Current Environmental Crisis and Indigenous Medical Practices." *Social Science & Medicine* 40, no. 3 (1995): 321-9.

Arvigo, Rosita. *Sastun.* New York: Harper San Francisco, 1994.

Burkhardt, Margaret. "Healing Relationships with Nature." *Complementary Therapies in Nurisng and Midwifery* 6, no. 1 (2000): 35-40.

Cassell, Eric. "The Sorcerer's Broom: Medicine's Rampant Technology." *Hastings Center Report* 23, no. 6 (1993): 32-39.

Davis, Ruth. "Understanding Ethnic Women's Experiences with Pharmacopeia." *Health Care for Women International* 18 (1997): 425-37.

Dossey, Larry. "Being Green: On the Relationships Between People and Plants." *Alternative Therapies in Health and Medicine* 7, no. 3 (2001): 12-6, 132-40.

Ellis, Peter Berresford. *The Druids.* Grand Rapids, Mich.: W.B. Eerdmans Pub. Co., 1995.

Erlen, Judith. "Technology's Seductive Power." *Orthopaedic Nursing* 13, no. 6 (1994): 50-53.

Felter, Harvey Wickes and John Uri Lloyd. *King's American Dispensatory.* 18th ed., 3d rev ed. Sandy, Oregon: Eclectic Medical Publications, 1983.

Freeman, Mara. *Kindling the Celtic Spirit : Ancient Traditions to Illumine Your Life Throughout the Seasons.* San Francisco: HarperSan Francisco, 2001.

Harmer, Bertha. *Text-Book of the Principles and Practice of Nursing.* New York: Macmillan Co., 1924.

Jung, Carl G. *Dreams*, Bollingen Series. Princeton, N.J.: Princeton University Press, 1974.

Kleffel, Dorothy. "Environmental Paradigms: Moving Toward an Ecocentric Perspective." *ANS: Advances in Nursing Science* 18, no. 4 (1996): 1-10.

Lewis, Charles A. *Green Nature/Human Nature: The Meaning of Plants in Our Lives.* Urbana, IL: University of Illinois Press, 1996.

Libster, Martha. *Herbal Diplomats: The Contribution of Early American Nurses (1830-1860) to Nineteenth-Century Health Care Reform and the Botanical Medical Movement.* Thornton, CO: Golden Apple Publications, 2004.

Libster, Martha, and Betty Ann McNeil. *Enlightened Charity: The Holistic Nursing Care, Education and Advices Concerning the Sick of Sister Matilda Coskery, (1799-1870).* Farmville, NC: Golden Apple Publications, 2009.

Louv, Richard. *Last Child in the Woods : Saving Our Children from Nature-Deficit Disorder*. Chapel Hill: Algonquin Books of Chapel Hill, 2005.

Matthews, John. *Drinking from the Sacred Well*. New York: Harper Collins, 1998.

Meleis, Afaf I. "Culturally Competent Scholarship: Substance and Rigor." *ANS: Advances in Nursing Science* 19, no. 2 (1996): 1-16.

Merchant, Carolyn. *The Death of Nature: Women, Ecology, and the Scientific Revolution*. New York: Harper & Row, 1989.

Nadkarni, Krishnarao Mangeshrao. *Indian Materia Medica*. 2 vols. Bombay: Popular Prakashan, 1976.

Roberson, Mildred H. "Home Remedies: A Cultural Study." *Home Healthcare Nurse* 5, no. 1 (1987): 34-40.

Sessions, Patty Bartlett and Donna Toland Smart. *Mormon Midwife: The 1846-1888 Diaries of Patty Bartlett Sessions*. Logan, UT: Utah State University Press, 1997.

Tracy, Margaret. *Nursing: An Art and a Science*. St. Louis, MO: C.V. Mosby, 1938.

Ulrich, Laurel. *A Midwife's Tale: The Life of Martha Ballard, Based on Her Diary, 1785-1812*. New York: Knopf, Distributed by Random House, 1990.

Wall, Steve. *Wisdom's Daughters: Conversations with Women Elders of Native America*. New York: Harper Perennial, 1993.

Wilson, Edward Osborne. *Biophilia: The Human Bond with Other Species*. Cambridge, MA: Harvard University Press, 1984.

World Health Organization. *The Conservation of Medicinal Plants: Proceedings of the International Consultation, 1988, Chiang Mai, Thailand*. Cambridge: Cambridge University Press, 1991.

———. *Guidelines on the Conservation of Medicinal Plants*. Geneva: World Health Organization, 1993.

the Air Element

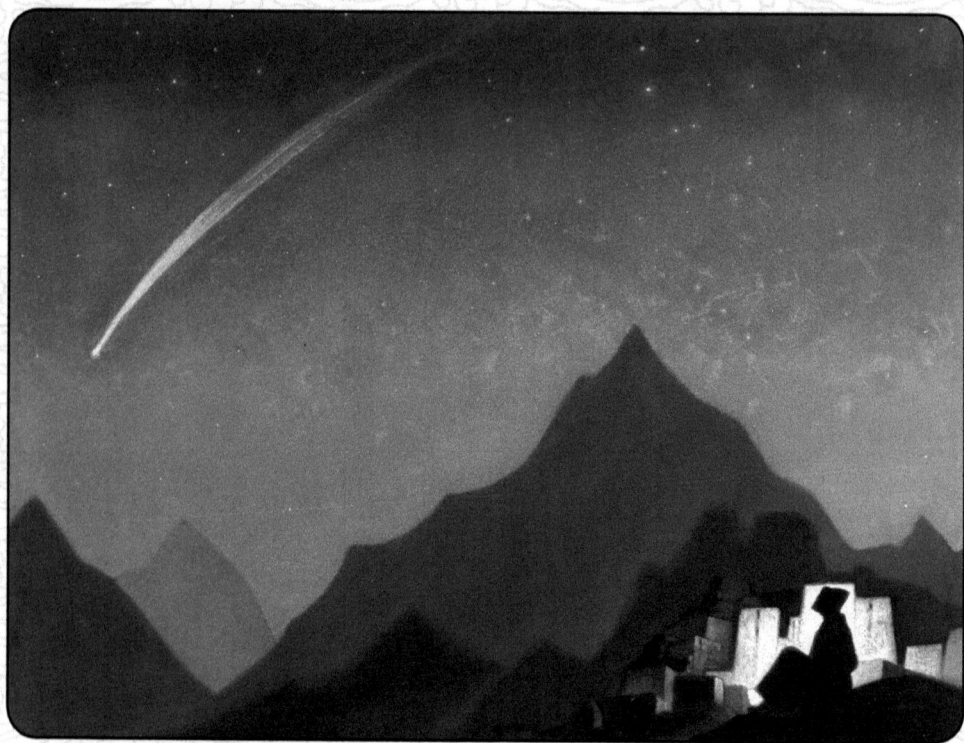

Star of the Hero
Nicholas Roerich, 1936

CHAPTER FOUR

Awakening the Air Element

The mind is a trickster, often casting illusion into the field of human perception. Ideas and mental impressions come and go like the wind. The mind alone should not dictate a nurse's work with clients and healing plants. It is a holistic model of care that includes accessing the spiritual, emotional, physical, and essential elements of Self through the senses, that provides a check and balance to the winds of the mind and mental body. Nature scientist Johann Wolfgang von Goethe once said that "the senses do not deceive; the judgment deceives."[1] Educating the mental body through study and skill development leads to organization of thoughts and a greater orientation to detail that can lead to improved "seeing," judgment, or analysis of health patterns. Education and study provide the platform for the grounding of intuition.

Intuition is the "form in which thought-content first arises."[2] In contrast to perception, which is an externalized orientation, thought-content comes from within us. Working with plants spawns intuitive internal experience. This may be due to the fact that plants are non-verbal living beings. When partnering with plants, we must be the non-verbal, pre-verbal selves that we were in early life, using different ways of communicating, knowing, and

---

1   Johann Wolfgang von Goethe and Jeremy Naydler, *Goethe on Science* (Edinburgh: Floris Books, 1996).
2   Rudolf Steiner, *Intuitive Thinking as a Spiritual Path* (Dornach, Switzerland: Anthroposophic Press, 1995), 88.

being in the world than exists after the eruption of language. Philosopher and nature-scientist Rudolf Steiner describes intuition as being to thinking as "observation is to perception. Intuition and observation are the sources of our knowledge."[3] Intuition is important in making connection with and ultimately knowing our environment and our clients. But, intuitive promptings without "roots" anchored in the mental body, thought, and intellect can lead to disturbances in the self of the nurse-herbalist and inappropriate care of the client.

The preparation of the mental body through study of any subject takes time and effort. People must first desire knowledge and have an abiding interest in the truth about the object of one's study. To sustain this interest, Goethe writes, "We must deepen our involvement in the objects of our attention and gradually become better acquainted with them. ... We will be compelled to distinguish, differentiate, and resynthesize, a process which finally leads to an order we can survey with some degree of satisfaction."[4] The purpose of this chapter is to provide suggestions for engaging the science mind in assessing and diagnosing health patterns of the clients who seek nurse-herbalist care.

Indigenous healers are often mentored their whole lives as they learn to work with plants. They learn from elder healers how to manage and interpret intuitive experience and then how to integrate that experience in a way that informs their knowledge of herbalism. Although my nursing education has always included teachings on spirituality, I did not receive my education on intuition and the psychic sense in nursing school or graduate nursing education. I received it from Oma and other healing elders who trained me in herbal care and comfort. Nursing programs typically support different ways of knowing, including intuition. There is also exceptional research contributed on the subject of intuition from nurse-scientists such as Drs. Lynn Rew and Lisa Ruth-Sahd. But there is an important intermediary step in translation of what is known about intuitive or psychic state and how, when, and where the nurse, particularly the nurse-herbalist who works with plants, puts that understanding into practice. This translation is important to the safety and efficacy of nurse-herbalist practice. I raise the issue here because the air element, and its

---

3   Ibid.
4   Goethe and Naydler, *Goethe on Science*: 32.

representation in the education of the mental body and continued study, is the antidote that can keep the trickster in check.

Intuition without rooting in the mental body is a "negative psychic state." I adopted this language from the work of Dr. Laurence and Mrs. Phoebe Bendit. Dr. Bendit was a Jungian psychiatrist and his wife, Phoebe, a clairvoyant. Psychic sense is similar to the other five senses in that it can be dull or acute. Negative psychism is uncontrolled, undifferentiated, and primitive. A person in a negative psychic state cannot differentiate the products of his own mind from that which is external to it. Reactions are most often unconscious. The Bendits locate the mechanism of action of the negative psychic state in the coeliac plexus, which is in the center of the body. The openness of the negative psychic state can be observed as leading to unchecked projection of thought onto clients ("I know more about you than you know about yourself"), spiritual boundary violations, and physical problems.

My first memory of my experience of a negative psychic state is when I was 2 years old. I was in my aunt's wedding as a flower girl. My mother tells the story that I walked down the aisle with Band-Aids up and down my legs and arms. I was a sensitive child who had numerous paranormal experiences. At that time, I was in a serious negative psychic state because I was very young and my parents, though religious, did not have an understanding of psychic energy or states and could not provide the education and protection I needed. When my mother told that story, I always intuited that there was an explanation for why I had those Band-Aids on my body. But it was not until I actively studied some of my own life history that I was able to transform the energy of the experience into a meaningful memory. You see, at the time, my mother's mother was very conservative. She did not believe that my mother, who was pregnant with my little brother at the time, should be in my aunt's wedding—a ceremony that for her represented "purity." The family was in the midst of a battle and my little sensitive self just needed the Band-Aids to plug up the holes in my energy field created by the hostility in the environment and rifts in the energy field. Understanding my early experience helped me to work with young children.

The positive psychic state, however, is controlled and consciously directed by a person. The mechanism of action of the positive psychic state occurs in the head. It develops with maturity as the person learns to exhibit greater and greater discernment and discrimination, and make deliberate choices in response to intuitive impressions. The Bendits explain that society is still very much under the influence of primitive "urges" and "only partly governed by the conscious mind."[5] The refinement of the positive psychic state informed by intuition begins when the intellect is engaged and applied in analyzing and making conscious choices about the intuitive or psychic promptings. In the case of nurse-herbalism in which healing plants and their powerful energy fields are routinely encountered by the nurse and the client, all intuitive promptings of the client and nurse about plant use would be informed and checked against the awareness born of experience and knowledge. Herbs should not be applied in the comfort and care of clients based on intuitive or psychic hunch. This is not a holistic approach and the risk to client, nurse, and plant populations is too great.

Here is one of the numerous examples I have witnessed over the years of the risk associated with negative psychic states driving herb use. I once worked with a chiropractor who "muscle tested" his clients for herbs and essential oils[6] of which he had little to no knowledge. There was a client who went to him for spinal adjustment and she came to my nurse-herbalist office after the visit for follow-up because he had prescribed 60 drops of tea tree (*Melaleuca alternifolia*) essential oil sublingually for her every day for her toenail fungus. He had put the bottle of tea tree oil near her body and used the science of body circuitry (aka "muscle testing") to determine that she needed 60 drops of the oil. But he did not know that essential oils should not be given orally without extensive knowledge of the oil and that the dose he intuited through muscle testing was very high. He did not factor into his decision that the oil of that plant is very cooling energetically and his client was thin and cold with a recent history of breast cancer, which is typically a cold condition of the breast. While the science of body circuitry can be a sound method of determining general effects of herbs on energy flows in and around the body, it is not safe to simply use muscle testing to determine which herbs should be applied in client care. It is a clear example of negative psychism. Fortunately, this client's

---

5   Phoebe Bendit and Laurence Bendit, *Our Psychic Sense: A Clairvoyant and a Psychiatrist Explain How It Works* (London: Quest Books, 1958), 109.

6   A plant's volatile oil. Essential oil is a processed herbal product, not whole herb.

common sense was still intact and she sought an herbalist's opinion about the oral use of the drops for her toenail fungus. It was her senses of taste and smell that also brought her to the clinic as the idea of taking 60 drops of tea tree oil sublingually made her nauseous. We worked together and came up with a solution that addressed her health patterns, including the resolution of the dampness represented in the toenail fungus. She actually did decide to use the tea tree oil for awhile but she used it topically.

Herbal Experiment: Opening the Channels with Cinnamon and Mint

Cinnamon Decoction
Purchase 5 small or 2 large cinnamon sticks (the bark of *Cinnamomum spp.*). Wash them thoroughly and place in small pot. Cover with spring or distilled water. Raise water to the boil and take off stove. Cover with lid and allow to sit for 4 hours as the herb expands. After expansion period, check water level and add enough water so that the level is about 2 cm above the herbs. Decoct (gentle boil) the herb for 45 minutes at a temperature where the steam just rises from the water – not a rolling boil. The water level should be about ⅓ of the original level after the cooking. Strain the decoction and discard or compost the herb. Sip the tea at room temperature. Cinnamon opens and warms the energy channels in the body. Record your experience of cinnamon decoction – body, mind, emotion, spirit.

Mint Infusion
Harvest or purchase fresh or dried mint leaf (*Mentha piperita*). Chop the fresh leaf or gently crush the dried leaf prior to infusing in boiled water. Put 1-2 teaspoons of fresh or 1 teaspoon of dried herb in a tea pot or tea ball. Pour one cup of boiled water over the herb. (Put the herb in the cup first and splash with the water rather than put the water in the cup first and try to submerge the leaf.) Strain and sip. Peppermint is energetically cold and opens and cools the channels of the head. Record your experience of the mint infusion.

It is not uncommon for a sensitive nurse to intuit a particular plant's benefit for a client. But this chapter provides the structure for the training and organizing of the mental body experience that is included in the holistic, integrative model for nurse-herbalism. Plants are such simple "folk." They are part of our daily lives and therefore it often seems silly to some to think that they should be studied. If we lived in the nineteenth century, I would agree. Peoples in all cultures have had intimate and powerful knowledge of their healing plants; but, nurses and other practitioners today do not necessarily grow up in rural areas where plants grow abundantly. Nurses do not have the connections with medicinal plants of their predecessors. Nor are they educated by their grandparents, parents, community healing elders, or nursing programs about healing plants. Nurses must have educational and mental preparation to partner with plants. And for those who have had the delight of being educated in the plant world, this chapter— as well as subsequent chapters—offers not only that preparation, but acts as a guide in leading you in the integration of nursing science and plant knowledge.

EDUCATIONAL PREPARATION FOR NURSE-HERBALISM

In professional nursing culture today, many call for evidence or the results of the clinical study of healing plants much as they would for the pharmaceutical drugs administered in nursing care. Because so many healing plants have been used by humans as food and medicine and are so prevalent in our culture, few want to spend the billions of dollars necessary to validate the actions of a medicinal plant that may have been used safely and effectively for centuries. Although there are clinical trials for any number of plants, educational preparation for nurse-herbalists also focuses on the traditional evidence for the safe and effective application of the herb and any laboratory studies on the plant constituents that may broaden the knowledge base of the nurse's understanding of herbs.

The focus of the education and research that is most helpful for nurse-herbalists is that which has a strong focus on the application of herbs in the comfort and care of an individual or family with an illness as opposed to the herbal applications in eradication of disease. The focus of care, as in nursing, is on the health pattern. Disease-focused care is the domain of physicians. While nurses and advanced-practice nurses can learn from the research and experience of herbs applied in the eradication of disease, a focus on the study of this must include the translation or decoding of that data into healing plant and nursing frameworks. Other botanical data that is helpful in nursing practice is the evidence for the healing traditions surrounding the application of the herb in various cultures with differing health beliefs and practices. There are herbal education programs that complement nursing practice quite well, such as TCM.

The focus of nurse-herbalist education and study is also to help the client find a greater sense of personal wellness through self-care and nursing care. Nursing practice includes an integration of the biomedical, traditional, and holistic nursing perspectives of plant applications in health care. All three paradigms allow the nurse-herbalist to "walk between the worlds" of science and tradition, producing holistic, synergistic plant therapy solutions to include in individualized plans of care. The three perspectives are a foundation for care that is pluralistic and diplomatic. Integrative care, as discussed in Chapter 2, is a diplomatic approach that uses knowledge and wisdom from different perspectives when helping clients make health care choices. The study of healing plants should parallel nursing's focus on the healing relationship as the platform for clear assessment and diagnosis of health patterns related to the actual and potential responses to disease and interventions for care and comfort that address those responses. When the focus is clear, the practice of nurse-herbalism is strongly differentiated from the use of herbs in medical practice and traditional practices of herbalism.

This book *The Nurse-Herbalist: Integrative Insights for Holistic Practice* as well as the curricula for my courses on nurse-herbalism and the Herbal Diplomat™ are based on nursing science, art, and practice. They are also rooted in nursing history in which the emphasis of nature care and herbalism for centuries has been the application of herbal teas (includes liquid alcohol extracts), syrups, and topical applications in patient care.

The syrups, teas, and topical applications such as compresses, poultices, plasters, and baths that are traditional nursing remedies may be applied in care as simples[7] or formulations. My choice to continue the nursing heritage of "teas and topicals" was not a nostalgic one. My research shows that nurses have been experts in these specific applications that are still appropriate today in any health care setting. There are also spiritual and legal reasons for staying close to a documented heritage of practice as will be discussed in more detail in Chapter 6. In essence, teas, syrups, and topicals are our professional strength. There are hundreds of nursing remedies in these categories that have centuries of traditional evidence of safe and effective application.

Nurses may learn about certain herbs or herbal supplements in their nursing programs, but this is not the study of *nurse-herbalism* per se. Nurse-herbalism courses should include nursing history, nursing applications as described above, and nursing science. Nurse-herbalism is translational science by definition. Nurses draw from the research of plant scientists, physicians, nurses, ethnographers, and ethnobotanists, to name a few, to gather knowledge of the plants that they choose to partner with in practice. Then the challenge begins! How can that data be "decoded" in such a fashion as to be applicable in the holistic care and comfort of clients? Decoding or translating science is not an easy task. It is only more recently that the National Institutes of Health has stressed the importance of translational science in health care research. I, like many herbalists, have for decades translated or applied the data from varied herbal research at the bedside of clients. When I was the director of the Herb Research Foundation's National Healthcare Hotline service in the late 1990s, I was positioned well to be able to glean snippets of research here and there that could be readily integrated into nursing care. I listened and looked specifically for research that supported the traditional herbalism I had learned from Oma and others as well as the intuitions I had experienced growing, harvesting, processing, and applying hundreds of medicinal plants in my practice as a nurse-herbalist and director of Herb Programs and gardens for a health center in the early 1990s.

---

7   "Simples" is a common term used in herbalism to describe an application with one plant. Examples of a simple are a cup of chamomile tea, a chamomile steam for the sinuses, an onion poultice, or a coffee footbath. See a Nurse's Herbal in Appendix A for details about these applications.

Given our nursing heritage, it is not surprising to me that I was able to readily build a momentum in study and application of herbs in nursing practice that is completely independent of the work of physicians, naturopaths, or other prescribers and practitioners. That momentum begins and ends with knowledge of nursing science, art, and the boundaries or scope of practice, which will be discussed further in Chapter 6. Over the years I have found pockets of nurse-herbalist development around the globe. Schools in Germany that are affiliated with state-of-the-art Anthroposophical hospitals offer their nursing students herbal education as part of a six-month certificate program on healing from the Anthroposophical perspective. At the hospitals I visited, the students grew the herbs in the gardens at the hospitals as well as learned to apply them in hospital care. For a number of years in Australia, Dr. Pauline McCabe had national funding supporting an educational program for nurses to receive dual baccalaureate degrees in nursing and naturopathy in which they studied herbal medicine.[8] In China, some nurses learn herbalism from the perspective of TCM. They may even administer intravenous herbal remedies in hospitals. In all of these programs, nurses work under the auspices of the physician; however, there are nurses and midwives around the globe who continue to explore herbal care options that fall solidly within the scope of nursing care. Herbal remedies are a natural addition to nursing education, which historically has included the fundamental modalities of touch, nutrition, communication, energy, and environmental interaction as ways of demonstrating care.[9]

Decoding Herbal Data

A background in nursing research, which includes an understanding of qualitative, quantitative, and blended methodologies, is helpful in the practice of nurse-herbalism. The nurse-herbalist must be able to discuss their practice and the gentle remedies they apply in terms of scientific study because so much of the culture requires that ability. I have had many instances when my abilities and knowledge were challenged

---

8   Pauline McCabe, "Naturopathy, Nightingale, and Nature Cure: A Convergence of Interests," *Complementary Therapies in Nursing & Midwifery* 6, no. 1 (2000).

9   Martha Libster, *Demonstrating Care: The Art of Integrative Nursing* (Albany, N.Y: Delmar Thomson Learning, 2001).

by nurses, physicians, administrators, and the public based upon the demand for evidence.

A nurse-herbalist does not need to have a research degree or experience to be able to decode scientific data, but in the current nursing climate and the state of herbalism, I recommend that nurse-herbalists have at minimum an undergraduate course in research. Bachelor of Science in Nursing-level courses in research address national standards of preparing graduates for research *utilization*. The language of research and how to find and apply published studies is typically the focus of the course. Course assignments often allow students to focus on their own clinical topics of interest related to their practice areas. This means that you could take a course in which you could actually learn to apply all research utilization concepts to herb research. When I teach research, I often use herb research publications for students' practice sessions and assignments. Here is the citation for one of the articles I have used to illustrate some of the concepts involved in decoding herbal scientific data:

Berthold, H., Sudhop, T., & von Bergmann, K. (1998). Effect of a garlic oil preparation on serum lipoproteins and cholesterol metabolism. JAMA, 279(23): 1900-1902.

This is the study that I will use later in this chapter to illustrate my steps for decoding data. (See Page 174).

There are a number of reasons that the nurse-herbalist should decode the data for him/herself or for clients as opposed to relying on others, particularly those in the media. Data are often used in advertising and by journalists in their media reports, but they may not be reported accurately or completely, leading to misunderstanding. In addition, the reports often reflect the values of the dominant biomedical culture and what types of data about healing plants are important within that culture. When a nurse-herbalist understands the basic research process for different methods from epidemiological studies to clinical trials to historical research, they are better equipped to contribute to the public discourse about plants using an integrative model. Providing traditional and nursing evidence of herbs as well as biomedical data can lead to a more complete understanding of plants and their healing applications. It is also a more accurate report of the character and characteristics of the plant that promotes and models healthy consumerism.

Responsible reporting and writing about medicinal plants should include the plant perspective. First, a review of the literature should include the botanical literature such as is published in journals on botany, ethnobotany, phytopharmacy, and folklore. International publications should not be excluded because herbs are researched by scientists all over the globe. This is particularly important if the plant in question is not indigenous to the investigator's or author's country of origin! Botanical databases such as NAPRALERT and HERBCLIPS (American Botanical Council) should be accessed. Book publications should be included in a literature review as plants are often most fully represented by those who have done extensive research and then published on a single plant.

Second, the data reported should include evidence of a plant perspective. The scientific name of a plant, genus and species, should accompany all common names. Scientific credibility is immediately questionable when research is conducted or reported without clarity as to the exact plant used in the study. Whole plant should be distinguished from plant constituents and the specific applications should be clearly identified. Third, bias should be controlled. The investigators and authors should respect cultural tradition and ritual. Slurring of healing traditions, plants, or peoples that use them is not permissible in other scientific endeavors and no exception should be made in the case of healing plants. Instead, it is customary to call for further research rather than seek to debunk herbs or herbalism. Gross generalizations or overstating the significance of data should be avoided.

In my experience, journalists in particular often inflate the significance of data, such as that which is gathered through simple surveys, one of the least rigorous forms of research. Journalists often discuss the "lack" of clinical trial evidence but neglect to discuss other forms of data available on healing plants. They report only from the standpoint of the biomedical culture and focus on the clinical trial method as the "gold standard." It is the gold standard of pharmaceutical research but does not always lend itself to answering the questions associated with herbal applications, particularly traditional and holistic nurse-herbalist applications. Clinical trials are not necessarily appropriate for illuminating the questions of herbal science. WHO, for example, recognizes records of historical and traditional use as relevant and important data for the safe and effective application of herbs in human health.

In Chapter 2, I outlined the three paradigms of health and healing that support the integrative process: biomedical, traditional, and holistic nursing. Those views also color the ways in which research or study of medicinal plants is or is not conducted and also how the findings of that study are interpreted and utilized in the health care arena. Typically, herb research that is conducted by those with biomedical values strives for the most rigorous clinical trial with the intent to establish causation and predict outcomes or determine the plant's mechanism of action for a specific effect in humans. Herbs are referred to as "products," "drugs," and "constituents" or "constituent groups." Scientists with biomedical and traditional values may study herbs using ethnographic, historic, or folkloric methods. In the traditional paradigm, herbs may or may not be studied at all. When they are studied from a traditional perspective, herbs are usually examined as whole plants or whole plant parts such as roots or flowers rather than plant constituents such as phytosterols or antioxidants.

The views of holistic nurse-herbalists are informed by both biomedical and traditional ways of knowing as well as how the plant has been applied historically in nursing care and comfort. Because the herbs that have been used by nurses are often common, it is rare that time and resources are applied to study them. In industrialized nations, research is often performed to increase knowledge and marketability of a particular product as a means to reimbursing the cost of research to further scientific knowledge. In the discipline of nursing, ingenuity and entrepreneurial insight are needed to be able to fund scientific study of nurse-herbalism that may or may not include a product that is the return on investment. There are possibilities of creating holistic studies in nurse-herbalism that improve quality of care—a measurement that can be tied to economic outcomes for a health care organization. Some examples of the questions that can propel that research are included in this book.

To review: This is a list of sample questions about herbs from a biomedical view.

- What makes this plant work?

- Are there any clinical trials on the use of this plant drug?

- How safe is this herbal drug for human consumption?

- How efficacious is this herbal drug in *curing* specific disease?

- What is the proper dose?

- What are the active ingredients/constituents in the crude herb drug and can they be synthesized and standardized? (Protect plant populations)

The nurse-herbalist reframes the questions to be more plant-focused:

- What type of research questions need to be asked about plant therapies and nursing care, and what methodologies will best answer these questions?

- How is safe use determined in the use of plant medicines?

- Do plants "cure disease" or do they act in other ways?

- How are the plants used, how long have they been used by people and practitioners, and is dosing possible?

- What are the healing properties, characteristics, and personality of the plant?

The plant-focused scientific perspective is often lacking in the research literature. There are any number of examples in which scientists, scholars, and public officials have rendered opinions on herbs publically without any plant knowledge whatsoever. They may base their opinions on the results of a single event or research study. Some people simply do not realize that they have no knowledge of the actual plant and that this impairs their perspective. One of the most important roles of the nurse-herbalist is as an advocate for plants and ensuring that science and publications include a plant perspective. As Associate Editor for Botanicals for the *Journal of Holistic Nursing,* I have had many opportunities to raise the level of plant awareness and knowledge among members, readers, authors, and potential authors. In 2008, I was invited to write a review and commentary on an article, a literature review and analysis of "St. John's Wort" (*Hypericum perforatum*) in the treatment of depression. I gave a plant perspective on the study and analysis.[10] The article was inspired by my feeling of dismay that nurses would consider a review of the biomedical literature on a plant's constituents sufficient for submission to a "holistic" journal. I was also saddened that nurses would use a simple literature review to render such a general conclusion that St. John's Wort not be used.

Let me be clear at this point that I am not an *advocate* for the use of St. John's Wort in depression. Nor am I the advocate for any herb. Whether an herb is applied or not rests squarely with the assessment and diagnosis of the health patterns of the unique client. I am an Herbal Diplomat™ who does want to ensure that healing plants are at least represented at the "table" of any discussion about them, particularly if that discussion is going to contradict centuries of traditional evidence for safe and effective partnership in human health. Nurse-herbalists facilitate that diplomatic process and dialog, often by asking questions from the plant rather than the human perspective. The following are examples of questions that can help decode any herbal scientific data:

1. Be sure to note the exact herb and/or the herbal preparation used in the study. Is the genus/species of plant reported? Did the study focus on plant constituents or the whole plant? Whole-plant studies are rare. Is the plant preparation described in detail?

    a. Berthold et al. Garlic Oil Study – The herbal preparation is a central issue for the decoding of this study. Garlic *oil* has not been known for its effect on cholesterol levels because steam-distilled garlic oil may not contain one of the active compounds, allicin, known to affect cholesterol metabolism unless it was prepared fresh each time it was used.[11]

---

10 Martha Libster, "Commentary and Plant Perspective on 'Hypericum and Nurses: A Comprehensive Literature Review on the Efficacy of St. John's Wort in the Treatment of Depression,' " *Journal of Holistic Nursing* 26, no. 3 (2008).

11 http://cms.herbalgram.org/press/061898press.html

2. Does the published study identify the type of study such as *in vitro* or *in vivo* – animal/human? *In vitro* studies are conducted in the laboratory. Herbal remedies from living plants are not typically applied in the laboratory environment.

3. Who are the subjects involved? Human? Animal? Cells? This is also important. The ways in which the bodies of animals metabolize herbs is not the same as in humans. For example, birds eat raw elderberries (*Sambucus nigra*) right from the tree. Raw elderberry is toxic to humans. I always cook my berries into a syrup for use during cold and flu season.

4. What are the data results and the limitations of those results? Every study itself has pros and cons in terms of its design and implementation. These are referred to as "limitations of the study." One example is whether or not the data from the one study can be "generalized" or applied to a larger group. There are certain parameters of scientific research that must be met for a study to be generalized. This is not so easy to establish and yet the media often report studies on herbs and other health-related issues as if the data can be generalized to the general public.

5. Questions to ask:
    b. What data or evidence are the investigators basing their advice / concerns / recommendations upon?
    c. What is their knowledge and experience with this herb either in their own care or in client care?
    d. What are the benefits and risks of trying or not trying an herbal solution?

In general, herbal data are only data. They may have no relevance to the care and comfort of the one client for whom a nurse is caring. Yet, data have the potential to help or harm the practice of the nurse-herbalist especially when data that are shared or communicated person to person or through the media take on the energy of public health policy. The most common example of concern is when data from a single study or event surrounding a particular plant are utilized to ban the use of a plant in health and healing. One such example is in the case of ephedra (*Ephedra sinensis*) in the United States, a plant that in formulation has been used safely for hundreds of years in Asia. The purpose of the scientific process in herbalism is to mindfully explore questions we have about the plant world and generate new knowledge. The meaning of data lies in the minds and hands of the people who use it. Responsible decoding and reporting of herbal data is an important responsibility of nurse-herbalists who are often in position to assess the knowledge level of the public who come to them for herbal care.

ANCHOR OF ASSESSMENT – THE PRESENCE OF PLANTS

The anchor of the nursing scientific process is assessment. Proper holistic assessment is the focus of much of nursing education and care. Nurses are educated to understand the importance of conducting a full assessment prior to creating a plan of care so that the plan solves the problems unique to the client. Nurses learn all types of methods of assessment that ensure a systematic scientific approach to problem solving. There are head-to-toe and systems assessments and methods associated with particular nursing theories such as the Roy Model of Assessment. Each nurse has his or her own preferred method of assessment. I have included the basic outline of my assessment in Appendix B. Since 1991, I have used an integrated East – West assessment strategy. I was taught the Roy Adaptation Model of nursing for three years while in nursing school from 1984-1987. The four modes lend to thorough, holistic assessment of the self in relation to others and the environment.

From 1992-1993, I studied Traditional Chinese Herbal Medicine (TCM without the acupuncture focus). The basis for Chinese herbal science is the principle that to promote health and longevity one must understand the fundamental principles of change in the universe. TCM herbal science is much like nursing in that health is viewed as a product of our inherent constitution, our interaction with the environment, and our ability to adapt to change. The methodology applied in TCM to assist a person to adapt to change is called heteropathy in which hot problems are cooled, cold problems are warmed, deficiencies are tonified, and excesses are dispersed or drained. In addition to the detailed history and visual and auditory assessments made in nursing (Roy Adaptation), the TCM practitioner determines the energetic nature of the person's constitution, called the "symptom-sign pattern," through tongue and pulse diagnosis. (See Appendix B) Neither of these assessment models diagnoses the cause of a problem or tries to eliminate a symptom as is the purview of the practice of medicine. The Roy Adaptation Model teaches that the goal of nursing assessment and intervention is to assist a person to adapt to change and restore balance. The goal of TCM is the same.

What is more important than the particular form of holistic assessment is that the nurse-herbalist start the assessment with a solution-focused, plant-based orientation. After centering, there are two parts of the assessment process that should be added to any regular assessment method. They are assessing the client's real concern and the presence of plants in the life of the client. The assessment of the client's real concern answers the question "Why now?" This is a technique common to solution-focused counseling that will be discussed further in the next chapter. Solution-orientation immediately begins to differentiate the model of care from medicine, which is problem based. Why has the client come to you, a nurse-herbalist, at this moment in their life? If you have never assessed this question, try it. Nurses are often surprised at how much they learn about their client and the purpose of the healing relationship from the answer to such a simple question.

Indications of the real problem, often not expressed during initial communications about an appointment, come up in the history of how the client found their way to you. This point of connection that the client identifies is, in my experience, the best starting point for assessment. Although it is always good to have a list of issues to cover in the assessment, the nurse-herbalist's list or method of head-to-toe is not efficient or necessary. Nurse-herbalists move more quickly into deep levels of assessment of health patterns when they follow the client's lead. I liken the experience to unraveling a skein of yarn that has gotten tangled up. To unravel the yarn, one has to start with a tangle that is ready to be sorted out. Using a mental script about how to approach the untangling of a skein of yarn and being "systematic" does not work. There is no how-to guide. But there are principles of sorting out problems, one of which is to follow the client's lead.

Clients have answered the "Why now?" question in many different ways. Some have started to weep and express relief at finding a different kind of care for an illness; some have family reasons for seeking a nurse-herbalist. Some say they love herbal remedies and some are seeking a cure for disease. These are just a few examples. It is in the detail of the story that you can assess many things quite easily about the primary concerns as well as any reservations the client has. Nurse-herbalists can work only with people who are actually their clients. If a person is not really interested in what you can provide them as a nurse, they will go elsewhere. It is important in the beginning to assess "why now?" as this will most often give you the opportunity to clarify what you do and do not offer as a nurse-herbalist. For example, the client will learn in the beginning dialog that nurse-herbalists work with health patterns though they are interested in and understand diseases that the client has been discussing with another practitioner. The client becomes clear with initial assessment that the care they are about to receive is nursing, not medical or some other form of care.

Secondly, it is important to assess what the client's relationship with the plant world is like. Rather than asking specific questions, ask a broad open-ended question such as, "What plants do you like?" They may tell you that they have a garden or that they are vegetarian. People often mention plants as a matter of course and do not consciously identify the plants in their history as their medicine. I often take the opportunity to reflect back to the client any plant they mention in conversation. I also note in my assessment what plants they talk about, encounter in their lives, interact with or dream about.

It is sometimes amazing how disconnected people have become from the plant world. I remember one time when I had been teaching herbal remedy making at a high school senior's health class for a few weeks and one of the students brought a vegetable snack with a dip to class. I noticed the change and said, "Oh, I see you have changed to plant snacks." Her response was, "No, it's just broccoli." I quietly told her that broccoli was in fact a plant. She smiled. The plants are everywhere and often taken for granted. Adding a plant focus to nursing assessment serves to raise each client's awareness about the presence of plants in their lives.

Many people apply plants in their self-care practices. They may bring their herbal remedies with them to their appointment. That makes it easier to identify what plant or plants they are partnering with. It is important when discussing plant remedies with clients that nurse-herbalists consider the following plant-focused questions when using a consumer, herbalist, or integrative model of care:

1. **Are we talking about the same plant?**
   Be very careful to be sure that you and the client are clearly discussing the same plant. Have the client bring in the plant material or the packaging of a plant product. Do not give information about the herb or herbal remedy without clarifying the genus and species of a plant.

2. **What is the traditional, biomedical, and nursing evidence?**
   Be knowledgeable of the traditional, biomedical, and nursing evidence that exists regarding the herbal remedy the client is considering. Assess the paradigm of the client. As clients speak about the herbs they are using, they will discuss their knowledge of the plants from one or more of these paradigms. People historically value different ways of knowing about plants and like having practitioners who talk about herbs from more than one paradigm.

3. **Listen to the history—What is the story of why the client is using the plant medicine or therapy?**
   Often clients have important reasons for taking a particular herbal remedy. Demonstrate genuine interest and welcome the client's reasons and thoughts. Do not correct the client. Listening to the client's story and the way they make a health decision during an assessment can provide many clues about how to guide the client in their healing process.

4. **How long has the client been using the plant remedy?**
   In general, most herbs can be safely taken as self-care measures for common everyday concerns for less than thirty days.

5. **What is the plant's history of use for the way the client is taking it?**

   Does the client have any experience in using the herb? Is the client treating their disease (biomedicine) with herbal remedies? What is known about the method or application of the herb for the way the client is intending to use it? For example, clients may be planning to ingest herbs in capsules that are not meant to be eaten and have historically been decocted or extracted. Being knowledgeable about historical applications can help the nurse provide the client with options as to how the herb might be taken.

6. **How is the client partnering with the plant? Simple or Formula?**

   It is important to determine how the client is partnering with the herb. Are they having an occasional cup of beverage tea or taking a standardized extract? How a client discusses this information can demonstrate their level of understanding of herbalism. Many people in Western countries have no knowledge of herbs that they see in the supermarket or pharmacy and may believe that the only way to take herbs is in pill or capsule form. I have had clients say to me, "Is it OK to just use fresh garlic or ginger that is in the store?"

7. **Does this client want information about biomedical evidence?**

   Nurses often have close relationships with their clients. Building rapport is not always easy. When a client shares that they are using a plant remedy from a traditional approach, describing the biomedical data about the plant may or may not be appropriate. Information giving on any topic necessitates an assessment of client readiness to listen and learn. It also means that the nurse needs to be sensitive to cultural and paradigm differences. I have seen clients withdraw immediately from caregivers who respond to their use of herbs in a manner that the client could interpret as being condescending or disrespectful. For example, questions such as, "What proof is there that the herbs work?" or saying, "There may be some drug interactions with those herbs so you better check with your doctor before taking them," are not helpful, especially since few physicians are herbalists. People know that biomedical practitioners do not routinely have knowledge of herbal remedies, so referring them to their biomedical practitioner may be an inappropriate next step. Instead nurses can best help clients by providing helpful questions that the client can use in self-monitoring and self-care. Nurses can make statements such as, "I'm not aware of any research on that herb but I'd be happy to get some information," or, "That herb has not been thoroughly evaluated by biomedical standards," rather than, "That herb is ineffective." Think of ways to demonstrate support for the client, regardless of what you may think or believe about herbs.

Whether a nurse approves or disapproves of herbal remedies, the ethical approach is to find a way to support the client. This is true for any client scenario. Nurse-herbalists follow the client lead and respect client choice as they provide information, education, and nursing care. It is sometimes a delicate balance. Preserving the nurse-client relationship should be a factor in the decision as to whether or not the nurse intervenes in self-care activities.

8. **Does taking this herb help the client and make them happy?**
   Assessing the relationship the client has with their choice of modality in self-care is critical to maintaining the healing relationship. Does the client have a relationship with the herb they are using for healing and does taking that herb make them happy? Clients' choices must be respected. Even if a client is experiencing a placebo effect from the herbs they are taking, it may not be worth discussing if the client then thinks that the nurse is implying that their remedy is really worthless and their choice is somehow insubstantial.

   Self-care with herbs makes people happy. Some people like to make their own medicines and remedies. People trust the herbal remedies that have been used by their families for generations. People like to smell and taste the herbs. They like being given a cup of tea to sip when stressed or rubbed with an aromatic oil when being massaged. Herbs make people happy, an emotion so often lacking in a troubled world. Happiness and comfort are part of the healing. Memory of a simpler, less technical world is comforting to many, especially those in the West. Herbal therapies often remind people of simpler times when there was a strong connection with the earth.

Talking about plant remedies with clients over a cup of tea and some plant-based snacks is a great way to assess the client's connection with the plant world. It is also an opportunity to start the process of a more conscious connection with the green world. I typically introduce liquid chlorophyll to the client in the first session. I may offer them a few drops in water at the beginning of the assessment intake session or at the end. I also recommend that clients take liquid chlorophyll in their water while they are working with me. I call this "talking plant." The chlorophyll connection was described in Chapter 3. Preparing a chlorophyll drink is the way I encourage the client's body to start talking plant. They make the water whatever shade of green is pleasing to them. Dose is determined by desire in this case. Increasing numbers of drops of chlorophyll liquid turns water black. Because I state that the color must be green, people stay within, typically below, manufacturer recommendations. For the past five years, I have been recommending a liquid chlorophyll product derived from stinging nettle (*Urtica doica*) rather than alfalfa (*Medicago sativa*). Nettle is a plant that I work with to assist transition and change a common phenomenon encountered in life and the focus of nursing care.

Referral Beyond Self-Care

Practitioners of herbal medicine, such as nurse-herbalists, physician-herbalists, doctors of Oriental medicine, naturopathic physicians, and clinical herbalists, have extensive education and experience in individualizing herbal therapy for clients. If a person using herbs in self-care has a concern, the most prudent action is for them to work with an experienced herbalist. In general, a person should self-refer or be referred to a herbal practitioner when they are considering taking the herb for the treatment of a health concern or taking any particular herb for more than thirty days (perhaps less, depending upon the individual), the client is taking medicinal amounts of herbs (more than beverage teas) and is pregnant, elderly, or is an infant less than 15 months old and/or the client is taking pharmaceutical drugs and herbal remedies simultaneously to treat a specific biomedical condition. The herbalist community often refers to others in the community especially when an herbalist has a particular area of expertise. Nurse-herbalists can join their local and national communities in responsible referral by declining to see a client whose needs, identified through thorough assessment and observations, do not fit within the nursing scope of practice or the arena of the nurse-herbalist's expertise.

Referral to a nurse-herbalist or another herbal practitioner is similar to the referral process used in sending a client to any type of specialist. During the assessment, the nurse-herbalist can identify an appropriate practitioner to refer a client to if the nurse-herbalist did not feel comfortable providing care for the client for any reason. My experience in referral was different early on after setting up my first nurse-herbalist practice than it is today. I have provided a lot of education over the years about nurse-herbalism and I have honed my explanation of my services and approach in such a way that people don't seek me out for biomedical care anymore. Clients who contact me may, in fact, have biomedical conditions such as cancer, depression, or infertility but they typically come to me for complementary holistic herbal care. The guideline to follow when referring to others involves four questions:

1. What is the herbal practitioner's education and experience?
2. Do they have a specific model for practice that they follow, such as TCM?
3. Is the practitioner certified from a formal education program or does the practitioner hold a national certification, if available? Educational programs require a greater level of commitment to study and therefore may demonstrate potential expertise as well as commitment to knowing the state of the science.

4. Does the herbal practitioner belong to any professional organizations and demonstrate a professional demeanor to which you would expose your clients?

5. Does the practitioner to whom you are thinking about referral communicate well and will s/he talk with you?

When clients seek care from a knowledgeable herbal practitioner, they often do not know what care to expect. The common frame of reference for care is that of the biomedical culture, which, as was said earlier, is disease focused. During the assessment phase of the nursing process, the nurse-herbalist involves the client in new ways of approaching care. Although, nurse-herbalists still take pulses and check blood pressures and tongues, the assessment is a dialog facilitated by plants. Adults and children alike have told me that it is "fun" to participate in this type of health care assessment. The fun continues into the diagnosis phase, when the nurse-herbalist synthesizes the patterns into a comprehensive picture of the client's state of health and well-being.

DIAGNOSIS: INTEGRATING THEORY AND PRACTICE

The nurse-herbalist diagnosis is a descriptive summary and synthesis of impressions and observations about the unique health patterns of the client or family. In my practice, I use nursing and TCM theories and diagnoses to "frame" and describe the client's symptom-sign patterns. Like medicine, diagnosis in nurse-herbalism is simply a way of organizing observations from the assessment. Unlike medicine, diagnosis in nurse-herbalism is descriptive of behaviors and energy patterns. The diagnosis emerges when the symptom-sign pattern is clear. In the intuitive state I "see" the client's patterns initially with clouds or fog. But after I have listened mindfully to the client's descriptions and perceptions of problems, observed them, assessed their pulse and tongue, and accessed the knowledge and experience stored in my mental body, the diagnosis becomes clear just like a pure lake on a beautiful sunny day. It is best to make diagnostic conclusions when one has real clarity about the pattern. All diagnoses are "working" diagnoses until the clouds over the lake clear.

All of the activities of the nurse-herbalist during the centering and assessment phases help clear the clouds and fog. It sometimes takes a few visits before the health patterns are completely clear to me. I have found that diagnosis cannot be forced. Patterns emerge. The timing of that emergence depends upon the relationship and level of understanding and communication between the client and the nurse-herbalist. Solutions to identified problems also emerge in their own time. Solutions, as will be discussed in the next chapter on intervention, are the health activities that will bring balance and harmony to the present pattern. They may start to be revealed during the diagnosis phase or even before. As the nurse-herbalist develops skill and experience in recognizing patterns, the time for the assessment phase shortens. Some patterns, or parts of patterns, can be recognized when the client walks into the space.

For example, nurses can often recognize the pattern associated with the nursing diagnosis of "sleep pattern disturbance" when they see a client for the first time. They may have an altered gait, speech changes, and their eyes may look tired. Nurses know some potential interventions for creating balance in that pattern; however, the interventions are determined by the unique expression of the particular client's behaviors related to sleep pattern disturbance because there are many types of patterns and combinations of patterns associated with sleep pattern disturbance. This is the same for all nursing diagnoses. After using the nursing diagnosis system for years, I realized that it was not quite adequate in providing the framework for organizing the behaviors I was seeing in my clients. This is when and why I turned to TCM. TCM pattern recognition system is thousands of years old. It provides a complete language that serves as a frame for the energetic themes that are the foundation of symptom-sign patterns observed in clients.

TCM Language

There is an entire science related to health pattern recognition known as Traditional Chinese Medicine that I encourage nurses to study. For the purposes of this book on nurse-herbalism, I focus solely on the 8 Principle Patterns, a foundational part of the theory of this ancient system of knowing about and describing (diagnosing) health patterns. The 8 Principle Patterns alone can help inform the nurse-herbalist's deep intuitive understanding of the energetic patterns associated with health and illness. The four groups of terms that represent the 8 Patterns are heat/cold, excess/deficiency, interior/exterior, yin/yang. I was taught that the distinction between heat and cold would be the most challenging to assess correctly. After more than twenty years of applying this theory in practice assessment, I affirm the truth of the teaching that the thermal nature of the client is most important and often the most difficult to diagnose accurately.

The four groups within the 8 Patterns describe the client's general energetic qualities; however, no one group is sufficient to provide a holistic representation or diagnosis of the client's pattern. In TCM, the qualities are grouped together, such as in the diagnosis of "Interior Heat Deficiency" (Called Yin Deficiency). The purpose is to then assign interventions, such as the preparing of a formulation of the most appropriate herbs that will specifically move the pattern toward greater balance. For example, if someone has heat in the head, the nurse-herbalist might suggest peppermint (*Mentha piperita*) tea, an herb that is energetically cold and experienced in the head area.

The terms heat and cold do not refer to actual body temperature. They represent the opposite ends of an energetic continuum—perceptions of heat and cold—with neutral (neither hot nor cold) in the center. Like all symptoms, everyone experiences heat and cold and points in between. It is when a quality, particularly an extreme quality such as heat or cold, is consistently present that imbalance exists and the quality can be inferred. One of the best indicators of heat/cold pattern is the tongue. A normal tongue, such as that of a healthy school-age child, is typically pink with a white coating. That coating is neither too thick nor too thin or spotty. Cold pattern includes:

1. Person feels cold or dislikes cold.
2. Person prefers to drink warm or hot drinks.
3. Urine is light in color and stools are loose.
4. Application of heat relieves discomfort.

5. Movements and speech are often slow.
6. Person acts withdrawn.
7. Pulse is slow.
8. Tongue tissue is pale and the coating white.

A normal tongue coating is white. Therefore, that symptom alone is not sufficient for diagnosing cold. A number of symptoms must be present for coming to a decision that the pattern is "cold" but not all on the list must be present. It is also possible for a person to have symptoms of both heat and cold at the same time. For example: a person my feel hot in the head and cold in their feet. They may walk slowly but talk fast—a symptom of heat. Heat pattern includes:

1. Person feels hot and dislikes heat.
2. Person is thirsty and prefers cold drinks.
3. Urine is dark in color and they may be constipated.
4. Cold applications reduce pain.
5. Movement and speech are rapid.
6. Person is outgoing.
7. Pulse is rapid.
8. Tongue tissue is red and the coating yellow.

Excess and deficiency, like heat and cold, are points on a continuum and can exist simultaneously in one person. The thickness of the tongue coating is one of the most important symptoms differentiating excess and deficiency. Excess pattern includes:

1. Uses energy forcefully.
2. Person's breathing is heavy.
3. Pressure and touch aggravate pain.
4. Movements are forceful and speech is loud.
5. Person is outgoing and sometimes aggressive.
6. Pulse is strong.
7. Tongue coating is thick.

Deficiency pattern includes:

1. Person is fatigued and perspires easily.
2. Person's breathing is shallow and they may be short of breath.
3. Pressure and touch help relieve pain.
4. Person's movement is weak and speech is quiet.
5. Person is often passive.
6. Pulse is weak.
7. Tongue coating is very thin.

The terms "exterior" and "interior" refer to the relative depth or superficiality of an illness in relation to the entirety of the symptom-sign pattern rather than to the physical expression in the body. Interior, for example, is not a literal term referring to the center of the anatomy, and exterior does not exactly refer to the skin. Exterior pattern includes:

1. Sudden onset of acute illness; chills and a low fever.
2. Sinus congestion and discharge.
3. Dull pain in the head and muscles.
4. Pulse is floating (a specific profile in which the pulse is felt more strongly at the surface of the skin and diminishes with increasing pressure).
5. Tongue typically has a normal tongue coating and tissue.

Interior pattern includes:

1. Chronic illness; acute illness that has become more severe.
2. Sensations of excessive cold or heat; high fever.
3. Abnormal changes in breathing not related to exercise.
4. Abnormal urination and bowel symptoms.
5. Pain in the trunk of the body.
6. Changes in speech and behavior.
7. Abnormal pulse.
8. Any abnormality in tongue tissue or coating.

Yin and yang are central concepts to Chinese philosophy. They are relative concepts that are explained in relationship rather than absolutes. In TCM, yin is the ability of the body to calm and cool itself and yang is the ability of the body to heat and energize itself.

The 8 Principle Patterns are, in so many ways, the most helpful theory in organizing observations, and identifying and naming patterns common to human health and illness. Clear energetic pattern recognition leads to proper herb choice or herb formulation and, in my experience, simplification of interventions. For example, one client with a medical diagnosis of uterine fibroids had persistent pelvic pain made worse with palpation (excess-interior). Her tongue coating was thick in the back of the tongue, suggesting excess, specifically "dampness," in her lower abdomen or "burner" as it is called in TCM. The purple hue of her tongue tissue and menstrual history suggested "blood stagnation" also in the lower burner, which would result in accumulated dampness.

When I asked her about her diet, she mentioned that she ate a sweet potato every day. The young woman was basically healthy, very active, and very health conscious. Sweet potatoes would not seem to many in the biomedical field to be a risky food. But from a TCM symptom-sign pattern perspective, the food was clearly a concern for this woman.[12] Think about sweet potatoes for a moment. They are orange (warm color as opposed to blue or green), sweet, and a bit gooey (damp). They may not be as damp as a block of cheese or a scoop of ice cream (more cold), but they are damp all the same. Part of the pattern diagnosis for this client was "Blood and dampness stagnation" in the "lower burner" potentially aggravated by daily ingestion of sweet potato. The potato had not "caused" the dampness, but it was a part of her daily lifestyle that was clearly supporting and aggravating rather than moving and draining the dampness. I suggested that the client do an experiment and abstain from sweet potato for one week and monitor her pain levels. Her pain diminished exponentially within a few days. In this case, simple abstention from a food rather than herbal intervention or formulation was all that was necessary for creating greater balance and harmony in her pattern. After the clearing of the effects of the sweet potato, which was aggravating the damp heat, I gave her an herbal formula that she took for a few weeks, after which she achieved a full-term pregnancy.

---

12   For additional study of TCM diet therapy, a foundational subject for the study of TCM herbalism, I recommend Bob Flaws, *The Tao of Healthy Eating : Dietary Wisdom According to Traditional Chinese Medicine*, 1st ed. (Boulder, CO: Blue Poppy Press, 1998).

During the assessment and diagnosis phase, it is good to have clients experiment with herbs and foods that they know. The sweet potato abstention experiment told me a lot about my client with pelvic pain. I learned not only that my assessment of pattern was most likely accurate but that the client's belief that plants/herbs would help her was correct. She responded to a simple diet change involving a plant food. These first experiments and the time spent in assessment are critical to accurate and efficient recognition of symptom-sign patterns.

In addition to TCM and the Roy Adaptation Model discussed previously, there are three additional nursing theories that are particularly helpful in supporting the nurse-herbalist's development of the ability to recognize symptom-sign patterns in their clients. These theories are Erickson, Tomlin, and Swain's *Modeling and Role Modeling*, Peplau's *Interpersonal Relations Theory*, and Margaret Newman's *Health as Expanding Consciousness*. All three theories warrant significant consideration and study; but, for purposes of this chapter, I will include only a simple summary about how I have applied the theories to nurse-herbalist practice. Applying nursing theories in practice can often "awaken" awareness and strengthen the nursing process, particularly assessment and diagnosis.

Modeling and Role Modeling

One of the most important contributions of the Modeling and Role Modeling theory to the nursing process is the suggestion that the nurse not "predetermine the sequence, quantity, and categories of data"[13] collected from the client. Instead, the theorists suggest that the nursing process is an "interactive, interpersonal process that nurtures and supports the person's self-care."[14] The client's concerns rather than the nurse's identified problem list are the primary focus of the theory. As discussed in previous chapters, it is important in nurse-herbalism that the client's relationship with plants be the primary focus of the assessment. Modeling and Role Modeling are skills that support the choice to be fully client-centered while attempting to solve tough problems *with* the

---

13 Helen Erickson, Evelyn Tomlin, and Mary Ann Swain, *Modeling and Role Modeling* (Englewood Cliffs, NJ: Prentice-Hall, 1983), 114.
14 Ibid., 112.

client through recognition of their unique symptom-sign patterns.

The concept of modeling refers in the theory to the nurse's process of developing an image and understanding of the client's perspective of their environment. Using communication skills, the nurse enters or "models" the client's world that is rich with thoughts, beliefs, and perspectives that are not the nurse's own. They may be quite foreign to the nurse. Assessment and diagnosis as modeling provide a framework for the nurse that in my experience nurtures a mental platform of receptivity to unique health patterns. Together with the energetics of TCM and the integrative approach and preparation through "entering the earth element," the nurse-herbalist can collect "data" from clients in the true spirit of partnership between persons and plants.

Communication that occurs during a therapeutic relationship that is modeled after the client's world is very different in terms of intention. Intention is subtle yet very important to the process of assessment and pattern recognition because intentions are quickly translated through the body of the communicator into non-verbal and verbal expression. Congruence between intention and expression is not a given. For example, I have often talked with people who say the word "yes" but their head may actually be shaking "no." Centering often helps the nurse-herbalist to become more aware, if not congruent, in verbal and non-verbal communication so that the client receives a clear message.

Active listening is a concept often discussed in nursing. Though common, it is not an easy task if one is committed to modeling the client's world. There are three aspects to the client's communication that I suggest nurse-herbalists pay attention to when creating the model of their client's world. First, listen for the *exact words* used by the client. Try not to edit their story and make the language fit your model. Second, listen for the *emotions* or *feelings* supporting the words that are said. The emotions will be stated or demonstrated in observable behaviors. Again, do not dismiss or edit the feelings that you observe. Because feelings are often expressed non-verbally, it is natural for the nurse-herbalist to experience some of what the client is feeling. That is called empathy. But while you stay true to the purpose of modeling the client's world, you also must maintain your own worldview, which includes the purpose of assessing for health patterns in that moment. If a client expresses emotion and you join them so fully in their world as to lose sense of your own world on your "side of the fence," you alter the relationship for which they have sought your care. The ability to demonstrate empathy while retaining professional purpose is an important skill. Setting intention sets in motion the skill training necessary for being able to integrate the client's emotions into the model of their world that is a part of the larger health pattern. Third, assess the *essence* of what the client is communicating to you about their world. Research has shown that appreciation expressed from the heart supports the ability to perceive the essence of someone else's communication.[15] Try expressing appreciation during your communication with an herb client and the channels of communication open. Try expressing appreciation toward a plant and watch the communication open too!

I learned the importance of plant to human appreciation when I was studying for my master's degree in psychiatric nursing. My teachers had me doing a lot of work, at one point monitoring my own self-talk—that is the thought dialog that goes on in the mind. I had an African violet plant in my living room and every time I walked by it I caught myself thinking "why don't you ever bloom?" The tone of my thought was really critical toward that little plant. So I stopped and apologized. You see, I have been told that I have always talked with plants since I was a small child. But I had never examined my thought communications with them. I went to my library and pulled out a book on the science of plant communication that I had read years back called *The Secret Life of Plants*.[16] It was clear that I had been ignorant, if not cruel, in my communication with my African violet. I decided to make amends and demonstrate how much I really appreciate that African violets continue to fill me with great joy on a daily basis whether or not they flower. I decided to buy some presents for my plants. For the African violet, I bought a set of silk African violet flowers. I put the silk flowers among the leaves of the plant and, do you know, that plant started flowering within one week of receiving its present! The plants taught me a wonderful lesson in communication and the ability to *model* the plant world as well as the human world.

Once the channels in the relationship are open, the ability to

---

15 See the research and publications of scientists at the Institute of Heartmath. http://www. heartmath.org/

16 Peter Tompkins and Christopher Bird, *The Secret Life of Plants* (New York: Harper & Row, 1973).

understand meaning in the client's world is much more accessible. I find that the *essence* or underlying meaning of whatever people communicate often can be summarized as, "Can you help me?" Because of this, I typically ask any assessment questions beginning with the words "how" or "what." I rarely, if ever, ask a client "why?" For example, I might ask "What is your concern about that?" or "How do you feel about that?" instead of "Why do you say that? or "Why do you feel that way?" "How" and "what" questions seem to convey a nurse's active listening skill and helpful attitude rather than "why" questions do. I think that "why" questions may be perceived as confrontational. There is one "why" question that I typically ask myself and sometimes verbalize to the client and that is the question "why now?" as discussed above.

The concept of role-modeling is applied in the theory in a different way than in its vernacular use. The theorists describe role-modeling as the "essence of nurturance" and the "basis for the predictive and prescriptive component of nursing practice."[17] Role-modeling requires unconditional acceptance of the person and their perspective. Role-modeling is applied in interventions that occur within the client's own model and at their own pace. Role-modeling will be discussed further in Chapter 5 on planning, interventions, and solutions. Modeling occurs as the nurse accepts and understands the client as the unique person that they are and role-modeling begins when the nurse moves from assessment and diagnosis to planning and intervention phases of the nursing process.

Interpersonal Relations Theory

Erickson, Tomlin, and Swain relate the modeling and role-modeling process to Peplau's Interpersonal Relations Theory. Nurse-scientist Dr. Hildegard Peplau (1909-1999) developed her theory in the 1950s. Published as *Interpersonal Relations in Nursing*,[18] her theory was one of the most significant works of twentieth-century psychiatric nursing. The work emphasized the nurse-client relationship as *the* foundation for practice. In the book, Peplau defined all nursing— not just psychiatric

---

17 Erickson, Tomlin, and Swain, *Modeling and Role Modeling*: 95.
18 Hildegard Peplau, *Interpersonal Relations in Nursing: A Conceptual Frame of Reference for Psychodynamic Nursing* (New York: G.P. Putnam's Sons, 1952).

nursing—as a "significant, therapeutic process." She held two guiding assumptions for her Theory of Interpersonal Relations: "The kind of person each nurse becomes makes a substantial difference in what each patient will learn as he is nursed throughout his experience with illness" and "Fostering personality development in the direction of maturity is a function in nursing and nursing education; it requires the use of principles and methods that permit and guide the process of grappling with everyday interpersonal problems or difficulties." In other words, nurses engage in relationships to solve problems within the context of that unique relationship. The holistic nurse-herbalist's foundation for offering creative solutions to problems is the understanding that emerges from the healing relationship. The nurse-herbalist client cannot be separated from the historical context of their relationships with past experiences, the environment, plants, others, and the nurse-herbalist. Assessment, which is strongly rooted in context, is an expression of mindful action.

Mindfulness, Reframing, and Non-Judgment

Erickson, Tomlin, and Swain's and Dr. Peplau's writings on the healing relationship inspire an approach to care that is highly non-judgmental and therefore preparatory to the Herbal Diplomacy™ work, which will be described later. There is one other communication skill that the nurse-herbalist can use to actively demonstrate a non-judgmental approach to modeling the client's world. That technique is known as reframing. The nurse-herbalist can assist the client in reframing their perceptions of events, others, plants, self, and anything. Reframing is exactly as the term suggests. The nurse-herbalist consciously places a different frame or context around a client's belief, thought, or experience. For example, I often *reframe* how my clients and my colleagues view herbalism. As I talk with people, it becomes very clear that when I mention that I am a nurse-herbalist, they often draw upon a definition of herbalism that for them means work with the herbal supplements found in grocery stores and pharmacies. Through dialog and modeling their world, I come to realize that they often think that my role is to prescribe herbal pills and capsules for diseases much the way they have experienced in a doctor's office with physicians and pharmaceutical prescriptions and over-the-counter drugs. That model of care is the dominant model and therefore is not surprisingly the "default" understanding of herbalism by much of the public.

Reframing, however, can assist in changing expectations and habits. By discussing what I do in partnering with plants and people to create wellness solutions, the public and my colleagues go through the process of reframing their premature cognitive commitments—mental habits. Social psychologist Ellen Langer writes, "Changing of contexts generates imagination and creativity as well as new energy. When applied to problem solving, it is often referred to as reframing."[19] Reframing generates innovation and creates the space for non-judgment and pattern recognition. It is also an antidote to breaking down habits of unconscious momentums of mindlessness that do not support the goal of providing holistic care.

Langer defines the nature of mindlessness as "automatic behavior" and "acting from a single perspective."[20] She differentiates the Eastern concept of mindfulness meditation from her work on mindfulness as the opposite of mindlessness. She writes that in Eastern mindfulness meditation, a person is encouraged to quiet the mind whereas in the mindfulness work that she describes in her book, the mind is actively engaged. The nurse-herbalist who applies the theories of Modeling and Role-Modeling and Interpersonal Relations in establishing healing relationships with clients with an openness of mind toward learning about who that person is and is not practices mindfully. S/he becomes comfortable with the uncertainty of working with people and plants. Nurse-herbalism is a field for mindful exploration of the nuances of nature science.

Health as Expanding Consciousness

The third nursing theory that I apply in the practice of nursing and nurse-herbalism is Dr. Margaret Newman's *Health as Expanding Consciousness*. Newman states that clients are our "partners in revealing the evolving pattern."[21] She is absolutely correct. In the ancient healing traditions such as Tibetan, Unani, and Chinese medicine, it is well known and taught that the cause and cure are at some level known to that person

---

19   Ellen Langer, *Mindfulness* (Reading, MA: Perseus Books, 1989), 138.
20   Ibid., 10.
21   Margaret Newman, *Health as Expanding Consciousness* (New York: National League for Nursing Press, 1994), 85.

experiencing the symptoms of illness. The role of the healer is to assist in the client's exploration of the cause and health patterns that are their teachers. Newman's theory, like the theory of her predecessor Martha Rogers, represents a distinct paradigm for *nursing* as science. Nursing science is pattern recognition. The person's pattern unfolds like a delicate flower before our very senses if we are open to the revelation and also ask the question that "solicits from individuals what was most meaningful in their lives."[22] As Newman states emphatically, "meaning is pattern."[23] This question is an important one to be sure to ask of your clients as it adds a depth of dimension to the understanding of the pattern that does not seem to be elicited by a simple analysis of physical and emotional symptoms.

I also ask this question in a way that relates to plants. "What plants are meaningful to you?" Or I might ask if they mention a particular plant, "What meaning does that plant have for you?" Making meaning is also an antidote to mindlessness. As we assess and diagnose—that is, create a picture of the health patterns of clients—we often mindfully reframe their understanding of self as well as health concerns that they bring to us for resolution. Clients often remark that the nurse-herbalist's mindful, thoughtful, intuitive approach to assessment and diagnosis is, in itself, healing for them. Throughout the reframing process and recognition of patterns of self, they become acutely aware and mindful of their own self-imposed barriers to health, healing, and longevity. Many experience the sparks of freedom that loose them from the bondage of disease for the first time as they prepare to move toward herbal solutions.

---

22 Ibid.
23 Ibid.

AIR – INTEGRATIVE INSIGHT –
BREAKTHROUGH BREATH & INSPIRATION

Breath can lead to breakthrough. That is a simple insight I received not as an herbalist or a nurse, but as a dancer. By breakthrough, I mean moving beyond the mental trappings that would have us believe a certain notion as true. The insight came when I was dancing with Sachiyo Ito's dance company in the 1980s. We performed national treasure dances of Japan that involved the intricate use of a fan. I was in rehearsal on a beautiful sunny day in a studio in New York City. Sachiyo modeled the dance and then showed me the hand movement that would make the fan swirl in a beautiful pattern in the air. But I could not get it.

Sachiyo taught by movement not by words. This is common in the art of dance. That was not the problem because I had been dancing since I was 7 years old and learning through watching a pattern was and is my preferred style of learning. The problem was not that I was an American trying to perform Japanese dances. Sachiyo had told me that she picked me for her inaugural company even though I was European-American because of what she had seen in my movement style when we took a class at New York University together. Evidently I had a natural movement pattern that communicated the essence of Japanese dance. But on that day in rehearsal, it was not working. The problem was just me.

I tried and tried but could not mentally force my fan to move correctly. So I stopped and walked over to the window. I just stood in the sun for a while and this voice like the wind said "breathe!" So I did and the fan magically carved through the air as if I had known how to do it all along. It was a breakthrough moment in my dance life. The insight I had from inspiration was profound. I realized that I am not really in control and that surrendering to the element of air—breath—just as I had been taught since childhood classes in Denishawn Ballet, was a key to understanding and embodying a movement pattern. I have always remembered that experience. Later when I entered private practice, I would sometimes experience the anxiety of ambiguity at not knowing if I would be able to help people find solutions to their problems. But I know that the pattern always becomes clearer when I remember to breathe. So I do, regularly. And when my client needs a breakthrough, clarity, or inspiration, I remind them to breathe too.

REFERENCES

Bendit, Phoebe and Laurence Bendit. *Our Psychic Sense: A Clairvoyant and a Psychiatrist Explain How It Works*. London: Quest Books, 1958.

Erickson, Helen, Evelyn Tomlin, and Mary Ann Swain. *Modeling and Role Modeling*. Englewood Cliffs, NJ: Prentice-Hall, 1983.

Flaws, Bob. *The Tao of Healthy Eating : Dietary Wisdom According to Traditional Chinese Medicine*. 1st ed. Boulder, CO: Blue Poppy Press, 1998.

Goethe, Johann Wolfgang and Jeremy Naydler. *Goethe on Science*. Edinburgh: Floris Books, 1996.

Langer, Ellen. *Mindfulness*. Reading, MA: Perseus Books, 1989.

Libster, Martha. "Commentary and Plant Perspective on 'Hypericum and Nurses: A Comprehensive Literature Review on the Efficacy of St. John's Wort in the Treatment of Depression.' " *Journal of Holistic Nursing* 26, no. 3 (2008): 208-11.

———. *Demonstrating Care: The Art of Integrative Nursing*. Albany, N.Y: Delmar Thomson Learning, 2001.

McCabe, Pauline. "Naturopathy, Nightingale, and Nature Cure: A Convergence of Interests." *Complementary Therapies in Nursing & Midwifery* 6, no. 1 (2000): 4-8.

Newman, Margaret. *Health as Expanding Consciousness*. New York: National League for Nursing Press, 1994.

Peplau, Hildegard. *Interpersonal Relations in Nursing: A Conceptual Frame of Reference for Psychodynamic Nursing*. New York: G.P. Putnam's Sons, 1952.

Steiner, Rudolf. *Intuitive Thinking as a Spiritual Path*. Dornach, Switzerland: Anthroposophic Press, 1995.

Tompkins, Peter and Christopher Bird. *The Secret Life of Plants*. New York: Harper & Row, 1973.

the Water Element

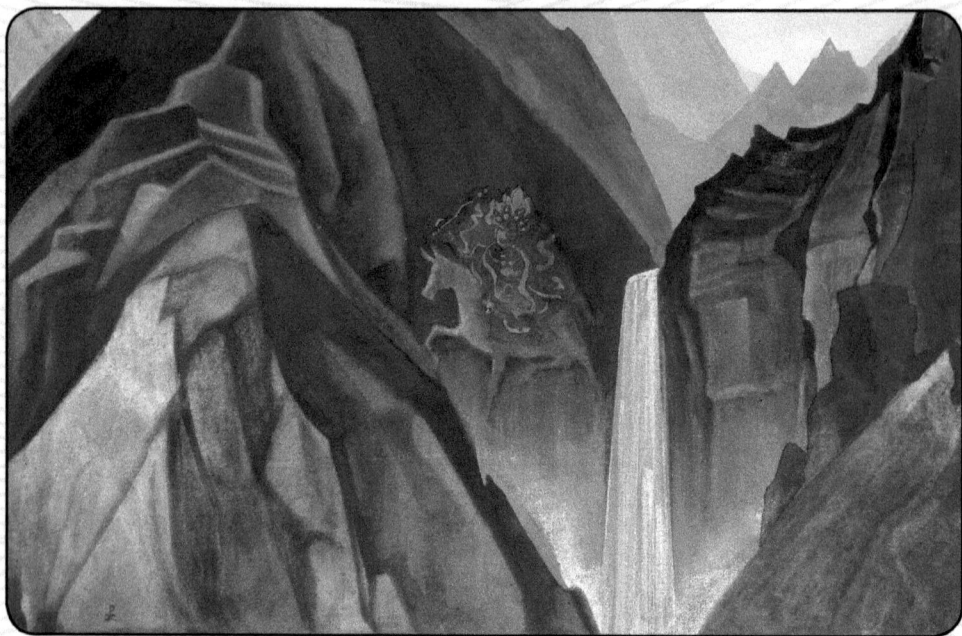

Palden Lhamo
Nicholas Roerich, 1931

CHAPTER FIVE

Welcoming the Water Element

To seek solutions to health problems is a common part of the human experience. That is why people contact a community healer. But a request for help never means that the person does not have a solution or multiple solutions of their own. People often try many remedies prior to approaching another for assistance and insight. People "self-medicate" with many types of interventions, substances, techniques, and activities. They may not even realize that they are self-medicating with certain behavioral choices. One example of a common choice is drinking coffee (*Coffea arabica*) to boost energy and mental clarity.

The most prevalent philosophy and historical pattern related to sorting out health problems that seems to undergird health care choices from self-care to biomedical invention is the *belief* that there is one cause and one cure for any health problem. This notion of one cause, one cure dates at least back to eighteenth-century Europe. The dominant biomedical system and the culture that surrounds it reinforce this belief. However, holistic assessment and diagnosis reveal that there is typically more than one health pattern underlying disease, discomfort, and illness. There are often multiple possibilities and solutions that will help and heal, create change, or restore balance related to a person's health patterns.

Nature holds answers to questions of human health. The body, like plants and all parts of nature, is made of matter—the five elements of Self. To study nature is to study Self. To study Self is to study nature.

Throughout this reciprocal quest, there is an abiding natural beauty deposited by the Creator. The ancient Greeks knew this. They built the Parthenon as a reflection of the architecture of the human body with its curves, *symmetria*, and seeming imperfections. Symmetria, as the harmonious relationship of one part of the body to another, was, for the Greeks, the definition of beauty. Their medicine, remedies, and solutions to discomfort in the body beautiful were drawn from the elements of Self—ether, fire, air, earth, and water.

Water is itself a solution to many health problems. It flows through the human body as it does Mother Earth. Without the flow of pure clean water, there is no life. Studies by scientists such as Viktor Schauberger demonstrate that the purity of water depends on its ability to *flow*. By modeling rhythm and flow in nature, specifically of the spiraling action of moving water, Schauberger[1] created ways of coursing water so that impurities could be removed and the water revitalized. Water and flow are also important in nurse-herbalism.

Seeking herbal solutions is nothing new. There is "nothing new under the sun." For centuries, nurses have made and administered water extracts of plants in many forms. Many of the solutions that make up the nurse-herbalist's materia medica are remedies that involve the use of water. The hot water bottle is one of my favorite caring solutions. Hot water bottles provide gentle, even-flowing heat because water is in perpetual motion. From a traditional perspective, pain in the body is often related to cold. Hot water bottles gently and deeply warm the body even when the client does not necessarily feel the pain as "cold." Typical cold areas include the back near the kidneys, joints, and the abdomen. When I was a school nurse, I had a policy that young children with tummy aches were to hold a hot water bottle to their abdomen while they lay down on their side. I would also offer them their choice of teddy bears to help hold the water bottle too. They always felt better within a few minutes. What magic in the hot water bottle...and the bear!

Nurses have also administered cups of herbal teas as a matter of course, formulated herbal broths for the hungry, and applied herbs to the body as baths, compresses, and other topical remedies in the care and

---

1   Olof Alexandersson, *Living Water: Viktor Schauberger and the Secrets of Natural Energy* (Bath, UK: Gateway Books, 1997).

comfort of clients young to elderly. Herbalism is a full body of science and a healing art that produces many health care solutions for the public. These solutions are time-honored remedies that hold potential for promoting greater health in individuals, families, communities, and nations. Nurse-herbalists offer access to a fountain of flowing plant- and water-based solutions. In herbalism, people can find multiple solutions to their health concerns just as water flowing downstream gathers soil from the banks of many lands.

Solutions in nurse-herbalism continue to grow and evolve. Gardens change with every new growing season. Likewise, the herbs with which nurses partner and the ways in which herbal solutions are applied in nurse-herbalism change over time. This chapter covers some of the most enduring of healing traditions in nursing—herbal medicine making—and how to create a plan of care that welcomes the water as nature care solutions that include achievable, client-centered goals and the creative means for implementing the plan. This chapter includes instruction in preparing time-honored nurse-herbalist solutions, many of which include the application of the water element: the creation of herbal teas, liquid extracts, soups, and juices and the application of topical herbal remedies, such as baths, foot baths, steams, and compresses.

The water element is traditionally associated with the emotional self. Nurse-herbalists recognize the importance of the feelings of clients and plants, and demonstrate a respect for the role of feelings in building meaningful healing relationships and partnerships between the worlds that are the platform for nature care. This chapter also includes counseling techniques that complement the nurse-herbalist, solution-focused assessment model. Planning, setting, and implementing goals as nurse-herbalist intervention are the focus of this chapter. The frame for this chapter is role-modeling as defined by Erickson, Tomlin, and Swain in their nursing theory, Modeling and Role-Modeling.

In the previous chapter, we discussed the concept of modeling as it related to assessment and diagnosis. We entered the clients' world to better understand them, their beliefs, thoughts, and desires. While modeling may be an ongoing process, role-modeling begins after the nurse-herbalist has *modeled* the client's world and synthesized understanding of that world as a diagnosis or health pattern. Role-modeling is the "facilitation of the individual in attaining, maintaining, or promoting health through purposeful interventions. These interventions are planned based on the data analyses."[2] While role-modeling throughout the planning and intervention phase of the nursing process, the nurse-herbalist is nurturing and promoting the client's strengths and solutions.

GOALS

One of the best platforms for identifying and promoting client strengths from which the most appropriate solutions can be created is the goal-setting process. During the discussion of the client's goals, the nurse-herbalist may experience a "check and balance" of how well s/he has actually modeled the client's world. If the nurse's and client's ideas about goals are really different, the nurse may not have fully completed the modeling yet. I also have found that the biomedical culture often creates certain expectations of health care providers that are unrealistic. When clients seek the services of a nurse-herbalist, they often still have many habits and thoughts related to health care in the biomedical culture that they project into the relationship with the nurse-herbalist. Managing client expectations is the responsibility of the nurse-herbalist during the planning phase. Managing expectations is one of the most important parts of the healing process not just for the client's well-being but for the well-being of the nurse-herbalist as well.

I have taught solution-focused counseling tips to nurses and herbalists for many years and experienced their relief in learning skills that can remove the burden of expectation placed upon them from the client. A certain level of expectation is natural given that they are paying for help with creating a plan of care with meaningful solutions. But some expectations of the nurse-herbalist and the solutions created with the client place the client at emotional risk and the nurse-herbalist and their practice at professional risk. One example is working with couples experiencing desire for conceiving a child. In the biomedical world, the couple is diagnosed as "infertile." I have worked with many

---

2   Helen Erickson, Evelyn Tomlin, and Mary Ann Swain, *Modeling and Role Modeling* (Englewood Cliffs, NJ: Prentice-Hall, 1983), 95.

couples diagnosed with infertility. After spending time getting to know them and their concerns, modeling their world and assessing health patterns, we move to the planning phase of the consultation. A typical response when I ask them to tell me about their long-term goal is, "We want to have a baby." Because neither the couple nor I have any ability to assure the attainment of that goal, I simply redirect and reframe it toward more specific concerns related to achieving pregnancy. Often, typical of parallel process, the goal of the herbal consultation work becomes managing the couple's own expectations about achieving pregnancy and learning to live with the process of working on conception in such a way as to make life bearable. Many of my "infertile" couples have come from the biomedical world where they describe the treatment of their health concern as unnatural (constant technological monitoring), pressured, stressful, depressing (failures from intercourse or technological attempts at creating conception), and expensive.

Often the nurse-herbalist needs to negotiate reasonable, solution-focused goals that reverse the patterns of negativity and problem-orientation and reframe the health concern or challenge as the life lesson to be learned. I often reframe the health problem or disease as the person's and my "Teacher"—that which will lead us to solutions if we observe carefully. I have witnessed that the knowledge of the problem as "Teacher" gives many clients great peace and comfort because the student and the teacher always talk. When the problem is simply a teacher rather than a death sentence or a failure of the body, the client realizes that there is then room for negotiation and the possibility for even small increments of change to occur.

Negotiating Planned Change

Those who provide health care are change agents as discussed in Chapter 1. During the planning phase, the nurse-herbalist negotiates the pacing and timing of the changes s/he and the client envision so that they both come to agreement about the focus of care and the outcomes the client expects to see in certain time increments. Herbs are catalysts for change but the changes related to herbal intervention are most often more subtle than what the nurse or client would know from their experience in the biomedical world with its powerful pharmaceutical and therapeutic interventions. A surgery is a powerful and immediate change in the body. Drinking a cup of herbal tea or engaging in an herbal steam does not have the same impact or power on the body. Herbal solutions are more subtle. Their effects are often powerful in terms of the client's patterns but the immediate felt experience is not. Therefore, nurse-herbalists must have a memory of the bodily experience of each of the herbal solutions they recommend to clients so that they can guide the client in application and, ultimately, evaluation of the effects of the herbal intervention. Based on their understanding of how plants "work" in general and certain herbs behave in particular, nurse-herbalists also negotiate the pacing and timing of the planned change with their clients.

As in any nursing plan of care, the nurse-herbalist should create with the client short- and long-term goals that are measurable and client-centered. Goals that are client-centered are those that the client verbalizes as important to solving their problem and promoting health and well-being. The nurse-herbalist needs only to provide the structure for creating measurable goals. Other than that, whatever the client requests is utilized in the plan. I start the goal-setting process with a solution-focused technique.

Solution-focused counseling is a form of Brief Therapy. The Brief Therapy Model, which started in the 1950s, states that problems are maintained by a person's attempted solutions. The goal of Brief Therapy and solution-focused counseling is to break up the escalating cycle of the attempted solution that has not moved a person toward solutions. Usually people and their caregivers, especially in the biomedical world, ask the common question, "What is the cause of the problem?" and "Can I/we fix it?" These questions are focused on the past rather than the now. Problems often continue because they serve a purpose in the person's life. Reframing the problem with the intention of working toward solutions inspires hope as the cycle of habit is interrupted and redirected as the movement pattern of an upward spiral or helix rather than the downward spiral of the water flow in a toilet bowl.

Solution-focused approaches support integrative nurse-herbalist practice. The simple process of working toward solutions diminishes the disease-orientation of the biomedical culture and therefore significantly reduces the risk of the nurse-herbalist slipping into a mode of practicing *medicine* with herbal interventions. To start the solution-focused process, ask the client the goal-oriented question, "How will we know that we have achieved what you want?" I also suggest a timeline that is typically three to six months. I ask, "What will you be doing differently or how will you be feeling differently in three months if we are successful in our plan?" Visualizing themselves as successful at solving their problems helps them imagine the positive outcome. We work backward from that vision of success, setting detailed short- and long-term goals that will end in their realization of their vision of success. Going through this process gently calls to mind in the client what they are doing or thinking that maintains the problem.

Occasionally the client has a hard time imagining a positive outcome. When this occurs, ask them what they are doing in the present time that is "working" and then create goals that encourage them to do more of what is working. There are some counseling tips discussed later in this chapter that are helpful in identifying and encouraging what works. If the client is not able to identify anything as "working," such as they experience their pain "all the time," then simply identify some different solution as an "experiment" to shift the energy from focusing on the problem toward beginning the process of creating solutions and envisioning wellness. Solution-focused counseling is part of a wellness strategy that is fully embraced in the behavioral health system and in public health arenas. It is an important intervention used in consulting with those in chronic pain, those dealing with chronic illness, and those seeking lifestyle changes and greater well-being and balance.

A solution-focused plan of care identifies and organizes goals that promote the client's strengths and ideas for solutions. Clients are often completely unaware of their own strengths. The nurse-herbalist becomes the reflecting pool of calm water that shows the client how they are in the world. Reflecting strengths with a client needs to be done carefully from within the client's model because for some, strengths are not always perceived as safe. The nurse-herbalist links the client's strengths to their health patterns. So in the example of one of the infertile couples with whom I worked, I reframed the biomedical experience with the clients this way: "You both clearly have great love already for the 'child' you wish in your hearts to create. ...You have set aside your lives for years to follow medical advice and are already 'parents' in the spiritual sense of the word." Their strength was their loving commitment to having a baby. We worked with that commitment and they decided to channel it into community action while working with herbs, counseling, and other healing modalities to prepare their bodies for conception. That couple conceived after six months of care.

Timing, Type, and Tuning

In 2003, I published an article on integrative care and the "3 T's of timing, type, and tuning".[3] I did not know about solution-focused care or Modeling and Role-Modeling at that time. I had been working in integrative care and as a nurse-herbalist for many years and simply gave my own language to the process of client-centered care. The three T's can be used to complement other skills and strategies for setting goals and documenting a plan of care.

Timing, knowing when to intervene or not, is one of the most important aspects to the *art* of nursing care. Again, it is the client's health patterns that really provide the answers as to when an herbal remedy should be applied. Knowledge of the plant's constituents and characteristics also drive the decisions about timing of interventions. Oftentimes I recommend that simples (single herbs) be taken at night before bed. In general, herbs should be taken at a time when their benefit or risk can be easily observed. I will often say, depending upon the herb or herbs, that the clients drink their tea thirty minutes before breakfast or one to two hours after supper. If a person is taking a pharmaceutical drug for short-term use, I have them wait to take herbs until the drug is finished. If the person is taking the drug every day and there is no plan for them to go off the drug, I do some research about the drug and its mechanism of action. I also study the potential interactions with each herb I am using in medicinal amounts so that I can make an informed decision as to whether or not I will recommend herbs for the client.

The *type* of herbs given is critical to the success of the achievement

---

3   Martha Libster, "Integrative Care--Product and Process: Considering the Three T's of Timing, Type and Tuning," *Complementary Therapies in Nursing and Midwifery.* 9, no. 1 (2003).

of the goals recorded in the care plan. Health patterns drive the selection of general categories of herbs based on their energetic qualities, but sometimes there may be a number of plants that my knowledge tells me would be correct for the client. It is in these moments that I allow my intuitive understanding of the plant to line up with the client's story and observe which herb fits the unique client profile best. Herbs are always chosen in context. I have also chosen *not* to give herbs on many occasions. I may give a foot reflexology treatment first and wait one week and reassess the tongue, pulses, and health patterns before starting herbs. Most often, I give Bach flowers for a few weeks at least and counsel the client to clear the pattern before giving herbs or a formula.

Lastly, *tuning* the herbs is important. This means that the nurse-herbalist determines how much herb to give and how often. In general, I do not give the same formula or herbal simple for more than thirty days. This was the parameter I gave for self-care but I, too, have found that if I give the right herb at the right time I rarely have to give any one remedy in the care plan for an extended period of time. This is one more reason why herbalism is not the practice of medicine. Physicians and nurse-prescribers often give a prescription to a person without any thought to how long that client might be taking the medicine. Typically, the answer is that the client takes the medicine "for the rest of their life." I know of no client who would knowingly agree to that. This is especially true of children and teens. They have an episode of epilepsy and are given a medication, and they and their parents are quickly looking for a way to go off the medication. It is common sense to weigh the benefits and risks of medications and find that long-term use of drugs is a major risk to health.

Deciding what the right herbs are for a person, what the right time is to give them, and what the right amount would be in that particular moment in time requires patient assessment of health patterns and study of the plant and biomedical literature. It is best for the nurse-herbalist to wait to give any herb medicinally (that is not as a culinary herb or food) until they have a clear picture of the health patterns and enough understanding of the herb to make the proper decisions for matching plants with people. While going through the process of clarifying the pattern(s), the nurse-herbalist can provide interventions for the client that help prepare the client's body to receive the herbs. Reading the cues for herbal readiness is sometimes a challenge.

CUES FOR HERBAL ACCESS

In my experience, adults who seek the care of a nurse-herbalist have health habits and patterns, thoughts and beliefs about their bodies and possible solutions to change and healing that are more often entrenched. Infants' and children's patterns are typically easier to identify because they have purer lifestyles and have not been introduced to the environmental factors, such as recreational drug use, consumption of alcohol and tobacco, sexual activity, and life stressors, that can significantly alter health patterns and create imbalances. Over the years, I have found that spending more time clarifying patterns while offering simple herbal and counseling interventions often leads to more effective care. My working hypothesis is that the nurse-herbalist uses simple herbal remedies as a way of *cueing* the body to remember its relationship with healing plants. It is not clear if the relationship is energetic, cellular, or genetic or all three. I have had conversations with and read the writings of plant scientists, such as Jim Duke, and biologists, such as Rupert Sheldrake, that still leave me wondering.[4] But my observations are shared by other herbal teachers. The body does not always need more herbs or formulations to initiate healing. Often a simple will do. Taking time, applying theory to practice, and getting the understanding of the patterns right is important.

There are two phenomena within the science and tradition of herbalism that I have explored as influential in the development of initial rapport with clients, introduction of their bodies to herbal remedies, and clarification of health patterns. I call the two phenomena "accessing cells" and "accessing dreams." Accessing cells is a concept that is discussed in the science on human consciousness. Physicist Fritjof Capra defines consciousness as "a special kind of cognitive process that emerges when cognition reaches a certain level of complexity" that he

---

4   Rupert Sheldrake, *The Presence of the Past: Morphic Resonance and the Habits of Nature* (Rochester, VT: Park Street Press, 1995).

likens to an "ever-changing stream."[5] Every cell is living and conscious. Current science focuses tremendously on DNA, yet dead cells also contain DNA. In working with life energy in plants and humans in relationship, we focus on the consciousness. Capra suggests that in seeking to understand life, we also describe cell metabolic processes or the patterns of relationships between the macromolecules in the cell.[6] The cell is viewed as whole. The cell membrane, like human skin, is the boundary that distinguishes self from other in the environment. The cell membrane is essential for distinguishing cellular life because cells exist in water or fluid environments. Without a membrane, they would be absorbed into the fluid environment. Membranes, unlike cell walls, are flexible and are always active, opening and closing all the time. The membrane sometimes lets substances into the cell and, at other times, keeps things out. "At the cellular level, the cell membrane regulates molecular compositions and, in so doing, maintains cellular identity."[7] It is the cell membrane that scientists have identified as providing the boundary for the action of metabolism—chemical and energy flow.

Cell membranes seem to *know* when to open and when to close. Cell consciousness adds a fourth dimension to the timing, type, and tuning of nurse-herbalists' plans and interventions. It is a common observation that a plant can affect seemingly opposing types of change in the body. For example: Some people who take ginseng *(Panax ginseng)* experience an increase in blood pressure, while others experience a decrease, depending on *their need*. I do not use this plant in practice because it is generally too warming, but when I was the Natural Health Care Hotline director at the Herb Research Foundation, my staff and I recorded calls about herbs like ginseng regularly. This effect noticed in ginseng and other plants is an adaptogen action in the body.

American herbalist Dr. John Christopher called herbs that work with the body's ability to adapt by opening and closing to herbal effects, "thinking herbs." He specifically wrote about the ability of lobelia *(Lobelia inflata)* to "think" during threatened miscarriage: "Where the baby is strong, the lobelia seems to have the knowledge to assist in healing a

---

5   Fritjof Capra, *The Hidden Connections: A Science for Sustainable Living* (New York: Random House, 2002), 38.
6   Ibid., 7.
7   Ibid., 9.

tearing and bleeding condition and stopping the bleeding. But if the baby is dead and should be aborted, the lobelia has the intelligence of directing the spontaneous abortion."[8] Dr. James Duke theorizes that, "All herbs are adaptogenic in giving your homeostatic body a whole menu of phytochemicals, and exposed to a choice, the homeostatic human body grabs those it needs, excluding to a degree those it doesn't need" (personal communication, February 2001).

Other examples of "thinking" plants with an adaptogen action are black cohosh (*Cimicifuga racemosa*) and angelica (*Angelica sinensis*), which contain phytoestrogens. Recent research has focused on the ability of plants with phytoestrogens to "think." "Phytoestrogens are weaker than the body's own estrogen. In premenopausal women, phytoestrogens compete with women's own, more potent estrogen, reducing the total effects of estrogen. As women's estrogen production falls, phytoestrogens supplement this hormone. When women have too much biological estrogen, phytoestrogens lower the burden; when they have too little, phytoestrogens pinch-hit."[9] What seems to be involved in the thinking process during the plant-person connection is the lock and key phenomenon in which receptor sites on certain cell membranes seem to be able to determine the effect of the herb needed to help the body adapt so as to bring about greater balance.

Adaptogen action of plant remedies is one door to a new world of science that explores our world at a cellular level where there exists a pattern of relationship—a metabolic network that includes, but is also more than, DNA. DNA may be part of our physical code but it is not the only expression of our consciousness. The work of psychoneuroimmunologist and scientist Candice Pert on the *Molecules of Emotion*[10] documents the cellular connection network through neuropeptide communication. Pert researches ligands, natural or man-made substances that selectively bind to a specific receptor on a cell. Ligands include neurotransmitters, steroids, and peptides. Pert recognized thinking or consciousness of cell membranes in her research. She found that drugs that are nearly identical in molecular structure can fit the same receptor but have opposite effects.

8   John Christopher and Cathy Gileadi, *Every Woman's Herbal* (Springville, UT: Christopher Publications, 1987), 47.
9   James Duke, *The Green Pharmacy* (Emmaus, PA: Rodale Press, 1997), 323.
10 Candice Pert, *Molecules of Emotion* (New York: Scribner, 1997).

"Both agonist and antagonist were believed to bind to the same opiate receptor, but somehow their 'intrinsic activity'—the effect they had on the cell—was different."[11]

Access to the cell membrane, its receptivity to herbal care, also becomes an important factor in the plan of care. Pert showed in her research that emotions have a clear impact on the cell membrane. She notes that conscious breathing is one example of how we can connect mindfully with and even create change in the peptide network within.[12] This research can be translated to practice in two ways. First, the client must be prepared holistically to enter the green world. All of the suggestions from earlier chapters about preparing a healing environment and modeling the client's world take on greater importance in light of this science. Second, the nurse-herbalist's work with breathing techniques during centering with the client can open cellular channels for herbal interventions. The nurse-herbalist who has a clear reading of the health patterns has, in my experience, clear access to adaptogen and other herbal action. During the planning phase of care, the client's receptivity to adaptation and change is documented. The goals that are created in relationship with the nurse-herbalist reflect and role-model the level of adaptation for which the client is ready.

The client's readiness as a receptor to adapt occurs at both the level of their whole being and at the cellular levels—the world within. Herbal remedies affect both levels. They may present the body with tens, if not hundreds, of phytochemicals, but something else happens. The body seems to know how to choose whether or not receptivity to those substances will bring about greater balance. As with the lock and key phenomenon, if there is no lock for the key, then nothing happens, and vice versa.

Within every plant and every human is a seed of potential for adaptation. When humans and plants come together to *share* an adaptation response, one of the most fascinating and possibly elusive parts of plant medicine science occurs. Pharmacognosist Dr. Norman Farnsworth, who has researched the adaptogenic effects of plants in humans, such as black cohosh and eleuthero (*Eleutherococcus senticosus*), taught me once, "The term adaptogen is used loosely. Some use it to

---

11   Ibid., 81.
12   Ibid., 187.

describe a 'tonic' effect and some use the term to describe a stimulant action to the immune system. The adaptogen effect of medicinal plants is related to the secretion of corticosteroids and the anti-stress effect but there are probably other effects as well that are not completely understood" (Farnsworth, personal communication, February 2001).[13]

Nurses know that no two people respond to the same intervention in the same way. Similarly, no one person responds to the same intervention in the same way at different times. For example, one woman taking a shower after giving birth might become lightheaded and need assistance to get back to bed, whereas another woman might not. An individual patient might have no pain during a dressing change one time and another time find the intervention agonizing. People change constantly, inside and out. Clients are in constant state of adaptation and their behavior is influenced "both by the environment, that is, the world within and around the person, and by the person's abilities to deal with that world."[14] Therefore, we realize that any plan of care that expresses relationship with healing plants is not a static but dynamic document.

"In our dreams," Paracelsus stated, "we are like the plants, which have also the elementary and vital body, but possess not the spirit."[15] Dreams are a part of traditional herbalism in many cultures. Herbalists, healers, and those who seek healing may dream about healing plants that are important to plans of care. Carl Jung states that dreams are "the direct expression of unconscious psychic activity" and are "not an integral component of conscious psychic life, but seem rather to be extraneous, apparently accidental occurrences…and are a remnant of a peculiar psychic activity taking place during sleep."[16] Dreams occur as helpful tools to living a full life that includes access to the reflections of the unconscious. Accessing and remembering dreams can help solve tough problems. Like all parts of the client's health pattern, symptom-signs from the dream world are analyzed within the context of the greater pattern.

Understanding the potential health benefits associated with naturally

---

13 Dr. Norman Farnsworth, world-renowned Professor of Pharmacognosy, died on Sept. 10, 2011
14 Heather Andrews and Callista Roy, *Essentials of the Roy Adaptation Model* (Norwalk, CT: Appleton-Century-Crofts, 1986), 7.
15 As cited in Helena Blavatsky, *Isis Unveiled* (Pasadena, CA: Theosophical University Press, 1998 (Originally published in 1877)), v. I, 170.
16 Carl G. Jung, *Dreams*, Bollingen Series, (Princeton, N.J.: Princeton University Press, 1974), 88,23.

occurring altered states of consciousness such as sleep and dreaming is fundamental to holistic nurse-herbalist practice. Clients often mention plants in various forms that present themselves in dream states. While the nurse-herbalist may not be a psychotherapist, s/he is licensed to counsel clients. Plants are part of race memory. They may also be part of the client's personal memory. Accessing that memory though dreams or waking states is as significant to the client's potential for healing as is accessing cell membranes. Dream states as well as other altered states of consciousness have been accessed in traditional healing rituals as a means of "communication" with the non-verbal plant world. It is often helpful if the client and the nurse-herbalist keep dream journals that identify plants and the context within which they appear in the dream state.

In general, it is important for the nurse-herbalist to know that there are different types of dreams. There are prophetic dreams of an upcoming event, retrospective dreams of past lives, allegorical or symbolic dreams, warning dreams, confused dreams, and chaotic dreams due to indigestion. There are also dreams of great insight and direction that come from our higher Self or sent by Adepts.[17] Modeling the client's world gives insight as to the type of dream that the client experiences at a given time. The nurse-herbalist does not interpret the client's dream. That would be incongruent with the approach to assessment laid down in Chapter 4. Asking the client general questions about their dreams can help the client interpret the meaning of their dream experience.

Herbs, plants, trees, and flowers can also affect dream states and other forms of consciousness. I have had numerous dreams of plants of great beauty from which I awoke feeling refreshed. My clients dream about plants too. I suggest that they always note any plants that come into their life, waking or dreaming. One client, who knew I would be checking her tongue at her next visit, said that she just *had* to have a "hot ball" on her way to my office. She came in and her tongue was all red from sucking on that *cinnamon* hot ball. Cinnamon became an important herb in her formula and care plan. This is the unconscious mind at work. Once the person associates plants with the nurse-herbalist, plants become ready symbols that the unconscious mind uses to communicate the needs of body, mind, and spirit for healing.

---

17 Blavatsky on Dreams. See http://www.theosociety.org/pasadena/sdcommnt/sdc-ap.htm

There are a number of soporific herbs such as hops (*Humulus lupulus*) and lemon balm (*Melissa officinalis*). There are also some that have been known traditionally to stimulate dreams. Bay leaf (*Laurus nobilus*) is one. We grow bay at our medicine house. It actually greets our guests, standing as a sentinel by the front porch. At a certain point in the year, the bay exudes the most exquisite fragrance. We wait for the peak of fragrance to do our harvest. A few years ago, we decided to preserve the beauty of the harvest. We made a medicinal bay cordial called Laurino for holiday gifts. The recipe included cinnamon and lemon. We gave the Laurino as gifts that year to inspire dreams of victory in the New Year. People reported amazingly beautiful and inspirational dreams as well as a good night's sleep.

It is also important to take care with some plants in regard to dreams and sleep. One time I was in Edinburgh, Scotland, where my husband and I found an excellent Chinese restaurant. I ordered a vegetable dish that appeared with a number of types of mushrooms in it. I did not eat very much of those mushrooms but when I went back to the B&B and started to go to sleep, I had a night terror dream about a woman terrorist. I was screaming in my sleep and finally woke up to find my husband deeply concerned. I spoke to a sleep specialist physician when I returned to the States and he thought I was experiencing jet lag, but I had been in the UK for over a week when I had the experience. I always thought it was the effect of the mushrooms. I did actually see the woman of the dream at the airport a few days later. A chill went up my spine so I said a prayer asking for protection for the airport, the people, and the country.

Clients can partner with plants to create rituals for sleep. Rose and lavender (*Lavandula angustifolia*) are excellent for dream pillows. Fragrant flowers make beautiful baths that surround and calm the nerve endings in the skin after a long day of work. Taking time for tea or a bath creates a period of transition before accessing the dream world where we have the potential to partner with plants in another dimension.

The Gentle Healer Within™

The nurse-herbalist partners with the client to create a plan of care that is meaningful for the client. This is most often a new experience for the client who has been treated in biomedically oriented facilities. Clients typically need assistance in making the transition from biomedical to holistic nurse-herbalist care. They often go through a period of subtle or blatant prescription "withdrawal." It is important to help the client during prescription withdrawal to address any ambiguity associated with being increasingly responsible for their health. Nurse-herbalists work in the biomedical world and therefore can empathize with the client.

It is helpful to also *model* the client's connection to the methods of planning and intervention in the biomedical culture when assessing them. There are a number of ways that nurses can help the client make the transition to nurse-herbalist care. I use "prescription pads" that my mother makes for me. I write a list for the client of any remedies or self-care homework I "prescribe" for them. I sometimes wear a white lab coat, such as when I do foot baths and foot reflexology treatments. All clients sign a consent for treatment/confidentiality form and we discuss the fact that my practice is licensed. I may also talk with their biomedical practitioners and share health records. These kinds of "normal" nursing behaviors often help balance out the new experiences of tongue diagnosis and herb tastings.

I also invite most clients to enter into a dialog with their Gentle Healer Within™. As an Advanced Practice Nurse-Psychotherapist, I have for many years helped clients establish through imagery a psychological safe place within their own heart where they can access their Gentle Healer Within™. There are many facets to this mind-body work for the nurse in counseling practice but the basic technique can be easily applied by nurse-herbalists. The purpose is to help the client establish a safe place that they can go anytime, anywhere when they need help in sorting out tough problems related to their health.

Begin with centering with eyes closed to move the attention inward. Then, with eyes still closed, invite the client to take their pulse on their wrist. After they establish a connection with their heart through the pulse, invite them to move their awareness to their heart in the center of the chest. I often have the client place their hands crossed over the heart for protection. This hand gesture is an ancient healing mudra of protection. Then I ask them to move their awareness to the secret chamber of the heart—the place in the heart that beats the heart. The physical point for

Herbal Experiment: Connection through Comfort with a Ginger Compress

Grate 4 to 5 ounces (150 g) of fresh ginger root. Put the ginger into a small cloth bag and add it to 1 gallon (3.8 liters) of simmering (not boiling) water. Allow the decoction to steep gently for five minutes. Holding both ends of a hand towel, dip the middle into the ginger water. Wring it out and fold it to the size of the client's mid-back where the kidneys are. Take care in applying the hot compress, making sure that the skin does not burn because of the heat. The compress should be applied as hot as is tolerated. Place a dry towel over the compress and a blanket over the towel, tucking each layer around the client so that air does not enter the compress and cool it. Prepare a second compress as the first. Replace the first compress after three to four minutes. Remove the blanket and dry towel. Place the second hot compress on top of the first and flip the compress over, making sure that the temperature is tolerated. This technique ensures that the connection with the ginger and moist heat is maintained.

The compresses should be flipped every three to four minutes for twenty minutes. The ginger compress will create increased circulation of blood and body fluids and move qi and blood stagnation that usually manifests as pain, inflammation, swelling, or stiffness. Many people with chronic pain benefit from ginger compresses to the kidneys as a systemic remedy rather than applying the compress to individual joints. Ginger compresses should not be used when high fever is present (too warming), on the head area, on the abdomen in pregnancy, for infants or the very old (too stimulating), or on an area of the body experiencing infection (heat) such as chest/lung area during pneumonia. I taught this to teenage women who were preparing to go to nursing school. They were taking NSAIDS every day for "pain." They were so surprised and happy to experience such pain relief with the ginger compress to the kidneys. They asked me if the effect was due to "the ginger, the hot water compress, or the loving kindness with which they had received the compress?" I asked them what they thought was the answer. They said, "All three!" Yes, the ginger is warming and stimulating as is the hot water. But the love with which the ginger compress is administered is just as important to the connection through comfort that can be made between nurse-herbalist, client, and plant.

this heart energy is thought to be associated with the Bundle of His. Ask the client to let you know when they get "there" by saying "OK." I do not give any more instruction than this and clients seem to have no problem finding this special place in their own hearts.

I then ask the client to begin a creative process. They imagine a place that is completely safe. It can be a real or imaginary place but it must be completely safe and they must be there alone (at least to start). I then walk them through the five senses and invite them to notice and then remember the safe environment that they are in. It is important to name all five senses (touch can be stated as kinesthetic awareness or sensations) since people typically have one or two preferred senses for imagery work. Knowing the client's preferred senses also helps the nurse-herbalist create a plan of care.

After the client has spent time noticing their safe place, ask them to "ask" their safe space for a name. I often ask the client to say the name when they are ready and I record the name and reference it in subsequent sessions. The client will notice that objects, sensations, sounds, etc. change in their safe place. Assure them that this is natural and ask them to pay close attention to those changes and feel free to follow those changes as they occur to see what "story" unfolds. The client can also "ask" the space about anything occurring in the space. I encourage the client to dialog with their inner space, which they come to realize as symbolic of their Gentle Healer Within™. I often instruct the client to ask their Gentle Healer for *one* suggestion to take back with them regarding a specific action they can take as the next step in the healing of whatever concern they are working on. The nurse-herbalist takes notes and reflects the highlights of each imagery session to the client. Clients typically find their experiences to be very powerful.

SOLUTION-FOCUSED COUNSELING TIPS FOR NURSE-HERBALISTS

Counseling is the most important complement to the skill of nurse-herbalism. In Celtic and other ancient healing traditions, the skilled healer always had the ability to counsel. While it is important to be able to listen, it is equally important to be able to counsel. The nurse-herbalist models the client's world so that they can effectively and specifically offer healing solutions that parallel the client's experience of making meaning of their heath challenges. The client does not simply seek the assistance of the nurse-herbalist to receive a list of herbs that they can try to suppress a symptom, though sometimes that is what the solution or intervention entails. Holistic nurse-herbalism includes all of the assessment and diagnosis skill discussed thus far and now also the skill of intervention that begins and ends with counseling—the ability to listen and mindfully guide and sometimes reframe thought, belief, and experience to move toward the dream of healing and greater wellness that the client envisions.

Counseling in nurse-herbalism serves a number of purposes. There are many counseling skills used in assessment. Modeling is just one. There are also a number of counseling skills utilized in creative and constructive solution-building with clients. Counseling skills help the nurse-herbalist guide and support the client in a way that inspires insight. These skills include teaching, coaching, inviting, guiding, and giving advice. Some counseling skills are more directive than others. As a general rule, there is very little call for being directive or prescriptive in nursing. All of the skills discussed throughout this book provide the foundation for *non-directive* or *non-prescriptive* counseling in nursing. Because of the close proximity between nursing and "physicianing" in hospital care, nurses often counsel and communicate with clients in a way that, like physician colleagues, is highly prescriptive.

Prescriptive or directional counseling is one technique, but it should not be the primary counseling mode in nurse-herbalist practice. The rationale for this is explained in earlier chapters on integrative insight, assessment, and diagnosis. Legal rationale will be explained in Chapter 6. The quickest and easiest way to learn to be non-prescriptive and non-directional in counseling is to practice from a solution-focused approach. The first rule is to observe thoughts and communication regarding "disease." Talk with clients about wellness and health patterns, and you will quickly be on the road to reframing your habit of prescriptive and directive counseling. Solution-focused counseling techniques build the nurse-herbalist's repertoire of non-directive approaches to care that enable the nurse to better model the client's world and pace with them.

Pacing with a client is so important. It is more than timing, type, and tuning. Pacing has to do with synchrony and harmony, a dimension beyond the physical plane but recognizable in it. That dimension is rhythm. Our bodies are rhythm. Flow of water or energy is rhythm. People's rhythms harmonize or entrain with other humans, animals, and plants. A newborn baby entrains with its mother. Their heart rate and respiratory patterns become similar. The menstrual cycles of women who work together often synchronize to occur on similar schedules. Pacing with clients occurs on the rhythmic plane. It also can be accessed intentionally when the approach toward the client is open. Questions and reflections are open-ended and non-directional. During assessment, the nurse-herbalist would say, "How are you?" or "Tell me what that is like?" rather than "Do you feel hot?" or "Did it hurt?"

During planning and intervention phases of care, the nurse-herbalist paces the client with non-prescriptive and non-directional communication such as, "Have you considered....?" or "You might want to try..." rather than saying, "Take this herb..." or "You should consider this..." There is a time and place for directional counseling. That is after assessment, diagnosis, and planning and at the end of the intervention phase. After the non-directional pacing is established and open-ended invitations have been extended to the client, they will most often make a choice. They might say something like, "That sounds great! I can't wait to try that. What do I do next?" It is at that point, when they have whole-heartedly invited me to tell them about a solution, that I become directional. However, I still rarely, if ever, become prescriptive and say, "You should do" this or that...or imply that the client should do anything. Any time the word "should" appears on the radar of your mind or thoughts, beware! *Should* means that you are in the prescriptive zone and are solidly in the biomedical paradigm rather than the holistic trail to integrative insight. The answers to the client's tough problems lie within him or her. The second that you enter their world as an expert on their model of the world, you effectively alter the expression of the voice and spirit of their Gentle Healer Within™. I encourage nurse-herbalists to test the validity of this observation. Nurses are human scientists. Observe the responses of your clients to the use of the word should. Observe the responses of your own psyche, body, and spirit when you stop using the word should…even for a day. It can be practice changing and life changing. It was for me.

It is within the client's historical pattern as progressive narrative that we find their solutions with them. They are often so close to those solutions that they do not see them, hear them, feel them, taste them, or smell them. During counseling and intervention, the nurse-herbalist has the opportunity to become a clear reflecting pool for the expression of the client's model of their world and the health patterns that have led them to seek care and comfort. The nurse-herbalist who wants to heal through simple counseling solutions purifies the pool of Self through self-care practices that prepare one to be able to reflect the pattern of another without personal agenda, need, or greed, but with a devotion instead to being as true to the need of another as possible. Solution-focused counseling techniques help the nurse-herbalist counsel the client while maintaining the boundaries of self that conserve the clarity of the reflecting pool. There are three techniques that can help support the creation of a successful plan for nurse-herbalist care.

Scaling

Scaling, the first technique, refers to numbers. The client is asked to assign a number on a scale of 1 to 10 to a particular experience they may be having. Nurses are familiar with pain scales. The client is asked, "How much pain are you experiencing now—on a scale from 1 to 10 with 1 being little or no pain and 10 being the worst pain." The client then assigns a number to the pain. But the solution-focused counseling technique goes one step further. The nurse-herbalist then asks a follow-up question. Starting where the client placed their pain on the scale, let's use 6 for this example, the nurse-herbalist then asks the question, "Your pain is a 6. I am wondering…if there was something that could be done to move that pain to a 5½, what would it be?" If the client has been working in their safe place or recalling dreams, they often have the answer immediately. If not, I give them some space to think. I may coach them to their safe place to answer the question from their heart's intelligence.

After the client identifies the intervention, I may make some suggestions for supporting interventions. For example, if a client said that they plan to put a hot water bottle on their neck every evening when they get home from work to lessen their chronic neck pain, I might suggest that they put arnica oil with lavender essential oil on their neck after they use the hot water bottle. Arnica and lavender both help with pain. Document the pain scale carefully and use it for evaluation of care.

Herbal interventions are often so gentle that clients may not clearly recognize the benefits of the herbal interventions from one week to the next. Scaling with numbers helps give them a "clear pool" perspective of their progress. The nurse-herbalist can reflect to the client who has said that they were not sure that they would get much benefit from simple herbal remedies, "Your pain was a 10 out of 10 when you first came to the office on the first of the month and now on the seventh, it is a 5 out of 10. It seems that your body is responding well, according to your scale. You have dropped five points in one week." Clients typically find this reflection intervention very meaningful.

Exceptions

Asking about exceptions is the second technique. When people first talk about their concerns to a nurse-herbalist, they typically do so from a problem-oriented perspective. If the client thought that they had a solution to their problem, they might not be seeking help. Their problem-orientation is normal. But as the nursing process moves forward, it becomes more important to work with the client to identify potential solutions. One way to do this is to ask the client if there is a time when the problem does *not* exist. This is an "exception question." For example, the nurse-herbalist might ask the client who states that they have chronic neck pain "all the time" if there is ever a time or place when they notice that the pain has subsided or gone away. This can really help identify solutions that the client has already noticed at some level and that can be repeated. Solution-focused brief therapy focuses on the repetition of what is working.

The nurse-herbalist must carefully time the presentation of an exception question. There must first be some rapport between the nurse and client before this question should be used. Consider what you might think and feel if you were to enter a nurse-herbalist's office and say that you have had chronic pain for many years and the first question you were asked was whether there had ever been a time when you did not have the pain. You might think that you had not been heard. Pacing and timing is important in the use of this technique, particularly with depressed clients who have extreme trouble seeing solutions.

The exception question is used after rapport has been established and the nurse-herbalist is refining the interventions such as deciding when a particular herbal intervention might best be applied. For example, the client with the neck pain stated that the pain was bad after a long day at work. The nurse-herbalist might recommend the herbal intervention for after work but also might then ask if there is a time when the pain does not exist. The client might say "when I went on vacation to the beach." Following solution-focused principles, the nurse-herbalist then would attempt to build a care plan that did more of what worked. In this case, the nurse-herbalist would want to help the client go on vacation to the beach. There are a few ways for the client to "go on vacation to the beach." First is to ask the client if they can go to the beach for a vacation. They may be able to go physically or not but even if they go away for a vacation, they still have to come back to their work, which they have tied to their pain.

I find the best solution is to re-create the exception with the client in the present moment. Using imagery, the safe place, dream work, and counseling, the client can re-create through their senses the memory and experience of vacation on the beach. As the nurse-herbalist listens to the client's imagery, they take note of any plants in the story. If the client does not mention them—they are, after all, such a subtle part of the environment that they often go unnoticed—the nurse-herbalist can ask the client what plants they noticed on or around the beach where they were "vacationing." Then be sure to integrate those same plants into the care plan. For example, instead of lavender or arnica oil, the client may mention coconut and papaya. Their plan could be adapted to include a coconut-based massage oil and they could sip papaya juice while putting their neck on the hot water bottle.

"The Miracle Question"

The third technique is called "The Miracle Question." This technique is often very helpful for those who cannot find any exceptions in their personal story. It can be framed simply as an "experiment" in *imagining* a miracle. The outcome of "The Miracle Question" is that clients often begin to realize that they do have some resources to heal and solve their tough problems. To begin, "The Miracle Question" technique must be done in relationship with a client. It is not effective if the nurse-herbalist uses the technique as a passing suggestion during counseling, such as: "What would happen if a miracle occurred and you no longer had neck pain?" That is not what the technique is about. The key to the miracle question is *process*.

The process for "The Miracle Question" begins with a statement of understanding. "I can understand now from your story how difficult this neck pain is for you." This is followed by an invitation to experimentation. "Because your pain is so (fill in the blank here with their word), I am wondering if you would like to participate in an experiment that I do with clients who have chronic long-standing problems such as pain?" If they say no, then this means that the pacing and timing of the counseling is off and the nurse-herbalist needs to do more assessment and modeling, which may or may not lead to asking "The Miracle Question"! If the client says yes, then this is the process:

1. Ask the client to state the problem they would like to solve. In this example, we will say "chronic neck pain."
2. Instruct the client to pick one day during the next week when they will wake up and a "miracle" will have occurred and their problem (chronic neck pain) is gone.
3. Instruct the client not to tell anyone about the experiment, but to keep a journal with them from the time they wake up until they go to sleep so that they can record their thoughts and feelings all during the miracle day.
4. Invite the client to act all day as if the miracle has occurred and journal along the way. If they need pain medication, etc., they should do what they normally would do but

also try to continue the day as if the miracle had actually occurred.

One of the first times I implemented "The Miracle Question" was with a woman who had a new baby and a 2-year-old. I was called to the home because of the newborn's pain with colic. After working on remedies for the baby, the mother became very concerned and told me that her biggest problem was that she realized she "hated" her 2-year-old. That realization was causing her terrible pain all over her body. She was most concerned and confused because she did not understand the origin of such "terrible thoughts" and she wanted to know why she felt that way about her older daughter. We followed "The Miracle Question" process after assessing that she was not homicidal and when I returned to visit her later that week, she was literally beaming with joy. I was shocked at the difference. We talked about what happened. What she journaled and learned on her miracle day was that she "really loved her daughter." She was able to articulate why she loved her and demonstrate that love to her. It was truly amazing.

"The Miracle Question" experiment can bring forward solutions from the Gentle Healer Within™ that are more meaningful than any remedy a nurse-herbalist or any other healer could conjure in their minds. As soon as the client begins to engage with the nurse-herbalist in dialog about visualizing a miracle, they have begun to practice what it would be like if they were to change and heal. Clients often start to feel more resourceful when they imagine the miracle. That simple feeling can lead very quickly to action that reinforces the next tier of feelings of being able and resourceful, and deeply knowing that they hold within them a simple power to heal.

THE POWER OF HERBAL SIMPLES

Herbs are remarkable partners for the nurse who counsels toward solutions. They are catalysts for the change that is needed to move toward solutions. So many solutions exist right at people's fingertips in their own homes, but the constructive discernment as to when, where, and how to use the herbal remedies based on health pattern recognition is in the hands of the nurse-herbalist. Many people have direct experience with the world of plants every day, even though they may not be fully aware of it. People who live in wood homes may never have had to grow or cut a tree, but they can experience the benefit of a sturdy home made from wood cut from the trunk of a tree. Many people wear clothes that have been made from natural plant fibers, such as cotton and linen. Members of industrial societies rarely make their own clothes from purchased fabrics, let alone spin their own cloth. The industrialization of society has created an easier life for many people, but it also has created a distance between people and the plants they regularly consume and utilize.

Although many people may not make their own cloth or cut the timber for their homes, they often make their own "medicine," sometimes on a daily basis. For example, many people enjoy making a stimulating cup of coffee *(Coffea arabica)* or tea *(Camellia sinensis)* in the morning. They may or may not know that the constituent known as caffeine found in coffee and tea is a stimulant drug, but they do know that when they drink their beverage of choice, they often feel more mentally and physically alert. When they need an energy boost, they know they have the option of making a cup of tea or coffee to help. They are making their own medicine—from a plant.

In addition to plant-derived caffeine, it has been estimated that between 35 percent and 50 percent of modern pharmaceutical drugs are derived from natural sources such as plants, and the majority of these products were originally used as traditional medicine or poison.[18] Some have put that figure closer to 60 percent. Although the pharmaceutical industry, like the lumber and textile industries, has assumed what used to be personal responsibility and now makes most of the prescription and over-the-counter drugs on the market, people continue to make their own medicines from plants. Self-care with plant medicines is not a new or old practice; it is an enduring healing tradition.

Plant medicines have evolved over time and are, with the help of technology, not just available in whole plant and extract forms or salves. Many plant medicines are now sold in capsules, tablets, and sprays,

---

18   Bo Holmstedt and Jan Bruhn, "Ethnopharmacology--a Challenge," *Journal of Ethnopharmacology* 8, no. 3 (1983).

and may actually look like pharmaceutical drugs. It is cumbersome to make our own cloth, our own homes, and our own medicines. Many welcome the relief of not having to attend to what used to be daily chores. Interestingly, with all the modern conveniences provided by the pharmaceutical industry, people still choose to make their own "medicine." They make that cup of coffee or tea in the morning and more!

People use plant remedies in their self-care practices, in part, because plant medicines are often more accessible and affordable. This does not mean that if drugs and surgery were more accessible and affordable that people would necessarily stop using the herbs. People use their own time-tested, native (or vernacular) healing methods that include the use of plant therapies because the plant medicines are known to be beneficial. Ethnographic research has demonstrated that vernacular health belief systems, of which plant medicine is a part, "have among their central values concerns for appropriate and timely intervention and for seeking the proper specialist. ... Combined use of conventional medicine and one or more vernacular strategies is extremely common. ...The persistence of vernacular health belief systems is not restricted to the ignorant, the desperate, the remote, the deprived, or the unacculturated."[19] People most often make logical and careful decisions about partnering with plants in self-care. Nurse-herbalists do also.

Nurse-Herbalism

Throughout this book, there are many herbal interventions as well as other types of remedies. The focus of this section of the book is nurse-herbalism as the application of plant remedies in care and comfort. Nurses have been part of the historical evolution of plant medicines for hundreds of years.[20] They have known about the plant medicines people apply in traditional healing practices. The plants that nurses and their clients partner with often provide the matrix and/or materials for the development of many of the drugs that nurses administer. But nurses

19 Bonnie O'Connor, *Healing Traditions: Alternative Medicine and the Health Professions* (Philadelphia: University of Pennsylvania Press, 1995), 21, 26, 32.
20 Martha Libster, *Herbal Diplomats: The Contribution of Early American Nurses (1830-1860) to Nineteenth- Century Health Care Reform and the Botanical Medical Movement* (Thornton, CO: Golden Apple Publications, 2004).

and the public rarely have knowledge of what goes into the making of the pharmaceutical drugs they encounter through prescriptions or over the counter. Nurses are taught the basics of pharmaceutical science with the goal that they safely administer medications under the direction of practitioners with prescriptive privileges. They are not expected to know everything about the production, source, and chemical composition of the drugs they administer or discuss with clients. Practitioners and clients trust the health care system, the federal regulatory bodies, and the educational system that prepares practitioners to support the development and administration of quality drugs.

In herbal medicine, there is a similar desire for quality remedies. Traditional healers and herbal practitioners often grow or wildcraft (harvest from the wild) medicinal plants themselves so that they can assure their clients that the plant is of the highest quality: it came from a clean source without pollutants, it was harvested according to proper planetary cycles, and the correct plant was grown and harvested. If their herbs are purchased, practitioners are mindful of the quality of their sources for plant materials. Practitioners who work with medicinal plants are expected to understand the plant in much the same way, and perhaps even in more ways, than nurses are expected to understand pharmaceutical drugs. Nurse-herbalists have a relationship with the medicine they administer and discuss with clients. This is rarely the case with the pharmaceuticals they prescribe and/or administer. Nurse-herbalists may grow the plant, harvest it, and prepare the medicine themselves.

American history includes several examples of nurse-herbalism using plant medicine skills. As previously mentioned, until the proliferation of pharmaceutical drugs, American nursing texts routinely included the plant medicines of the day. Nurses were taught plant medicine theory as a matter of course. As the rise of university-educated health practitioners continued throughout history, many treated only the wealthy, who expected something different from their university-educated healers. Poorer people were still treated by community healers and herbalists. For a time, the different systems existed side by side. But over time, as university education of health practitioners, including nurses in the twentieth century, became more associated socioculturally with biomedicine and its growing interest in technology, herbalism and natural remedies became marginalized from the biomedical sphere. My research[21] documents this transition as occurring in the United States approximately between the 1850s and 1950s. The herbal remedies that are easily accessible outside "the back door" became associated more and more with lay healers. American physicians marginalized herbs from their orthodox practice in the late nineteenth and early twentieth centuries. Nurses and midwives, however, have not fully severed the tie but certainly do not boast of a long tradition of expertise in herbalism as they could. There are some countries or parts of countries in which nurses are quite connected with herbal tradition, such as in China, India, and Germany.

But in general, those of the dominant biomedical sphere and much of the populace of industrialized nations think and perpetuate a myth that herbal medicine is "crude" and therefore lesser medicine. Herbal medicine science and traditional medicine making is often dubbed "unscientific." However, countries such as China have rejected a systemic focus solely on a biomedical scheme of primary care, which is well known to be the most expensive system in the world. During the government of Mao, it was recognized that the country could never have enough Western drugs or practitioners to provide health services for the entire population of the country. In 1929, the Chinese government outlawed the practice of TCM because the Kuomintang government had decided that TCM was "unscientific." Subsequently, Mao created a system of "barefoot doctors," traditional practitioners who had some training in Western biomedicine to care for the people, primarily the poor rural populations. Many people do not consider the care provided by traditional practitioners to be of less value. In fact today, the Chinese government values and markets its traditional system of health care to other countries, hence the steady flow of Western practitioners entering China for tours and education in traditional modalities such as acupuncture and herbalism. The socioeconomic drive to create a health care system for all Chinese people created an integrated system of traditional and conventional Western medicine that exists today.

As in China, the scientific and political leaders of many countries throughout history have attempted, and continue to attempt, to control

---

21   Ibid.

and even outlaw the traditional use of medicinal plants by the people and practitioners by labeling the practices unscientific, unproven, or potentially unsafe. Often these labels are applied without adequate study of the cultural practices or the centuries-old records of safe use of many herbs by humans. Because traditional healers, in many cases, have not been able to practice openly, the knowledge and wisdom associated with many traditional plant medicine practices and medicine making is on the verge of extinction. The traditional healers who use and teach the use of indigenous plants have gradually disappeared. In Hawaii, for example, the traditional healers, known as "kahuna" (or keepers of the secrets), like Aunties Anita and Marie, were driven underground in the 1800s when licensing of health practitioners occurred as a result of Westerners coming to live on the islands. Today, access to traditional healers is often still by word of mouth in Hawaii and the average age of traditional Hawaiian healers is 70.[22] Historical assessment shows the same potential with the nurse-herbalist caregiving and medicine-making tradition in both industrialized and developing nations throughout the globe.

The close relationship that nurses have with the people suggests that allowing the partnership with the plant world and our history of medicine making to decline, as did medicine one hundred years ago, would have the effect of distancing us from the people and communities for whom we care. This is because the people have never disconnected fully from the plant world. Although the people of industrialized nations may turn to processed supplements rather than whole-plant teas and compresses, studies show that herbal remedies in general are still important to many peoples and cultural traditions. The public's access to herbal remedies continues as part of an enduring, well-documented "hidden health care system."[23] One American study showed that even among the 44 percent of adults who regularly access the biomedical system of care with its prescription medications, "nearly 1 in 5 (18.4%) reported the concurrent use of at least 1 herbal product, a high-dose vitamin, or both."[24] Therefore

---

22 Nanette Judd, "Laau Lapaau: A Geography of Hawaiian Herbal Healing" (Unpublished Doctoral Dissertation, University of Hawaii, 1997).

23 Lowell S. Levin and Ellen L. Idler, *The Hidden Health Care System* (North Carolina: Golden Apple Publications, 2010).

24 David Eisenberg and others, "Trends in Alternative Medicine Use in the United States, 1990-1997: Results of a Follow-up National Survey," *JAMA* 280, no. 18 (1998): 1572.

nurse-herbalism and medicine making must endure as nurses continue to strive to meet the needs of their clients for holistic care.

Many resources are available on herbal medicine making. Nurse-herbalists learn directly from experienced nurse-herbalists, traditional healers, and herbalists. They also can learn from their country's formularies, pharmacopoeia, dispensatories, and historical texts on herbal medicine making. The recipes, remedies, and information on the preparation and administration of herbal remedies included here and in Appendix A focus on the areas of nursing tradition: herbal teas, syrups, soups and extracts, and the application of plants topically and in creating a healing environment. The information provided is derived from my many years of experience in partnering with plants as well as from traditional herbals, dispensatories, and textbooks.

The plant parts that are traditionally used in nurse-herbalism and medicine making are the bulb, bark, twigs, flower, leaf, fruit, skin, juice, pollen, root, rhizome, tuber, seed, and/or whole plant. The quality of a plant medicine is related to the way the plant is grown, harvested, and processed. Plants used for healing should be grown without the aid of pesticides and herbicides because the chemicals used in these products can be toxic to humans. There is a potential for chemical residues to remain with the plant even after processing. Medicinal plants should not be exposed to these strong chemicals. The plants used should be fresh. Dried herbs can maintain a fresh quality for certain periods of time, depending on the plant and plant part. Flowers and tiny leaves are fragile and therefore more susceptible to a loss of vitality than whole roots. Plant parts should be preserved as whole as possible to maintain freshness. They can be chopped or ground right before use rather than stored as such. Certain plant constituents, such as volatile oils, deteriorate or dissipate quickly. Freshly picked herbs can spoil or lose vitality in a matter of hours or minutes. In general, fresh plants are used immediately, and thoroughly dried plant materials are used as soon as possible but usually have a shelf life of approximately one year, again depending on the plant. Dried herbs for external use may be able to be stored longer, depending on the plant.

How and when the plant or plant part is harvested is very important to the quality of the remedy. Some nurse-herbalists, as some in the herbal medicine industry, continue the tradition of planting, harvesting, and preparing remedies according to specific lunar, solar, and planetary cycles, rhythms, and configurations. Attention to cosmic forces, as is scientifically noted in biodynamic gardening, is known to increase the hardiness of the medicinal plant and the potency and prevalence of medicinal components. Herb companies, such as Weleda and Dr. Hauschka Cosmetics, that use biodynamic principles pay close attention to how the medicinal plants used in their products are grown in relationship with the whole environment, including the flow of water near the plant, the balance of the soil, and the position of the planets.

The plants in one of the medicinal plant garden projects I coordinated in the 1990s had been planted originally by horticulturists who had used traditional astrological data regarding appropriate timing for planting and the positioning of plants in a garden. Laboratory testing of herbs grown in that garden revealed exceptional quantity and quality of known active constituents even after more than one year of storage. The astrological approach may have been helpful in harnessing the para-magnetic forces necessary for growth and quality.

The processing of the plant is also important to the quality of the medicinal plant preparation. While plants are known to contain healing constituents, the "medicine," according to many traditions, actually resides in the healer. Many plant medicine makers are aware of this and are very careful and meticulous about their preparations. Remedies are often thought to be best if hand-harvested. The purity of the menstruum (solvent) used to extract the medicinal constituents of plants, such as water (referred to as the universal solvent), alcohol, glycerine, vinegar, and oil, is very important. Some herbalists recommend using only distilled or soft water in making remedies to facilitate the extraction process because hard, well, or spring water may foster precipitation.

Making plant remedies is an opportunity for nurses to improve their understanding of the plant-human relationship and to develop their skills of exploring nature's way of assisting in the process of human healing. Being in nature—touching the ground, smelling the trees and flowers, looking up at the sun and the clouds—can be soothing and reassuring. Not only are medicinal plants potentially healing for the receiver of the remedy, but those making and applying plant remedies can also be healed because of the contact. Connecting with the natural world can be a way of reconnecting with one's roots. Roots anchor a plant deeply in the soil and protect it from being blown about by fierce winds or rain. Roots provide nourishment for the plant and are the point of connection between the soil and the plant. Direct interaction with the plant world through medicine making is one way to connect with nature and one's roots. When human beings connect with their own roots, they discover a source of security, protection, and nourishment. Nurses can benefit from learning what plant remedies are most prevalent in the local areas where they live. Herbal remedies come in a variety of forms. Making herbal remedies from plants is an art, a science, and a cultural experience. Making and taking tea in Japan is different from making and taking tea in England. So we begin with teas and tea tastings, one of the oldest nurse-herbalist traditions.

Tea Tastings

While taking tea is a global culinary tradition, "tea tasting" for medicinal purposes is best known in traditional circles and little known in biomedicine. Tea tasting is the scientific process used for centuries in determining the medicinal energetic qualities of herbs. I learned tea tasting when I studied Traditional Chinese Herbal Medicine. Over the course of about fourteen months, I was required to "taste" about 240 herbs. Tasting is an important part of herbal education. The term *tasting* is actually something of a misnomer as all of one's senses are actually engaged in the process of experiencing the herb, not just the sense of taste.

A tasting traditionally begins with sitting meditation and ends with reflection. The meditation period is a time of preparing the body to act as a barometer for the action of an herb in the body. Prior to meditation, an herb is cooked, extracted (decocted or infused) in water. The cooking and preparation of the tea for tasting is also a meditation for me. To begin, herbs are handled with awareness and gratitude. My source of gratitude stems from my awareness of growth of the plant and the effort and energy it took, human and plant, for the petals, twigs, roots, seeds, or leaves of any given plant to be on my table. It is a critical part of herbalism that the person applying plants in care have a first-hand understanding of what it takes to grow and produce herbs and herbal products. Growing and working with medicinal plants is a memorable experience. Whether that memory is of planting culinary herbs in a small home garden or directing the harvest of acres of red clover buds (*Trifolium pratense*) and long rows of valerian roots (*Valerianan officinalis*) while the deer lounge in the field nibbling the tender mugwort (*Artemisia vulgaris*) leaves, I remember. I can still see the shapes and colors of the herbs I have grown over the years and the weeds I have pulled. I close my eyes and can see the wild mustard plants we weeded out of the fields while lying down on a flatbed behind a tractor so that we could weed quickly. I recall plant story after story of harvests and medicine making. The details of herb production stay with us because plants are alive! Their life force is what makes meditation on their preparation for tea tasting and other remedies so vibrant and beautiful.

Gratitude and appreciation open the heart and all of the channels in the body. It is in this open state that a tea is tasted. Tasting can be simple. There are two primary questions to ask your body when tasting herb tea:

1. Where do I feel the effects of this herb enter my body?
2. What is the thermal nature of this herb?

Question 1, in the TCM tradition, is answered in terms of the three "burners": upper, middle, and lower. The upper burner is the head and upper chest area, the middle burner is the abdomen and chest area, and the lower burner is the lower abdomen. While the focus is the torso and head areas, you can also report any sensations in your limbs. Some herbs may be felt in more than one burner. Peppermint (*Mentha piperita*), for example, is typically felt in the upper burner, but many also feel the effect of mint in the middle burner. Take a moment to remember peppermint. It often helps to close your eyes to block some of the visual stimuli from the environment. What do you remember about peppermint entering your body? Can you remember it opening your sinus and head channels?

Peppermint is also one of the plants I use to teach about thermal or energetic nature of herbs, the second question posed during a tea tasting. The energetic scale for this experiment is a hot to cold scale. The scale is this: Hot ..…..Warm ….Neutral ….Cool …..Cold. Whether peppermint tea is served as a (temperature) hot or cold beverage, peppermint tea and the plant are considered energetically *cold*. Cayenne pepper (*Capsicum frutescens*), on the other hand, is energetically *hot*. Peppermint tea is energetically cold and enters the upper and middle burners. Ancient monks who conducted the tea tastings reached consensus long ago about the classification of peppermint. There are hundreds of herbs that are classified in a similar manner and are recorded in the TCM Materia Medica. Over time, people have reconfirmed the value of the empirical process of tea tasting.

Tea tasting and energetic classification of herbs results in a more proper use of herbs in care. The energetics of an herb is part of a profile or personality of a plant that is important to understand when attempting to create plant-person partnerships. "Personalities" have to match. One of the most poignant examples of energetic mismatch I have encountered occurred in a class I took in the 1990s. I remember it well. The woman came to the class saying that she suffered from "hypertension." When asked her symptoms, she said that she felt hot and that her body was "close to exploding" with tension. If we simply think about the energetics, it would seem clear that this woman is "hot"—thermally speaking. In fact, her tongue was bright red with no tongue coating, indicating that the heat in her organs had burned off the tongue coating considered normal. She craved cold beverages. Her eyes were bloodshot and her cheeks flushed even at rest. She was indeed hot! She was so hot that she was exhausted.

One of her self-care solutions was to go to her health food store where she found an herb product for increasing energy. It contained cayenne and ginseng, two very hot herbs. Although cayenne is known to move or invigorate circulation and ginseng does improve energy in the body, what the TCM system classifies as "tonifying Qi," the herbs were absolutely not right for this woman. They were too hot. Hot plus hot equals hotter. The TCM system, like nursing and life in general, is oriented to promoting balance, not imbalance. Therefore, this woman needed solutions, remedies, and herbs that would cool her down and result in improving her energy, which was being dissipated with the fluids and heat. I have found over the years that the energetics of a remedy is more important to positive outcome in care and comfort of clients, particularly in chronic conditions, and that the best way to begin to learn energetics of plants is by tea tasting.

Teas, also called "tisanes," are aqueous or water extractions of medicinal plants. Tea preparations, as is shown in Chapter 1 with the quote from Sister Matilda Coskery's book, *Advices Concerning the Sick*, are a well-established nursing intervention. Water extractions are often hot but can be cold, especially if the plant has highly volatile active principles. Infusions are water extractions of the plant material that is more delicate, such as leaves and flowers. The plant material used is allowed to steep in the water for a period of time. Fresh or dried plants can be infused, but because of the water content in fresh plants, more plant should be used per cup of tea than with dried (approximately 3 teaspoons [15 g] of fresh herb is equal to 1 teaspoon [3 to 5 g] of dried herb). The decoction method of making tea is used when the plant material is hard or woody (i.e., roots or barks) because more heat is needed to release the medicinal constituents in the plant (usually the mineral salts and bitter principles). For decoction, the plant material is simmered and/or boiled for at least fifteen minutes, sometimes longer. In TCM practice, the formulas often contain roots and harder parts of plants, and the usual decoction time is 1½ to two hours. If the plant material used is dried, the plant material is steeped in warm water for approximately four hours before simmering to allow the dried herb to absorb water and expand. Infusions and decoctions can be taken internally and used externally. External uses are discussed in the section on topical applications.

Infusions and Decoctions

To make a medicinal tea, boil the water and select the herb you want to use. When using large dried flowers or leaves, break up the amount of herb needed in the pot or tea net. If using fresh herbs, cut them into pieces and bruise them with a knife so that volatile oils will not be absorbed into the skin of the hands. Measure the herbs for the tea. The general rule for quantities is 1 to 2 rounded teaspoons (about 5 g) per cup of water. Pour the boiling water over the plant material, and cover the cup or teapot to prevent the volatile oils from escaping. These oils will accumulate with water on the underside of the lid. Be sure to shake the condensation on the lid back into the tea. For very thin and tender parts of plants, steep for approximately three to five minutes. For other plant materials, steep for approximately ten minutes. Strain and drink tea hot.

These are general guidelines and following a specific formula may be required, depending on the herb(s) being used. Infusions are made in small quantities on an as-needed basis because they often contain constituents that spoil quite readily after hot water infusion. Beverage teas are infusions. They are usually a *blend* of plant leaves or flowers and are steeped so that a person receives very small amounts of any one plant's medicinal constituents. The concept of a beverage tea is similar to a blend of herbs used in seasoning Italian foods, such as oregano *(Oreganum vulgare L.)*, basil *(Ocimum basilicum)*, and thyme *(Thymus vulgaris L.)*. Instead of making an infusion of thyme and using it medicinally, either drinking it or putting it in a bath, a small amount of thyme is blended with other herbs and put into a sauce for pasta. Likewise, the intent of the beverage tea infusion is for culinary purposes rather than medicinal use.

For a decoction, the same supplies are needed as are used in making an infusion. The plant material used is usually the harder part of a plant such as the root or bark. With roots, the pieces are often much larger than with leaves or flowers. Use approximately 30 g (1 ounce) of herb per 750 ml (1½ cups) of water. Place the dried, hard herbs in a pot and cover them completely with cold water. Bring the water almost to the boil, cover, and remove from the heat. Allow the herbs to stand for about four hours while the dried herbs expand. (This step can be skipped when using fresh herbs.) After standing, the herbs are simmered in a pot (not aluminum) for approximately fifteen minutes. Volatile oils will escape during simmering. These instructions are a generalization and specific instructions (as with TCM formulas where the herbs are cooked for two hours) should be followed whenever possible. The decoction is strained after cooling slightly and then taken warm or at room temperature. Decoctions are considered more potent than infusions. Larger quantities of decoctions often are made. The rule of thumb is that decoctions can be kept refrigerated for up to seventy-two hours and portions reheated, without boiling, for use during the day.

Medicine in Small Amounts

The medicinal constituents found in plants are most commonly acquired through ingestion in small amounts in teas, soups, broths, syrups, and liquid alcohol extracts. Some medicinal plants, such as saw palmetto *(Serenoa repens)*, have a history of also being eaten as staple foods. Herbs are used in many cultures in food preparation. Herbs such as dill *(Anethum graveolens)* and basil *(Ocimum basilicum)* are used in foods because of their supportive effects on digestion. They are used traditionally in small amounts determined by taste. Oral ingestion of herbal remedies through teas, juices, and foods enables the person to taste the plant. Taste is a good way to regulate oral ingestion of herbs because many medicinal plants and many plant constituents are not the most pleasurable to taste. Medicinal plants can be bitter, sour, pungent, astringent, salty, and sweet. Often, tasting a medicinal plant reveals a combination of tastes that is unique to that plant. The understanding of the importance of taste in herbal medicine is highly developed in the Indian system of medicine known as Ayurveda as well as the TCM system.

In the Ayurvedic system, bitter taste is said to restore the sense of taste. In many cultures, the use of medicinal plant bitters, a combination of bitter plants, is used in aiding digestion. Typical bitter plants include goldenseal *(Hydrastis canadensis)*, yarrow *(Achillea millefolium)*, and dandelion *(Taraxicum officinalis)*. My mother used to harvest dandelions in the spring to make a vat of dandelion wine that we drank at special dinner occasions to aid digestion.

Sour taste is helpful in digestion as well. Sour is associated with lemon *(Citrus limon)* and other citrus fruits as well as rosehips *(Rosa canina)* and hawthorn berries *(Crataegus laevigata)*. Pungent taste increases the appetite and promotes digestion and sweating. Examples are black pepper *(Piper nigrum)* and onion *(Allium cepa)*. Astringent taste is drying and constricting, and is used to promote absorption and restriction of fluid. The astringent taste, associated with the tannin constituents in plants, is experienced when tasting tea *(Camellia sinensis)* and raspberry leaf *(Rubus idaeus)*, and feeling witch hazel *(Hamamelis virginiana)* on the skin. In addition to its effects on digestion, the salty taste found in plants such as seaweed also promotes the body's ability to retain fluids.

Sweet taste, found in herbs such as licorice *(Glycyrrhiza glabra)*, kudzu *(Pueraria lobata)*, and psyllium *(Plantago psyllium L.)*, is nutritive and promotes growth of tissues.

Soups

One very common way of receiving the benefits of small amounts of medicinal plants is to make soups or broths with herbs. Soup and broth making with herbs is a nursing tradition that has been important to holistic care and comfort since the seventeenth-century work of the Daughters of Charity of St. Vincent de Paul. These early nurses and their foundress, Louise de Marillac, viewed broth making as an important intervention that strengthened the client. Broths and soups were made from meat, vegetables, and occasionally grain, such as barley. The nurses also used culinary and medicinal herbs in the preparation of their broths. The Daughters followed "Particular Rules" that included the section title "The Ordinary Diet to be Given to a Patient." The herbs that were considered best for a patient's broth were sorrel, lettuce, purslane, chicory, white beet, Chinese leaves or Chinese cabbage, and caraway. In winter, when aerial parts of herbs were not as available, the sisters used chicory, parsley root, and hulled barley.[25] They fed and healed thousands of sick poor in Paris and throughout France with broths and other herbal remedies.

Broths and soups are still an easy and effective herbal remedy to employ in the care of clients. For instance, I often suggest ginger *(Zingiber officinale)* and astragalus *(Astragalus membranicus)* added to chicken soup to strengthen the stomach and spleen energy systems because many people have sluggish digestion, particularly during cold months. One of my favorite winter soups is onion and watercress *(Nasturtium officinalis)*.

This soup was inspired by one of my favorite herbalists, a Swiss naturopathic physician named Dr. Alfred Vogel. The bioforce herb company was started by Dr. Vogel, who suggested that watercress is helpful for sore throat and health patterns related to colds and flu. He

---

25 As cited in Martha Libster and Betty Ann McNeil, *Enlightened Charity: The Holistic Nursing Care, Education and Advices Concerning the Sick of Sister Matilda Coskery, (1799-1870).* (Farmville, NC: Golden Apple Publications, 2009), 176.

stated that the watercress "boosts" the thyroid.[26] Here is my Winter Watercress and Onion Soup recipe:

- Slice two large onions and place in a 3-quart sauce pan or soup pot.

- Cover with 3-4 cans organic chicken or vegetable broth (or make your own!)

- Add 1-2 cups water.

- Add Braggs Liquid Aminos to taste.

This soup should be a little on the salty side to cut the phlegm in the throat. It will also be balanced out by the sweet taste of onions after they cook. Add freshly ground pepper to taste. Bring to a boil and then cover and simmer until onions are soft. Take 1 tablespoon of Kudzu (*Pueraria lobata*) powder (from macrobiotic section of health food store) and cover with a little water. Stir to paste. Add 1/4 cup of the broth to kudzu and stir until thoroughly mixed and then add to the pot. This mixture will thicken the soup slightly. Kudzu is a cooling herb that heals the gastrointestinal lining where the viruses that cause the common cold take hold, according to the research of Dr. Edward Bach. When the onions are soft and you are ready to eat, cut the watercress leaves gently and place 1/4 to 1/2 cup of leaves in a soup bowl. Cover with very hot soup and by the time you get to the table, the greens will be ready to eat. They are slightly spicy. Substitute chard, kale, or other chopped green leafy vegetable if you do not have cress available.

Syrups

The Rev. Simon Gabriel Bruté (1779–1839), chaplain to Mother Seton and the early American Sisters of Charity community, wrote of the importance of the sister-nurses' caring interventions, "Let us bless, love, serve with great joy, and expansion of heart, in the smallest things. Alas! What great things we can do for this Sovereign Master of

---

26 H. C. Alfred Vogel, *The Nature Doctor: A Manual of Traditional and Complementary Medicine* (New Canaan, CT: Keats Publishing, 1991), 162.

Heaven and earth, this King of Eternity! What? Anastasia, a broth—
Sally, the washing,—Jane, some ciphers,—Augusta, some crochets and
quavers,—Xavier, the medical syrup... what more?"[27] Nurses have been
expert fruit and medicinal syrup makers throughout history. The French
Daughters of Charity used fruit syrups to administer bitter-tasting herbal
extracts and powders. They made syrups from peach blossoms, cherries,
chickory [sic], water lilies and roses.[28] Louise de Marillac demonstrated
an extensive use of herbal knowledge employed in her nursing care. For
example, one recipe for a purgative "potion" is included in a letter from
Louise to Monsieur L'Abbé de Vaux in 1641:

> Forgive me, Monsieur, if I take this liberty as well as that of telling
> you that, if you have not already been purged, I would be pleased
> to render you this little service by preparing you a potion which I
> believe should be made up of the weight of three copper coins of
> senna steeped overnight in a good mixture of refreshing, pleasant-
> tasting herbs. To this add one-half ounce of cleaned black currants
> mixed with an ounce of peach syrup (the pharmacist here has
> given me some that is excellent) or, if this is not available, the same
> amount of pink rose syrup.[29]

To clarify, Louise's comment about the "pharmacist" referred to
a Daughter of Charity. Two centuries later, Shaker infirmary nurses
documented a number of syrup recipes in their receipt books, such as
a "Syrup for summer complaint"— a blackberry and clove syrup used
for dysentery that was recorded as being "an excellent medicine; and
has cured many"[30] and the Canterbury nurses' receipt for Onion Syrup:
"Slice your onions then put them in a vessel cover them with honey make
your vessel air tight then let it stew gradually till the onion is done. Strain
off the liquor & it is done."[31]

---

27 As cited in Libster and McNeil, *Enlightened Charity: The Holistic Nursing Care, Education and
    Advices Concerning the Sick of Sister Matilda Coskery, (1799-1870).* 45.
28 Louise Sullivan, *Spiritual Writings of Louise de Marillac: Correspondence and Thoughts.* (New
    York: New City Press, ed. and trans. 1991).
29 Ibid., 47.
30 Shakers, *Receipt Book*, Fruitlands Museum, Harvard, MA, Shaker Manuscripts - Reel 1.3.
31 Canterbury Shaker Nurses, *Infirmary Recipe Book*, Sabathday Lake, ME, Shaker Manuscripts
    (1841), 9.

To make a syrup, start with a strong herbal tea or the juice pressed from a plant such as the berries of the elder (*Sambucus nigra*). Elderberries *must* be cooked thoroughly for human consumption and then the seeds strained from the liquid. Sugar or honey is added to the tea or juice. Then the liquid is boiled, reduced, and thickened into a syrup plant remedy. I preserve my syrups with a small amount of organic vodka or brandy. Syrups make excellent children's remedies. My young clients like my thyme (*Thymus vulgaris*) syrup, in particular, during cold and flu season. I do not preserve my children's syrups with alcohol.

Liquid Extracts

Tinctures and liquid extracts are preparations in which alcohol is used to remove the medicinal components of a plant. Alcohol is an excellent menstruum (solvent) for most plant constituents, and it also serves as a preservative for the finished product. Because of the alcohol, the shelf life of an herbal tincture or liquid extract is approximately ten years. Tinctures of dried plants should be a 10 percent or 1:10 plant weight/volume of menstruum. Liquid extracts of dried plants should be a 20 percent or 1:5 solution, and fresh plant tinctures are 50 percent or 1:2 weight/volume solutions. Herbs that are potentially more toxic should be tinctured rather than extracted. In the marketplace, a tincture is often a 1:10 preparation, meaning one part plant is used to ten parts alcohol. A liquid extract is often a preparation of one part plant to five parts alcohol or less. When buying alcohol preparations, it can be somewhat confusing for the consumer because the words tincture and extract are not always used in a standard fashion by manufacturers. Understanding the preparation is important when buying alcohol products because cost comparisons should include how much plant constituent may actually be extracted.

Making your own alcohol preparations requires some research because some plants are best extracted dry and some fresh. Alcohol preparations are performed by either the percolation method or maceration. Because percolation involves the use of laboratory equipment that most people do not have in their homes, maceration, a simpler and effective method, is described here.

Supplies needed include:

- Fresh or dried herb

- Wide-mouthed jar with lid

- Food grade ethyl alcohol (Pure grain spirits up to 190 proof [e.g. Everclear] are used for maceration.)

Maceration begins with cutting up the fresh herb or powdering (coarse, not fine) dried herb and putting the plant material in the wide-mouthed jar. The appropriate amount and type of menstruum is then poured over the plant material and the lid to the jar is placed on tightly. The jar is then put in an accessible but dark corner of the kitchen or workroom. Shake the jar at least twice daily so that the menstruum can thoroughly penetrate the plant material. Shake and store the jar for two weeks. Heat is not necessary because of the longer maceration period. At the end of the two weeks, the plant material is strained into a bowl. Use cheesecloth to press out the remaining menstruum from the plant material. Take the alcohol extract, pass it through a coffee filter, and transfer the strained liquid to dark-colored dropper bottles.

Tinctures and liquid extracts lose potency when exposed to light and therefore are prepared and stored away from light. The bottles used to store tinctures and extracts should be dark-colored glass and have glass droppers. Dropper bottles are necessary because the dosages for the concentrated tinctures and liquid extracts are smaller and are given in drops. Although drops of extracts and tinctures may be taken directly under the tongue for fast action, I typically suggest that they be put in a small amount of boiled water, herb tea, or syrup. Historically, alcohol extracts have typically been taken in small amounts in a glass of wine or cup of tea. The bottles should be labeled with the name of the remedy and the date it was prepared.

The alcohol extraction process entails understanding the water content of the plant material used and then adding the appropriate amount of grain alcohol necessary to extract the medicinal constituents. Different amounts of alcohol are used for fresh and dried plants. Often alcohol is diluted with water for extraction—50 percent alcohol and 50 percent water, or 100 proof. "Diluted alcohol or proof spirit is employed, when the substance is soluble both in alcohol and water, or when one or more of the ingredients are soluble in the one fluid, and one or more in the other, as in the case of those vegetables which contain extractive or tannin, or the native salts of the organic alkalies, or gum united with resin or essential oil. As these include the greater number of medicines from which tinctures are prepared, diluted alcohol is most frequently used."[32]

If dry plant is used, then the amount of menstruum used to extract the plant material to make a 1:5 liquid extract is five times the weight of the plant material. Thus, if you have 500 g of dried plant, you will need 2,500 ml of menstruum for the liquid extraction. If a 1:10 tincture is to be made, then ten times the weight of the dried plant, or 5,000 ml of menstruum, is needed. Generally, the menstruum used for dried plant tinctures is 50 percent alcohol and 50 percent water, or 100 proof (vodka). If a fresh plant is used, then there is already a significant amount of water present and water is rarely added. A fresh plant can have as much as three times the amount of moisture as a dried plant. The water content can be measured by moisture analysis and then the correct amount of menstruum calculated. In general, for fresh plant tinctures, a 1:2 weight-to-volume calculation is made and the plant is extracted in straight 190 proof alcohol (such as Everclear). For example, if 200 g of fresh plant is collected, then 400 ml of alcohol is used for the maceration.

Many clients ask what the differences are between homeopathic remedies and herbal extracts. A fresh herb tincture made by extracting one part herb in two parts alcohol is often referred to as a "mother tincture." This mother tincture can be shaken and diluted 1:10 to give a "homeopathic" tincture with a potency known as 2X. Then that 2X tincture is shaken and diluted once again 1:10 with alcohol/water and that dilution is known as 3X. This shaking and dilution process is known as "potentization." Samuel Hahnemann, a renowned homeopathic scientist, described his observation of the effect of potentization as, "The more a substance is succussed and diluted, the greater the therapeutic effect while simultaneously nullifying the toxic effect."[33] The potentization

---

32   George Wood and Franklin Bache, *The Dispensatory of the United States of America* (Philadelphia: Grigg & Elliot, 1839), 1065.

33   George Vithoullkas, *The Science of Homeopathy* (New York: Grove Press, 1980).

process continues and the potencies are recorded carefully.

Homeopathic medicine includes the use of remedies that have been diluted as many as twenty-four times (Avogadro's number), which is the point at which there are no detectable molecules of the original mother (herbal) tincture. Homeopathic remedies are not only derived from plants. Minerals are also used. The remedies are then used based on the "Law of Similars" ("like treats like") in which the symptoms of a condition are actually treated with a homeopathic dilution originally made from a substance, such as a plant, known to cause the same symptoms. Thus, homeopathy, although it uses plants as mother tinctures, is not the same science or the same healing art as herbalism. Unlike naturopathy or medicine, the practice of nurse-herbalism does not include homeopathic remedies. Homeopathy is recognized in a number of countries such as the United States and the United Kingdom as the practice of medicine even though some Boards of Medical Examiners, such as in the state of North Carolina, have disciplined physicians for the practice.

Nonsynthetic vegetable glycerin also can be used for maceration of plants. Glycerin is a type of alcohol that also is known as glycerol or glyceric alcohol. Glycerin is not as effective as alcohol in preserving plants, so some plant medicines include a greater volume of glycerin or are a mixture of glycerin and alcohol. Glycerin also is more effective than water but less effective than alcohol in extracting resinous and oily plant constituents. Glycerites are often used with children, who may be repulsed by the smell and taste of alcohol. Some may recommend glycerites for those who are sensitive to alcohol, but I usually recommend teas for these folks and avoid alcohol and glycerin altogether. People who are sensitive to alcohol can be carbohydrate sensitive and do not do well with simple sugars, carbohydrates, or alcohol, which are metabolized quickly.

Standardized extracts are plant preparations in which some plant constituent, identified as an active ingredient, has been adjusted to ensure that the potency of the product is standardized. There is some debate as to whether or not the concept of standardization is misleading to the public because many herbs' healing benefits are not the result of one constituent or active ingredient, but rather the synergy between multiple constituents. Active ingredients have yet to be isolated in many medicinal plants. Standardized extracts are generally more expensive than other extracts and tinctures. Labels on products should disclose the plant constituent and percentage of that constituent to which the product has been standardized.

Comments about Capsules and Pills

Some standardized extracts are sold as capsules or pills. Herbs are often sold as capsules or pills. Because many people are used to taking pills prescribed from biomedical practitioners, they often prefer taking herbs in these easy-to-use forms as opposed to having to prepare their own medicine or take liquid herbal preparations. It is actually simple to prepare capsulated herbal remedies. An herb is crushed into a fine powder using a mortar and pestle, and the capsules are either filled individually or by using a capsule holder where the herb powder is spread into the open capsules and the excess scraped away. The other half of the capsule is then applied. In terms of safety, capsules that are self-prepared from herbs you have identified may be better quality than those bought in a store. When purchasing herbs in capsule form, the consumer must instead rely on the integrity of the manufacturer and the standards of the governing agency of the country where they live. Because the herb is powdered, it is not easy, if nearly impossible, to identify the herb by visual inspection, smell, and sometimes taste. The risk of adulteration (the wrong plant being added to the product) also can be greater with powdered medicinal plant products.

The plant in capsules and pills is not tasted. In traditional medicine systems, such as Ayurveda, taste and sensory experiences of the plant medicine are considered the beginning of the healing process because the nervous system is stimulated by the senses. When viewed from a traditional herbal paradigm, the consumer who ingests the herb in capsule or pill form may not be getting the full benefit of the plant that they would get by tasting the herb in decoction, infusion, or liquid extract preparations. Some traditional herbalists also consider the bulking agents used in making herb capsules and tablets to be unhealthy in daily quantities. In TCM, these filler materials can be stagnating to the liver energy system, an important issue for women who often have symptoms indicative of liver stagnation before selecting their herbal remedy.

Not all herbs are meant to be ingested as whole plant. Many herbs are now sold in pill or capsule form as dietary supplements. Some liken the expansion in the dietary supplements industry in America to the patent medicine era of the 1800s. Traditional herbal *Materia Medica* are specific about which herbs can be eaten after decoction. For example, in the Chinese *Materia Medica,* "dong quai" *(Angelica sinensis)* is said to be edible. Many people might find the taste of "dong quai" or any other herb repugnant and therefore may ask to take the herb in capsule or pill form; however, using an herb in a way that is unsupported by traditional history means that the herb's safety record as a capsulized whole plant must be established. A capsule or pill form may not be as safe or effective as when used in traditional forms such as decoction. In the case of dong quai, it is edible but is traditionally taken as a decoction in formulation with other herbs. Its centuries-old safety record is as part of a formulation. The capsule form of the herb may be safe as a single herb remedy but the traditional history of safe use is not the same and therefore does not apply.

Some practitioners believe that the benefit of using pills and capsules is that doses of specific plant constituents may be more easily controlled than in tea form. While this may be correct, whole plant dosages *can* be specifically measured out for teas. In TCM, we use a measurement system and dosage strategy with a precision to 1/3 of a gram or better that allows for the herbal remedy or formula to really meet the specific needs of a client on a given day. Yet, some practitioners and clients are more comfortable with pills. Comfort with one's medicine is an issue nurses know quite well. Nurse-herbalists educate clients regarding the benefits and risks of use of herbs in various forms. I do not recommend capsules or pills as a rule with one exception. I do suggest milk thistle (*Silybum marianum*) standardized extract for those who have experienced significant changes in liver enzymes, liver toxicity, or exposure to pollutants such as chemical spills, chemotherapy, or air travel.

Topical Remedies and Creating a Healing Environment

Topical herbal applications are also nursing practice. Nurses are already familiar with the use of herbal and floral creams, lotions, waters, packs, and other remedies to the exterior of the body. Topical application of herbal remedies is an area of nursing that is ripe for clinical research. Although the whole body can be affected by topical applications, the skin and the nervous system are most particularly affected. The skin, as the largest organ of the body, and the peripheral nervous system both have connections with the whole body. Topical remedies are used not only in skin care, such as care of a localized wound (an application called a vulnerary in herbalism), but also are used to address systemic discomfort and imbalances affecting body, mind, and spirit. The importance of skin applications is described by Anthroposophical nurses in Europe. They write, "A 'breathing' can take place between the external curative quality of a substance administered to the body and the body's reaction to it. This 'breathing' process also can be described in terms of question and answer; the questions usually come from the outside, the answer follows from within."[34]

Topical application of plant remedies to the skin allows a physical chemical reaction to occur and also creates a healing moment when the patient's attention is focused on that part of the body receiving the external application. The patient can use the moment to tune into the body and connect with the Gentle Healer Within™ to ask what is needed for healing, and then listen for the answer. People often have a very limited awareness of their bodies when they are healthy. When ill or in pain, it is human nature to want the discomfort in a particular area of the body to go away. Topical applications provide comfort and provide the client with an active outlet for participating in the healing process.

Historically, nurses have provided total patient care that has included the hygienic care of the body as well as administering treatments that involve topical applications. Some nurses, such as enterostomal or wound and skin nurses, specialize in topical applications to the body and care of the skin. Nurse-herbalists administer hot baths for soothing anxious patients and apply herbal remedies in the form of poultices, plasters, compresses, salves, ointments, lotions, and more.

Compresses

A compress, which nurses used to refer to as a "fomentation" or "stupe," is a folded piece of material made of a natural fiber that is applied

---

34   Tieneke Van Bentheim and others, *Caring for the Sick at Home* (New York: Anthroposophic Press, 1980).

moist to a part of the body so that it presses against that body part. Compresses combine the knowledge of the external use of herbs and the science of hydrotherapy or use of water. Natural fiber cloth, such as wool, cotton, silk, and linen, is used because it is more absorbent and allows the skin to perspire and breathe during the compress. A compress can be applied hot, warm, or cool, and in herbalism is saturated with an infusion, decoction, tincture, or herbal oil. The cloth is cut to fit the area where the compress is to be applied. For example, a compress for the eyes will be smaller than a compress for the kidneys. Some examples of compresses that can be used in patient care are arnica compresses for a sprained ankle, witch hazel compresses for puffy eyes, and mint compresses for fever or heat in the head, back, abdomen, or thighs.

Cool compresses are made by dipping the cloth into the infusion, decoction, or tincture, wringing out the cloth and applying it to the body part. The compress is not necessarily covered because the compress is changed as soon as the heat from the body warms the compress, as in the case of fever. With warm and hot compresses, the nurse must use a wrapping technique that prevents the compress from being exposed to air and cooling down. The cloth is dipped in the hot or warm infusion or decoction and is placed in a wringing towel so that the nurse does not have to touch the steaming compress directly and it can be wrung out thoroughly. Hot compresses are not applied wet and drippy because they cool too quickly. After wringing, the compress temperature is tested against the arm of the nurse and, if tolerable to the skin, is applied as hot as possible to the patient's skin.

After the compress is applied, it is completely covered with another cloth and then a thick cloth or towel to keep the heat in. Each successive cloth covers the previous one by a few centimeters to be sure to seal in the heat. The compress is left in place for about twenty minutes. It is possible to use a piece of plastic, like a plastic bag, to seal in the heat of a compress but this may not allow the skin to breathe fully. Consider other means of keeping the application warm, such as changing the compress during the application. If the compress turns cold, the patient will become uncomfortable and it should be removed and replaced with a warm one. If the patient relaxes deeply or falls asleep, the compress is left in place for the twenty minutes. Compresses that are secured and worn for longer periods of time are kept moist by adding a small amount of the infusion, decoction, tincture, or oil at intervals throughout the day. For certain conditions, hot and cold compresses using different herbs may be alternated.

One common cool compress used in nurse-herbalism is a compress with witch hazel *(Hamamelis virginiana)* infusion or tincture. Cotton bandaging is cut to the size of the eyes and dipped in the witch hazel infusion or tincture. The excess is squeezed out and then the compress is applied to the outside of the eyes to relieve puffiness. The hot compress with ginger was explained earlier in the Herbal Experiment.

After the nurse-herbalist prepares the plant infusion, decoction, tincture, or oil, s/he prepares for the timing and rhythm of applying compresses, packs, and wraps. Learning topical applications is similar to learning bed making. A certain "look" must be achieved, so that the patient associates comfort with the application. In bed making, the sheets should not be wrinkled because the bedridden patient's skin is better protected and patients are often more comfortable when their covers are straightened. With compresses and packs, the look of the application should be tight and tucked in. The patient should feel protected by the compress or wrap and not feel as if the pack or compress is going to fall off or move. The compress or wrap should be a comforting temperature, and the patient should be told when it will be applied to their body so that they will not be shocked by a temperature change.

My favorite herbal wraps and packs are for the feet. I have applied herbal wraps and packs to the feet for twenty-five years as part of the Science of Energy Flow® Foot Reflexology treatments I do. The feet are a holographic representation of the entire body with all of its organ systems and energy patterns. Herbal foot and body wraps are a wonderful expression of the science and art of nursing. Nurses have tremendous opportunity for growth, theoretically and clinically, in the area of external applications, especially in regard to herbal compresses, fomentations, and stupes. In my foot treatments, I typically apply castor oil *(Racinus communis)* and moist heat packs.

I first learned the castor oil pack application for the feet from Oma and later learned about the history of the castor oil pack from a healer who had been affiliated with the Edgar Cayce Foundation in Virginia

Beach, Virginia. Edgar Cayce (1877–1945) was a medical clairvoyant for forty-three years whose work includes the use of numerous plant remedies. Cayce recommended castor oil packs in such cases as impaired lymph flow; inflammation; congestion; constipation; gallbladder, liver, kidney and pelvic disorders; muscle spasms, and back pain. Castor oil is very viscous compared with other oils and when placed on the skin provides a protective coating that subsequently penetrates the tissues very deeply. With the assistance of heat, the oil is taken up readily by the skin and tissues, and provides a deep healing and soothing effect.

There are two ways of doing a castor oil pack for the feet or any part of the body. The Cayce method is to completely soak a wool flannel with the warmed castor oil and apply it to the feet or body part. In clinical practice, I use significantly less oil by applying the oil directly to the feet or body part and then applying the flannel soaked in very hot water. I use stretchy German cotton instead of wool flannel. After applying the moist pack, I put a thin piece of plastic over the flannel to seal in the heat of the pack. For the feet, large plastic baggies can be slid over the foot after the compress is applied and squeezed next to the foot so that all air escapes. After the plastic is applied, the small hand towel is wrapped around the foot in a way to keep air from entering the pack. After both feet are wrapped and tucked in, they are placed at the center edge of a larger towel, and a hot water bottle is placed at the bottom of the feet outside the small towels. The edge of the large towel away from the patient is folded up over the bottle and pack. Then the towel ends are wrapped up and around the feet, securing the bottle in place and keeping the warmth in. Then cover the patient with warm blankets. The castor pack can be kept in place for up to one hour. More typically, I leave a hot moist castor pack in place for about twenty minutes. After the castor oil pack is removed, be sure to keep warm the body part treated with the pack. People always comment that this herbal application is very comforting.

Poultices and Plasters

Herbal poultices, also known as cataplasms, are similar to compresses, except that instead of putting the cloth in an infusion, decoction, tincture, or oil, the cloth is used to hold a slurry or softened paste of the plant material, which is then applied to the skin. Nurses have historically applied flaxseed, bread, onion, or hops as poultices. In 1924, Bertha Harmer wrote that poultices "give the patient great relief and a sensation of comfort if properly applied."[35] They can be used as a therapeutic measure for pneumonia; to relieve distention in postoperative patients; and for painful, inflamed, and infected wounds.

According to historian John Haller (1985), poultices were an "essential element in effective therapeutics" throughout history until the later nineteenth century when "germ theory and knowledge of asepsis led to its gradual extinction,"[36] at least in biomedicine. Practitioners varied the temperature of the poultice based on the nature of the disease. They routinely used oats, cornmeal, arrowroot, carrots, chlorinated soda, and charcoal for poultices. With the advent of germ theory, the poultice fell into disuse by many, but not all, physicians because they were "found to be the source of pyogenic bacteria."[37] In some countries, nurse-herbalists continue to use the poultice, prepared fresh, with appropriate attention to hygiene and protecting the patient against the possibility of introducing bacteria and infection.

To apply a poultice, cut material to size and cut or chop the herb chosen for the poultice. The herb can be raw, cut, mashed, or lightly sautéed. A slurry of the raw or cooked herb is placed in the center of the cheesecloth or fabric. Then fold the fabric to enclose the herb. The poultice should be a size that fits the body part to be treated. The poultice is left in place for a certain amount of time determined by the nature of the herb and the tolerance of the patient.

Plasters are a type of poultice in which the plant material is applied directly to the skin or through a thin cloth. The plaster is often made of a plant powder that has been mixed into a thick paste. The most common plaster used in the past by nurses is the mustard plaster. More recently, nurses who work with lactating mothers have acknowledged the benefits of green cabbage *(Brassica oleracea)* leaf plasters to the breast in cases of engorgement. The cabbage leaf is applied directly to the breast, chilled,

---

35   Bertha Harmer, *Text-Book of the Principles and Practice of Nursing* (New York: Macmillan Co., 1924), 208.

36   John Haller, "The Poultice," *New York State Journal of Medicine* 85, no. 5 (1985): 207.

37   Ibid., 208.

without any cloth. [38] Another example is the use of aloe vera leaf plasters on first- and second-degree burns. My grandfather taught me as a child how to apply aloe plasters to my skin after being in the sun. Aloe leaf with its slippery gel is very cooling and moistening for the skin.

Infused Oils, Liniments, Salves, and Ointments

Herbal oils (also called oil infusions to distinguish them from essential oils) are made by saturating fresh plant material with a fixed oil such as sunflower, olive, sesame, or canola oil. An herbal oil is massaged into the skin for various reasons, depending on the plant used. For example, the flowers of *Arnica montana* are infused in oil and can be rubbed into sprains and sore muscles. To make an herbal oil, collect fresh or dried plant material. You may need to do some research to know whether to use dried or fresh plants. Some plants such as St. John's Wort (*Hypericum perforatum*) plant must be used fresh. I apply St. John's Wort oil to first- and second-degree burns, wounds, and for muscle and trigger point pain. To make the infused oil, the aerial parts of a *fresh* plant (flowers and small leaves) are collected, chopped, and placed in a wide-mouthed jar. Add a little oil to the plant material and then crush the flowers again with the back of a spoon. Then add more oil to cover the plant material completely. Shake the jar and place it in a warm location for ten days to two weeks.

The oil must be approximately 37.7°C or 100°F during the infusion time. St. John's Wort oil's signature is that it turns red. The red color is due to a constituent in the plant known as hypericin. After the oil infusion is completed, the plant material is strained from the oil. The residual oil is pressed out of the plant material with cheesecloth. Because fresh material is used, some water may still be in the herbal oil even though the cheesecloth covering allows for some evaporation. If allowed to stay in the preparation, the water could cause the oil to go rancid, so it is best to let the strained oil sit for one to two weeks undisturbed. The oil will rise above any water remaining and can be decanted off into brown glass storage bottles. The water can then be discarded.

---

38   Kathryn Roberts, "A Comparison of Chilled Cabbage Leaves and Chilled Gelpacks in Reducing Breast Engorgement," *Journal of Human Lactation* 11, no. 1 (1995).

If dried plant material is used to make an herbal oil (herbs other than St. John's Wort), grind the dried herb to a powder when you are ready to make the oil. Wet the herb thoroughly with oil and stir. Add oil to the jar so that the level is a few centimeters above the herb powder. Cap the jar tightly and put in a warm place. The same method is followed as used for fresh material except that the dried herbs absorb the oil. The oil level must be checked after the first twenty-four hours, and more oil is added if needed.

Liniments are lighter topical remedies than oils and are usually alcohol or camphor based for quick absorption by the skin. Liniments have been used traditionally to warm and stimulate muscles and ligaments. They evaporate quickly so that no oil is left on the skin as with herbal oils. Liniments are often used before physical exercise to warm up the body, but they also can be used for local inflammation after exertion. Liniments are used in specific areas of the body, not for full-body massage. The herbs traditionally used as liniments are the more warming herbs like cayenne and lobelia. One of my favorite liniments is a camphor-based liniment with lobelia that is applied to the temples for discomfort related to headache, migraine, and eyestrain. The camphor, as with all alcohol-based liniments, is cooling, while the herb is warming. Liniments feel initially cool on the skin and then quickly begin to warm. They cause a beneficial exchange of the blood in a specific area through this cooling and warming action.

Herbal salves and ointments are semisolid plant preparations that are absorbed into the skin. The base for an herbal salve or ointment is the herbal oil (already prepared above) and beeswax. Approximately 28 g per 250 ml oil or 1 ounce wax per 1 cup oil is used to change the consistency of the topical preparation from oil to a salve or lotion. Tincture of benzoin (1 drop per 30 ml or 1 ounce of oil) is added as a preservative. To make a salve, place the herbal oil and shaved beeswax in the top of a double boiler until the wax is melted. Test the consistency by pouring a small amount of the salve into a jar. It should harden quickly and be the consistency that you want. Add more oil if you want the salve to be softer and more wax if you want it harder, depending on the nature of the application. For example, in the care of an open wound, a hard salve would not be used because applying it takes a little more rubbing, which is not helpful when the wound is healing. A softer salve would be needed that can be smoothed over the wound easily. When the consistency of the salve is right, tincture of benzoin is added as a preservative.

Aromatic essential oils also can be used in making oils, liniments, salves, and ointments for topical application. Essential oils are single constituents extracted from aromatic plants. They make up a very small amount of the whole plant. Essential oils evaporate readily and therefore, once extracted, must be kept in sealed bottles. They are sold in small amounts because they are a highly concentrated plant constituent. For medicinal purposes, they must be used in pure form. Aromatic oils often are considered precious and valuable, and are used in small amounts. Like perfume, essential oils are meant to be used in amounts that do not overpower the sense of smell. Some essential oils are lighter in fragrance than others. For example, lemon verbena is lighter than cinnamon or basil. Herbal oils, often used for massage, are made with drops of essential oils in a fragrance-free carrier oil such as sweet almond oil. Create a 2 percent to 3 percent dilution (ten to twelve drops per 1 ounce/30 ml of vegetable oil for adults and a 1 percent dilution (five drops per 1 ounce/30 ml oil) for pregnant women, people with illness, and children. Essential oils I like to add to liniments include ginger, eucalyptus, and peppermint.

It is better to invite patients to participate in choosing their own essential oils to be added to massage oil or liniments. Essential oils represent the subtlety of plant consciousness. Therefore, I do not recommend purchasing essential oil blends created by others. Nurse-herbalists should carefully select the best-quality essential oils plant by plant. The individual essential oils can be used singly in a carrier oil or blended (three, five, or seven oils in a carrier oil) for each unique client so as to achieve a specific medicinal effect. The fragrances of essential oils are an *essential* contribution to the creation of a healing environment.

Inhalations and Steams

Partnering with plants to create a healing environment is very important in the care of clients. The personality or medicine of a plant is not only ingested orally or felt through contact with the skin. Plant medicine can be experienced through environmental interaction. It can be inhaled with the air as aromatherapy, steams and inhalations, absorbed with water through herbal baths, "taken in" through our vision and other senses, and experienced by direct interaction through a garden experience.

Aromatherapy, like homeopathy, is related to herbal medicine, but it is a specific science and art in its own right. The essential oils from aromatic plants can be used to affect the health of body, mind, and spirit. Throughout history, perfumers have known of the medicinal benefits of the aromatic volatile fragrances they used. Religious rituals continue to include the aromatic use of plants as incense, such as frankincense (Boswellia carterii). The olfactory cells are the only place in the human body where the central nervous system comes in direct contact with the external environment. Humans' sense of smell is one direct connection with their environment. Plants often provide that sensory experience. The essential oils from plants used in aromatherapy do not just provide a pleasurable or memorable experience, they have been shown through numerous studies to have specific healing properties as well. Studies have shown the antibacterial, antiviral, and antifungal effects of essential oils in the human body and other significant effects on mood, alertness, and perception. Scientists such as Dr. Alan Hirsch of the Smell and Taste Treatment and Research Foundation (www.smellandtaste.org) research the effects of odor from various plant sources on learning and behavior. Nurses have done research on aromatherapy on such health concerns as the inhalation of lavender essential oil to ease anxiety levels in women undergoing mammography screening[39] and angelica (Angelica archangelica) in the reduction of post-pump depression and promotion of sleep in postoperative patients.[40]

Medicinal qualities of herbs also are taken in with the air through smoking and steaming. Herbs such as mullein leaf (Verbascum spp.) may be smoked for their healing effect upon the lungs. The herb is smoked in much the same way a tobacco cigar or cigarette is smoked. Herbal steam inhalations are often used in the healing of the sinuses. Chamomile inhalations are commonly used for sinus congestion and pain. Chamomile has anti-inflammatory properties.

---

39 Cynthia Blake, "The Effect of Aromatherapy on the Anxiety Levels of Women Undergoing Mammography Screening" (Unpublished Master's Thesis, University of Phoenix, 1998).

40 Jane Buckle, Clinical Aromatherapy (London: Arnold Publishers, 1997).

The nurse-herbalist first prepares a warm room for the client. Have the client sit next to a table. They should dress warmly, with socks on and feet resting on a hot water bottle. The herb (such as chamomile flowers) is placed in the bowl and boiling water poured over the plant material to release the essential oils. Drape the client's head and shoulders with a large towel and then have them position their head over the bowl so that the vapors do not escape. The patient breathes in the vapors for about fifteen minutes, at which time their head is dried and covered with a small dry towel to prevent chilling.

Full Body Baths and Foot Baths

Some people may consider herbal baths a luxury and the reward for those who have the means to frequent a day spa. But they are really a necessity and an essential part of any nurse-herbalist's health promotion program or care plan. Hippocrates, the "father" of modern medicine, stated that the key to good health rested on having a daily aromatic bath and scented massage. During herbal baths, the plant medicine surrounds the body, allowing for the intermingling of plant and human in a deeply healing experience. Many herbs are used in baths for their aromatic effect such as raising spirits and calming the nerves. Plants can also be used to create other healing effects as well. Rose petals *(Rosa gallica),* for example, can be floated in a bath to heal and nourish the skin and soothe a troubled heart. Herbal full baths, sitz baths, and foot baths are all used in the care of clients.

To prepare an herbal bath infusion, use one handful of cut herb per liter or quart of water. For a full-body tub, make 3 quarts/L; use less for smaller basins. Steep the herbs in cold water for a few hours or overnight and then heat almost to boiling, cover, and allow the herbs to steep for ten minutes. Strain the infusion and pour into tub or basin filled with warm water. Adjust the temperature and then submerge the body. Baths should last at least twenty minutes because that is the amount of time the pores take to open fully. The largest pores in the body are in the feet. The feet, as mentioned previously, are also a holographic representation of the entire body—its organ systems and energy centers—and therefore a foot bath can be just as effective as a full-body bath in creating a healing environment with the client.

After the bath, the body should be wrapped warmly in towels and allowed to perspire for a short time. Even the feet will perspire after a foot bath. Dry the body and put on fresh clothing. Some essential oils such as rose, eucalyptus, and rosemary can be used instead of herbal infusions in a bath. Three to fifteen drops of pure essential oil can be used per large tub, depending on the type of oil. For a foot bath, five to ten drops per liter or quart of water are used. Taking an herbal bath and smelling fragrant oils can cause one to remember soothing moments of direct interactions with plants, either during a walk in the woods or through a fragrant garden. Engaging other senses while in the bath can accentuate the healing potential of the herbal bath. I often will invite clients to sip and smell an herbal tea while taking their bath. The herb may be the same or complementary to the herb or herbs in the bath.

Engaging all of the senses is possible when partnering with plants to create a healing environment. The plant in the relationship provides the chalice for healing, but the client and nurse-herbalist offer intent. This book emphasizes the importance of *how* the plant medicine is applied by the nurse-herbalist and client. There are so many herb books on the market that describe *what* plants to use for *which* conditions in the body. But without knowledge of *how* to apply those herbs for those conditions or health patterns, it is questionable if healing is possible. Nursing care represents the *how* of healing arts. How a person demonstrates care is the intentional catalyst for change and healing. Nurse-herbalist care begins with first contact with plant and client. The care expressed in the harvesting and processing of the plant is important to the potency of the resulting remedy. How a nurse-herbalist or client applies an herbal oil to the skin, prepares a bath, and serves a tea are just as important to the healing experience as the constituents and energetics of a plant remedy.

As nurses around the world grow in their understanding and re-discovery of herbal remedies and medicine making, they can share with others their experiences of how those remedies influence clients' health and illness and their own health and well-being. This sharing about plant therapies is helpful to the development of herbal remedies as part of nature care and their continued recognition as nursing practice. Nurse-herbalists can then teach and empower others in their communities to learn the art and science of herbal medicine making and establish plant partnerships that can be instrumental in healing illness, promoting health and long life, and connecting with one's roots.

WATER – INTEGRATIVE INSIGHT –
REFRAMING THE CLEAR LIQUID DIET

In 1986, when I was a new graduate nurse, I worked
on a medical-surgical unit in a hospital in Los Angeles.
I had been a professional dancer and teacher for many
years and therefore had a love for the body as a temple of
creative energy and potential. I just could not understand why after
significant surgical procedures, sick hospitalized patients would be
given "clear liquid diets" that were full of chemicals, preservatives, food
dyes, and stimulants such as monosodium glutamate. I have never been
able to shake the sadness of having to administer such "diets" to postoperative patients under my care. I did what I was taught in nursing
school and said a prayer. I visualized the gelatin, broth, juices, and hot
drinks as purified of all harmful substances and transformed into light
and healing energy. But I also knew that it would be much better to
serve a different clear liquid diet. It did not happen—at least during my
tenure in hospital care.

At the time, I did what I could and started the process of reframing
the clear liquid diet given to post-operative patients. I started talking
about new solutions. That solution is now in this book too. Instead of
MSG-ridden broth, I recommend that strained miso, organic chicken,
or beef broths be offered to patients. Pure organic clear juices can be
given as drinks and gelatins made from those juices can be offered
instead of the products with food dyes in them. Most importantly,
herbal teas could be selected by knowledgeable nurse-herbalists for
recovering patients just as in days gone by when nurses were experts
in dietary management of the sick. Just as water is essential to life,
reframing and recovering the power to administer proper sick diets to
patients is essential to the historical evolution of holistic nursing care.
Bring back the nurse's broths. Hereafter herbal teas!

REFERENCES

Alexandersson, Olof. *Living Water: Viktor Schauberger and the Secrets of Natural Energy.* Bath, UK: Gateway Books, 1997.

Andrews, Heather and Callista Roy. *Essentials of the Roy Adaptation Model.* Norwalk, CT: Appleton-Century-Crofts, 1986.

Blake, Cynthia. "The Effect of Aromatherapy on the Anxiety Levels of Women Undergoing Mammography Screening." Unpublished Master's Thesis, University of Phoenix, 1998.

Blavatsky, Helena. *Isis Unveiled.* Pasadena, CA: Theosophical University Press, 1998 (Originally published in 1877).

Buckle, Jane. *Clinical Aromatherapy.* London: Arnold Publishers, 1997.

Capra, Fritjof. *The Hidden Connections: A Science for Sustainable Living.* New York: Random House, 2002.

Christopher, John and Cathy Gileadi. *Every Woman's Herbal.* Springville, UT: Christopher Publications, 1987.

Duke, James. *The Green Pharmacy.* Emmaus, PA: Rodale Press, 1997.

Eisenberg, David, Roger Davis, Susan Ettner, Scott Appel, Sonja Wilkey, Maria Van Rompay, and Ronald Kessler. "Trends in Alternative Medicine Use in the United States, 1990-1997: Results of a Follow-up National Survey." *JAMA* 280, no. 18 (1998): 1569-75.

Erickson, Helen, Evelyn Tomlin, and Mary Ann Swain. *Modeling and Role Modeling.* Englewood Cliffs, NJ: Prentice-Hall, 1983.

Haller, John. "The Poultice." *New York State Journal of Medicine* 85, no. 5 (1985): 207-09.

Harmer, Bertha. *Text-Book of the Principles and Practice of Nursing.* New York: Macmillan Co., 1924.

Holmstedt, Bo and Jan Bruhn. "Ethnopharmacology--a Challenge." *Journal of Ethnopharmacology* 8, no. 3 (1983): 251-6.

Judd, Nanette. "Laau Lapaau: A Geography of Hawaiian Herbal Healing." Unpublished Doctoral Dissertation, University of Hawaii, 1997.

Jung, Carl G. *Dreams,* Bollingen Series. Princeton, NJ: Princeton University Press, 1974.

Levin, Lowell S. and Ellen L Idler. *The Hidden Health Care System.* Farmville, NC: Golden Apple Publications, 2010.

Libster, Martha. *Herbal Diplomats: The Contribution of Early American Nurses (1830-1860) to Nineteenth-Century Health Care Reform and the Botanical Medical Movement.* Thornton, CO: Golden Apple Publications, 2004.

———. "Integrative Care--Product and Process: Considering the Three T's of Timing, Type and Tuning." *Complementary Therapies in Nursing and Midwifery.* 9, no. 1 (2003): 1-4.

Libster, Martha and Betty Ann McNeil. *Enlightened Charity: The Holistic Nursing Care, Education and Advices Concerning the Sick of Sister Matilda Coskery, (1799-1870)*. Farmville, NC: Golden Apple Publications, 2009.

Nurses, Canterbury Shaker. *Infirmary Recipe Book*, Sabathday Lake, ME, Shaker Manuscripts 1841.

O'Connor, Bonnie. *Healing Traditions: Alternative Medicine and the Health Professions*. Philadelphia: University of Pennsylvania Press, 1995.

Pert, Candice. *Molecules of Emotion*. New York: Scribner, 1997.

Roberts, Kathryn. "A Comparison of Chilled Cabbage Leaves and Chilled Gelpacks in Reducing Breast Engorgement." *Journal of Human Lactation* 11, no. 1 (1995): 17-20.

Shakers. *Receipt Book*, Fruitlands Museum, Harvard, MA, Shaker Manuscripts - Reel 1.3.

Sheldrake, Rupert. *The Presence of the Past: Morphic Resonance and the Habits of Nature*. Rochester, VT: Park Street Press, 1995.

Sullivan, Louise. *Spiritual Writings of Louise de Marillac: Correspondence and Thoughts*. New York: New City Press, ed. and trans. 1991.

Van Bentheim, Tieneke, Saskia Bos, Ermengarde de la Houssaye, and Wil Visser. *Caring for the Sick at Home*. New York: Anthroposophic Press, 1980.

Vithoullkas, George. *The Science of Homeopathy*. New York: Grove Press, 1980.

Vogel, H. C. Alfred. *The Nature Doctor: A Manual of Traditional and Complementary Medicine*. New Canaan, CT: Keats Publishing, 1991.

Wood, George and Franklin Bache. *The Dispensatory of the United States of America*. Philadelphia: Grigg & Elliot, 1839.

the *Fire* Element

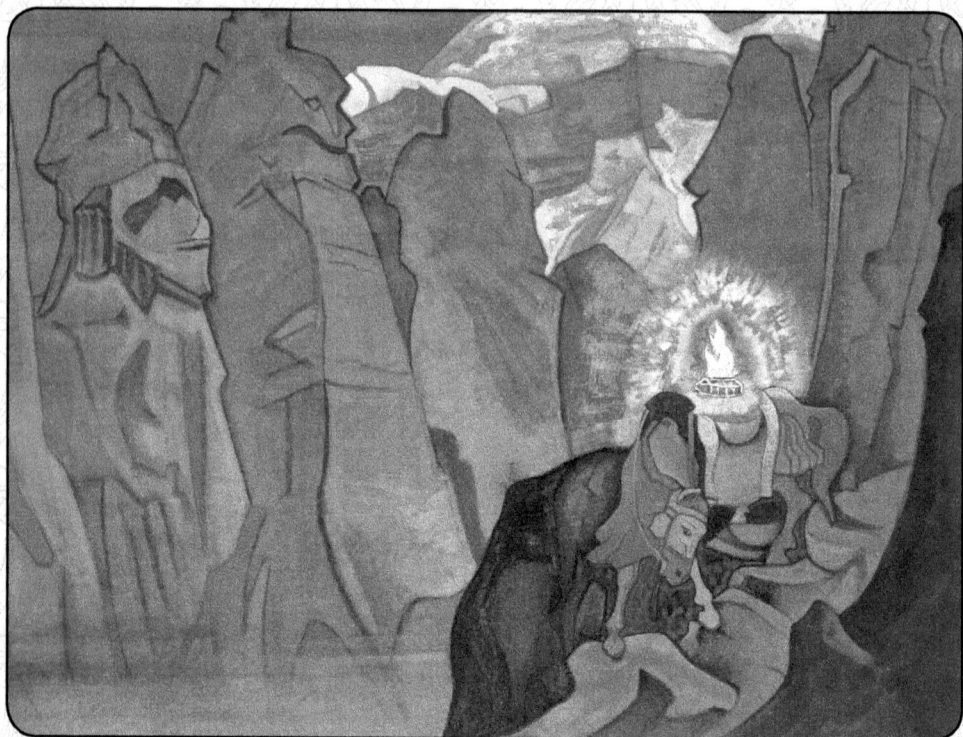

Treasure of the World
Nicholas Roerich, 1924

CHAPTER SIX

Fanning the Fire Element

Herbal interventions have the ability to catalyze major changes in body, mind, and spirit. To catalyze is to exert an effect in the body. Teas, poultices, alcohol extracts, soups, and other remedies made from healing plants extend a gentle but powerful action to the human world that is quite different from the interventions of the biomedical world, such as surgery, pharmaceutical drugs, and radiological treatments. The effects of herbal interventions are all able to be evaluated and measured in some way. This chapter is about evaluation of outcomes and the responsibilities nurse-herbalists have to society and the profession to examine, review, and protect the heritage and evolution of the science and art of nurse-herbalism.

Herbal remedies can be strong medicine. However, they are not drugs or surgery. They have their own power and therefore come with their own caveats. It is neither scientifically nor culturally appropriate to equate herbs with pharmaceutical drugs when they are applied in their whole form. This means that unless an herb has been processed into an herbal drug or a supplement that is very close to a pharmaceutical drug—standardized extracts that will be discussed later in this chapter—it needs its own rules and regulations for application. This chapter demonstrates how current regulations, statutes, and professional guidelines can be readily applied in the practice of nurse-herbalism. The specific legal content of this chapter concentrates on rules that guide practice in the United States of America where I have been a nurse-herbalist for more than two decades. However, this content focuses primarily on the *principles* of safe and effective nurse-herbalist practice that are the foundation for establishment of laws, statutes, and best practice guidelines. These principles reflect the standards for the evaluation of a given intervention. Herbal interventions such as compresses and teas are different from biomedical interventions. While expectations of high standards for evaluation of effectiveness may be present, the method or means for that evaluation is often quite different from evaluations found in the biomedical paradigm.

Biomedical interventions are often very powerful, sometimes overshadowing and overwhelming a client with their chemical and energetic intensity. This power is often evidenced in the body as heat or fire. For example, the fire of a chemotherapy or radiation treatment strips the body of fluids and dries tissues and hair. All instruments of healing are necessary in a health care system that would serve the whole community. Yet, in industrialized societies there has been such emphasis on the biomedical that other treatments such as herbal remedies are often marginalized and may even be dismissed all together.

Throughout history, people have requested strong medicines to overcome their ailments. The "chemotherapy" of the nineteenth century was calomel[1] and the "radiation" bloodletting and blistering of the skin. Health beliefs have included the notion that to heal serious illness, one needs to first take remedies that will propel one to the brink of death where the body will then overcome the illness and health will rise as a phoenix bird. But in the nineteenth century, the people, with the support of many physicians, began to reject such notions of medicine that harmed as well as healed. Criticism of traditional therapeutics such as calomel and bloodletting had "become cliché in sophisticated medical circles: physicians of any pretension spoke of self-limited diseases, of skepticism in regard to the physician's ability to intervene and change the course of most diseases, of respect for the healing powers of nature."[2] Our history suggests that we have had periods where our health beliefs

---

1   Mercury chloride
2   Morris Vogel and Charles Rosenberg, *The Therapeutic Revolution: Essays in the Social History of American Medicine* (Philadelphia: University of Pennsylvania Press, 1979), 15.

changed and we no longer thought of healing as a need to stick our hand into a fire but realized that the healing warmth and beauty of the fire could be had without having to actually stick our hand into the flame. Heat, power, and fire are a matter of degree. While some herbs such as mustard (*Brassica alba*) and cayenne (*Capsicum frutescens*) certainly have the ability to scorch the body inside and out, the power of herbal remedies is, in general, different from the biomedical.

Gentle is defined as "free from harshness; kind; delicate."[3] The delicate expression of symmetria and beauty in the plant world is powerful. Colors, shapes, and structures are often intensely engaging. Tasting a plant can be a powerful experience for a person. The gentleness of a healing plant's presence and its healing action is its gift. Herbal medicine is living medicine. Each plant contributes its gentle, powerful essence to the healing relationship. People are often well aware of the healing powers of plants. Yet the gentle but powerful properties of plants sometimes elude those in biomedical science:

In the developed world, the active constituents of medicinal plants are of major importance; plant extracts are of minor importance as drugs. It is known that ca. 119 drugs of known structure are still extracted from higher plants and are used globally in allopathic medicine … 10-15% of the 250,000 species of flowering plants on the planet have been used medicinally. However, only a fraction of these are of sufficient importance to be considered as candidates as registration as drugs in developing countries based on widespread and continuous use and with some type of experimental confirmation of their biological activities.[4]

Healing plants often defy human science and drug development. To appreciate their power, their *fire*, one must enter *their* subtle world.

Plants, like humans, are all unique. The face of one pansy (*Viola tricolor*)

3   Merriam-Webster, *Merriam-Webster's Collegiate Dictionary*, 10th ed. (Springfield, MA: Merriam-Webster, 1999).
4   Norman Farnsworth, Preclinical Assessment of Medicinal Plants. In Shigeaki Baba, Olayiwola Akerele, and Yuji Kawaguchi, "Natural Resources and Human Health: Plants of Medicinal and Nutritional Value. Proceedings of the 1st WHO Symposium on Plants and Health for All: Scientific Advancement, Kobe, Japan. August 1991," (Amsterdam: Elsevier, 1992), 87.

is not the same as another. The exquisite violet buds of the paw-paw tree (*Asimina triloba*) are shaped differently than the buds of the fig (*Ficus carica*). How fortunate we are to have such partners who, like the St. John's Wort, are not only ready to help and heal but actively seek opportunity to connect with the human domain. Seeds ride on our pant legs and flowers appear in our dreams. The thorns of a rose let us know that the most etheric beauty in the plant world is often protected in this dimension and often surrounded in mystery. *Urtica doica*, commonly known as "stinging" nettle, is a plant that reminds us that receiving the fire—the benefits of a medicinal plant—is still a mystery to scientists[5] and comes with a price that, in the case of nettle, is a sting to remember. If we are to receive the chlorophyll, carotene, and vitamin C stored in the nettle leaf and experience its antihistamine action, we must know how to approach it, how to handle its stinging leaves, and how to make medicine with it.

The price for partnering with nettle and all healing plants is knowledge and a caring heart. We must have knowledge about the plants with which we partner and a caring heart that desires to use that knowledge for the healing of humanity. Knowledge and a caring heart are the keys that open the door to plant partnerships and the release of healing light. This may seem like a simple commonsense maxim, but the stark reality is that people, particularly those who live in industrialized rural and urban society, often think that they have knowledge of the healing properties of a plant when, in fact, all they have is *access* to that plant. That access may be a description of someone else's knowledge of a plant documented in a book or journal. It may be a ground-up leaf stuffed into a capsule. A person can have access or an invitation to ingesting and applying herbs in many forms and in many ways, some of which have no connection whatsoever to traditional, time-honored usage. A person may never have to go into the woods, be stung by a nettle, or grow their own plant medicines to receive some healing benefit from the green world. Greater access to herbs potentially means lesser knowledge of the healing plant itself. It is the responsibility of the nurse-herbalist who espouses holism to ensure the presence of the fiery element—knowledge and conscious awareness of the living plant—in the care and comfort of clients.

The fiery dimension of holistic care begins with the development

---

5   Varro Tyler, *The Honest Herbal* (New York: Haworth Press, 1993), 223.

of knowledge and a caring heart that would use this knowledge for healing humanity safely and efficaciously. To have knowledge of a plant means that the nurse-herbalist knows a plant's botanical and common names, where it grows, its physical characteristics, its smell and taste, how and when it is harvested, and how it is best applied in care and comfort. Knowledge of a plant also includes being with the plant in its habitat in the wild or in the garden. My most important knowledge and understanding of plants has occurred in relationship with the living plant. It is in relationships with plants that our "medicine" is made. The medicine of the healer is within. Access to a plant is only the first step in the development of the nurse-herbalist's medicine within. Knowledge of a heartfelt relationship to the plant leads to the development of the nurse-herbalist's unique medicine. Every nurse-herbalist has the potential to bring new knowledge of healing plants to their clients because their relationship with a plant or many plants is unique. To read about plant medicines and apply them in care is simply not sufficient. Medicine is made because the nurse-herbalist has first-hand knowledge and a heart connection with the plant with which s/he partners. This is *best* practice.

EVALUATING BEST PRACTICE

Best practice in nurse-herbalism is identified through consistent and thorough evaluation over time. Evaluation is the fifth step in the nursing process in which the nurse-herbalist compares the change or transformation of client behavior against their assessment and goals. Goals and interventions are then adapted based on the evaluation. Best practices in nurse-herbalism are developed with knowledge of medicinal plants as well as caring interventions of practitioners and supportive research. The nurse-herbalist can glean plant knowledge from many sources, including the experience and teachings of traditional healers and herbalists as well as the publications, teachings, and products of plant science specialists, such as pharmacognosists and ethnobotanists.

The herbalist, now sometimes referred to interchangeably as either a clinical or medical herbalist, studies some of the same theories of plant medicine as physicians and other scientists. Although some herbalists' roles in a community may be similar to that of a shaman or traditional healer, many herbalists study medicinal plants both from the perspective of the science of the time and the cultural traditions of the use of a particular medicinal plant. They often value and make decisions about which plant medicine they will use with a client based on both viewpoints. For example, the *Materia Medica* of the traditional Chinese herbalist contains information not only about the energetic qualities of the herb, such as whether the herb moves "qi" or drains dampness, but also contains information about laboratory data, such as the antibacterial or antifungal activity of an herb and what type of organism is affected by its activity *in vitro*. Herbalists also use medical language comprising terms applied by physicians and nurses.

Pharmacognosy is defined by some as the science of "descriptive pharmacology dealing with crude drugs and simples."[6] It is the study of natural drugs and their constituents. Pharmacognosists focus on plants as a source for the development of pharmaceutical drugs. They attempt to identify and isolate a single active principle from which a synthetic copy can be replicated. Some pharmacognosists also cross train in ethnobotany.

The ethnobotanist studies the relationships of people and plants. Ethnobotanists research "the way people incorporate plants into their cultural traditions, religions, and cosmologies," which leads to a greater understanding of the people themselves.[7] Ethnobotanists often study indigenous peoples' use of medicinal plants. One of the oldest forms of ethnobotanical research is the search for new drugs among the plants used in traditional practices. In the United States, Canada, and Western Europe, there is a "one in four chance that a medicine contains an active ingredient derived from a plant. ... 89 plant-derived drugs currently prescribed in the industrialized world were discovered by studying folk knowledge."[8] Ethnobotanists are key players in the conservation of plant biodiversity and indigenous plant wisdom.

Since early history, ethnobotanists of many cultures have recorded

---

6 Merriam-Webster, *Merriam-Webster's Collegiate Dictionary*.
7 Michael Balick and Paul Alan Cox, *Plants, People, and Culture: The Science of Ethnobotany* (New York: Scientific American Library, 1996), 4.
8 Ibid., 25.

the plants used for healing purposes. Historical writings and recordings such as the Ebers papyrus of the Egyptians, the *Shen Nung* of the Chinese, and the *Caraka Samhita* (the Sanskrit medical writing of India) have been results of the work of ethnobotanists of the day. Today, in addition to their observation and recording skills, ethnobotanists use the modern techniques and technology of the molecular biologist and the chemist to answer questions related to the behavior of plants, the human behavioral response to plants, and the relationship of people and plants. Many of the drugs administered by nurses today, such as aspirin *(Filipendula ulmaria)*, codeine *(Papaver somniferum)*, quinine *(Cinchona pubescens)*, and vincristine *(Catharanthus roseus)*, exist as a result of the tremendous successes of ethnobotanical researchers. Ethnobotanists go beyond simple observation in the charting of the various plants used in a particular culture and searching for what man can take from the plant world in the form of drugs. They are scientists who "walk" between both the scientific world and the world of the people and their healers, often serving as translators for both realms.

When I first began to formalize my practice of nurse-herbalism in 1989, I was working as a nurse in what today would be identified as an integrative care group practice. One of my roles was to work with horticulturalists to oversee the growth and harvesting of herbs grown on the farm. We had fields strewn with red clover and row-cropped areas of valerian *(Valeriana officinalis)*, borage *(Borago officinalis)*, and calendula *(Calendula officinalis)*. We also had a large greenhouse and a formal landscaped garden in the shape of a clock in which our "mother" herb plants were grown on one of the twelve clock segments associated with twelve astrological signs. Placement of the plants was chosen per Culpeper's classification of the herb according to astrological sign. I also oversaw the production of herb processing in the farm's food processing plant. I studied the science and art of high-volume herb production. My favorite memory was harvesting rows of valerian root on a rainy day when I had no staff and had to meet a production deadline. It was just me and two long rows of valerian.

Valerian taught me that fresh root is sweet and a little spicy. I smelled it all day through the gentle rain because it is that powerful. I felt its sedating effects after a few hours of handling and smelling the roots and flowers. But, like its stalks that were quite straight and tall, I had no problem staying upright. I was gently sedated, calm, and also somewhat nauseated from the heavy sweetness of the smell. A few years later, when I was a hotline service director at the Herb Research Foundation in Colorado, people would call the hotline stating that they were worried that their valerian capsules had gone "bad." They reported, as is well known in herbal community, that dried valerian root smells like dirty socks. But my valerian from that harvest never did and never has smelled like dirty socks. I still have some stored in a special place. My hypothesis is that valerian harvested in the gentle rain may release its sweetness for longer periods of time than that harvested in the drying sun. I have no scientific evidence but I do have some dried roots that still smell beautiful and inviting that I do not need to put in capsules.

Valerian[9] is also quite warming energetically. People who take the herb biomedically as a supplement often do so because they cannot sleep, but they would do better to try a cooling plant like chamomile. Inability to sleep is often caused by heat (imbalance) patterns that a warming plant would aggravate. In many herbalists' experience, including my own, some clients report that valerian causes a paradoxical effect in that it seems to act as a stimulant instead of a relaxant. It usually poses no health threat, just minor discomfort similar to strong coffee. Some traditional texts do identify valerian as a cerebral stimulant even while recognizing its sedative effects.[10] Working with valerian, and all healing plants, nurse-herbalists such as pharmacognosists, ethnobotanists, and herbalists become aware of the *complexity* of living medicine. People can respond to herbal remedies differently because their energetic patterns are unique. Also, the climate, soil conditions, altitude, and other growing conditions can greatly influence the power of the herbal remedy. The *consciousness* or awareness of the grower, harvester, and producer also influences the quality of the plant medicine. Some plants, like valerian, have a long history of highly attentive growers who consider the plant special and even sacred.

Spikenard, a precious aromatic oil used in Egyptian and Eastern

9 The name "valerian" is derived from the Latin *valere*, meaning "to be well." Valerian is a perennial and likes to grow in moist environments and is often found along streams, in damp meadows, and woodlands. Valerian can grow to a height of 2 to 5 feet (0.6 to 1.5 meters).
10 Harvey Wickes Felter and John Uri Lloyd, *King's American Dispensatory*, 18th ed., 3d rev ed. (Sandy, OR: Eclectic Medical Publications, 1983).

civilizations in spiritual practices such as anointing, comes from a plant *(Nardostachys jatamansi)* that is a close relative of valerian. According to legend, valerian was discovered by St. Panteleimon and has been revered in Russia for its calming properties for two thousand years.[11] The root was highly regarded for its healing properties by ancient Greeks and Romans, who considered it a powerful sedative. One of valerian's many uses in European folklore has been as a homemade cough syrup in which the root is boiled with licorice, raisins, and aniseed. This expectorant is for those that are short winded and have a cough. It helps to open the passages and to expectorate phlegm easily. In addition to being taken as a single herb, valerian works synergistically with chamomile *(Matricaria recutita)*, hops *(Humulus lupulus)*, and lemon balm *(Melissa officinalis)* to produce a calming effect. Valerian preparations are still a widely used nonprescription hypnotic and daytime sedative. It does not promote addiction and can be used during withdrawal from benzodiazepines with the guidance of knowledgeable health practitioners.

The nurse-herbalist's consciousness and carefulness lead to development of knowledge and a caring heart and nurture the integrative insight that can emerge from entering into the complexity of living plant medicines. Herbal remedies may be gentle and simple chalices for healing energy in their whole forms as teas and topicals, but they should not be construed as simplistic. All changes and transformations from partnerships with plants such as valerian are evaluated in the client within the fiery context of consciousness, carefulness, and complexity. It is from within this context that I have developed the following 10-point guideline for best practice in nurse-herbalism:

1. Know the plant. It is best to grow the plant with which you partner or have observed it and harvested it in its natural habitat over all seasons for a year. It is best to apply a plant medicinally only if someone has introduced you to the plant and shared their understanding and experience partnering with a given plant.

2. Use simples first. Start with culinary herbs. Very small

---

11 Igor Zevin, *A Russian Herbal: Traditional Remedies for Health and Healing* (Rochester, VT: Healing Arts Press, 1997).

amounts of herbs are used in cooking and beverage teas. They are common and yet their medicinal applications are rarely noticed by the public. *How* a plant is applied is what distinguishes it as "medicine" from food.

3. If an herb is applied according to traditional use, know the cultural context for that tradition. Traditional herb use typically refers to whole-plant applications.

4. If an herb is applied according to biomedical use, particularly as an alternative medicine to allay disease process, know the biomedical/clinical research on the whole plant or its constituents.

5. It is preferable to integrate both traditional and biomedical/clinical evidence when deciding how, when, where, and why to apply a plant in practice.

6. Learn how to formulate herbal remedies for a specific client need. This is discussed later on in this chapter and in Chapter 7.

7. Work with whole-plant applications as much as possible. In doing so, you will receive the benefit of a momentum of best practice embedded in nursing tradition.

8. Use herbal supplements rarely. Do not sell herbal supplement products. Instead, develop a relationship with a local pharmacist or health food store that can carry the products you recommend.

9. Growing and supplying the whole herbs you recommend in practice to clients is a quality control practice. It is best to grow them organically and test their quality occasionally by sending samples to a laboratory that does thin-layer chromatography.

10. Be mindful and scientific when including plants in the nursing process. Documenting observations and outcomes helps in the process of organizing experiences with plants into a body of knowledge that can be shared with other clients and clinicians.

Nurse-herbalism is rooted in knowledge developed at the nexus of the art and science of plant partnerships and applications along with nursing care within the social context of legal, ethical, and personal-professional standards of the *Five Rights* of best practice. The abilities of plants like stinging nettle and valerian to heal and the nurse-herbalist to facilitate that healing are evaluated within the framework of the five rights.

FIVE RIGHTS OF NURSE-HERBALISM

The rest of the chapter is organized according to the five rights of nurse-herbalism. These will be familiar to practicing nurses as congruent with the five rights of drug administration in nursing: Right Herb, Right Route, Right Time, Right Dose, and Right Person. There is one major difference between applying the five rights in nurse-herbalism and administering pharmaceutical drugs. In conventional practice the nurse, unless s/he is an advanced practice nurse working under prescriptive authority law, applies the five rights when administering the drugs prescribed by another practitioner. In nurse-herbalism, the remedy is created by the nurse-herbalist and administered most often by the client. The five rights of nurse-herbalism are applied when creating a remedy, teaching the client about that remedy, or actually administering the remedy to the client. These five rights can be utilized to evaluate conscious, careful practice.

The five rights promote a depth of knowledge in nurse-herbalism that leads to a "fire" of practice precision. My definition of quality care is precision. There is nothing more gratifying than providing care and comfort to a person or family with the right plant or formulation, at the right time, in the exact right amount, and as the perfect application. I am a minimalist and find great pleasure in providing care in which I can partner with plants and clients to identify the precise, that is, the smallest amount of herb, the fewest herbs, the fewest applications, and the shortest length of time for that application that must be used in client care that will achieve the goals we have established. Precision can lead to cost savings, plant conservation, fewer adverse effects, and improved client connection with the plant world. I am never just satisfied with knowledge of how to assess a client and how to apply herbs in comfort and care. The desire for greatest precision in herbal application has led me to a scientific exploration of the integration of the two. It is the fire of the heart and a dedicated vision of precision in the five rights that leads to the possibility of integrative insights in nurse-herbalism.

The fire element is under-utilized in holistic practice. It is easy to become satisfied with plant understanding associated with the first three elements: earth-physical, air-mental, and water-emotional. We can create beautiful healing environments, welcome the plants, learn about herbs, and apply them with caring hands and thoughtful communication. But to bring the fire element into practice and heal through transformation and transmutation with plants as partners, the nurse-herbalist must cultivate the fire of the spirit. Helena Roerich, an early twentieth-century spiritual writer and founder of the Agni Yoga Society[12], wrote of fire:

> The element of Fire, the most all-pervading, the most creative, the most life-bearing, is least observed and esteemed. The human consciousness concerns itself with a multitude of empty and insignificant considerations, but the most wonderful of all escapes it. … Much that has been told about the heart must also be applied to the Fiery World, but with particular acuteness. The impetus of Fire is as strong as the structure of a crystal. … Live embers are needed for the purification of the consciousness; the rainbow flame affirms the striving of the spirit. A multitude of applications of the work of Fire reveal themselves as the most striking conditions of existence. Beginning with the ordinary light formations visible to the open eye, up to the complex fires of the heart, we are led into the realm of the Fiery World.[13]

The fire element is reflected in the consciousness and awareness of the nurse-herbalist. Fire and consciousness are demonstrated by nurse-

---

12 Helena Roerich defines yoga as that "supreme bridge to cosmic attainment." Agni yoga is "a path not of physical disciplines, meditation, or asceticism—but of practice in daily life. It is the yoga of fiery energy, of consciousness, of responsible, directed thought. It teaches that the evolution of the planetary consciousness is a pressing necessity and that, through individual striving, it is an attainable aspiration for mankind." http://www.agniyoga.org/ay_info.html

13 Helena Roerich, *Fiery World 1* (New York: Agni Yoga Society, http://www.agniyoga.org/ay_frame.html?app_id=FW1, 1933).

herbalists in the precision of their plant partnerships, in their attention to detail when creating and applying herbal applications, in their love for a client that transcends basic professional duty, and in relationship with the laws of the land and the laws of being—human and plant manifest in the five rights.

Right Plant

In order to safely and effectively adhere to the five rights, nurse-herbalists become well acquainted with the plants they use in practice. A basic education in herbalism typically includes the didactic study and tasting of hundreds of plants over the course of months to years as well as clinical application experiences while under the guidance of a master herbal teacher. Acquiring depth and breadth of knowledge and experience with a particular plant or plants and their uses as healing remedies is one way that nurse-herbalists demonstrate their level of expertise. Nurse-herbalists must be able to scientifically discuss why an herb or formula of herbs is suggested in the care of a particular client and evaluate the effect of the herb in transforming client behaviors and health patterns.

There are many factors affecting a client's patterns. Being able to clearly identify the "rightness" or effectiveness of an herb requires one to be able to connect the herb and any change in pattern or behavior. Data from all five rights converge to create an understanding of changes in pattern. One way to evaluate the rightness of an herb is to introduce the herb and document a change in pattern. For example, the nurse-herbalist might recommend a cup of cool peppermint tea for a client with fever who was experiencing the heat of the fever in their head. The client might report the heat and accompanying discomfort as a 10 on a scale of 1 to 10 with 10 being the most discomfort and 1 being little discomfort. After drinking the tea, the client reports that the heat is a 3 and the discomfort "manageable." If the client continues to drink peppermint tea during the fever with similar results, then the nurse may conclude that the herb seems to be the "right" herb.

Another way to evaluate the rightness of an herb is to remove that herb. In the example of the client with fever, one might substitute plain water for a few hours instead of peppermint tea and note any change in fever. Over many years, I have scientifically confirmed that people who experience fever in their head feel better when drinking peppermint tea. But not everyone likes peppermint tea. Despite my evidence, I still practice according to the model of care discussed in this book. When practitioners, scientists, or the public call into question the validity of traditional evidence related to herbs such as peppermint tea, I often suggest that they try a cup of tea the next time they have a fever. The potential benefit of simple herbal applications often outweighs the risk.

Weighing the Benefits and Risks

Health decisions are made through an evaluative process of weighing the benefits and risks of an action. People's decisions to employ means other than biomedical interventions in the care and comfort of themselves and their families are rarely the result of a lack of education or comprehension or ignorance of orthodox medicine as the "best" care. Research shows that this assumption about people's decisions to use complementary or alternative medicine strategies to biomedicine is a stereotype designed to maintain the values of an official worldview.[14] There are also extensive studies demonstrating that even people who have access to and knowledge of biomedical interventions choose therapies other than biomedicine.[15] My historical research shows that people often choose herbs. My experience is that they choose herbs for many reasons, but in general they choose herbs because they have weighed the benefits and risks of different interventions and they prefer to use what nurses refer to as the "least invasive" treatment first.

Nurses can understand people's needs for simpler, less invasive solutions. People do not want to do more harm in the process of solving their health problems. It is almost instinctual for them to want to bring about greater balance in their lives. The nurse-herbalist supports the decision-making process by providing information and herbal opportunities that encourage an informed choice in care based upon

---

14 Bonnie O'Connor, *Healing Traditions: Alternative Medicine and the Health Professions* (Philadelphia: University of Pennsylvania Press, 1995).

15 Lowell S. Levin and Ellen L. Idler, *The Hidden Health Care System* (Farmville, NC: Golden Apple Publications, 2010).

the fullest understanding possible of the benefits and risks. Safety is a concept that can be oversimplified, leading to gross generalizations. As discussed in previous chapters, the nurse-herbalist offers perspectives on health patterns and plants, a skill that the public does not necessarily have. They weigh the benefits and risks of certain interventions but can benefit greatly from a nursing professional who can put the picture together with them.

Some people in their assessment of benefit and risk find that herbs are historically gentler medicine; however, this does not mean that they are without risk. The nurse-herbalist's attention to the five rights and timing, type, and tuning can really help the client determine risk at the moment of decision. When making health decisions, nurse-herbalists help their clients put benefits and risks of partnering with plants in context. For example, if a client just sustained a laceration to a hand, direct pressure is the least invasive intervention for stopping bleeding. Direct pressure and elevation of the limb (i.e. First Aid) is an accessible and inexpensive treatment. Suturing may be needed but is not the first concern. Herbs may be helpful for wound healing but they are not the first concern, either.

Clients weigh benefits and risks and make logical choices, but they don't always make the best decisions about herb use. I once had a community client who cut her finger. She worked in a vegetarian restaurant and knew about the healing as well as nutritional qualities of seaweeds. She knew that seaweeds can help stop bleeding. When she cut her finger, she wrapped it in seaweed. Unfortunately the cut was very severe and she did not really apply direct pressure. The blood pooled and coagulated under the seaweed as expected but, without pressure, the skin did not knit together at all. After a number of hours, she sought nursing care. The wound could not be sutured right away because there were so many tiny pieces of seaweed in the wound that we were concerned about infection. Infection is a big concern with a hand injury. So we weighed the benefits and risks of care and decided to soak off the seaweed bandage so that the laceration could be sutured as much as possible.

Although the client's understanding of seaweed's action was correct—that is, she was not ignorant or uneducated about herbs—she did not, in our estimation, realize the seriousness of her hand laceration. Herbs were not the best first choice in this acute-care scenario. I have many more examples of clients with acute and chronic illness, pain, and general discomforts in which herbs have been extremely valuable and safe, especially when compared to the risks associated with long-term use of pharmaceutical drugs or invasive surgeries. Nurse-herbalists are careful and thoughtful in their application of herbs and are often in positions where they can educate the public, too, about proper precautions. I recommend that nurse-herbalists utilize decision trees when triaging acute-care situations. There are wonderful books such as *Take Care of Yourself* and *Take Care of Your Child* that can be used in practice. I worked with Dr. Vickery, one of the authors of these books, in his company called Health Decisions in the 1990s. Dr. Vickery was a researcher on self-care at the National Institutes of Health Center for Disease Prevention and Health Promotion. He was expert in teaching the public about benefits and risks related to health decisions without instilling fear.

I do not subscribe to the fear tactics that I often read and hear from biomedical practitioners and nurses about herbs or any therapy including drugs and surgeries. Instead I support health pluralism and the notion that given the benefits and risks of a specific situation, any of these treatments may be best practice at a particular point in time. The nurse-herbalist determines the rightness of herbal applications based on the five rights and a thorough assessment.

Nurses are accustomed to working with the strong medicines and therapies of the biomedical world and must be careful not to describe herbs through the same lens. Cautions should first and foremost be based on knowledge of the medicinal plant. Biomedical and traditional healers alike give cautionary information related to the use of plants. For example, a nurse or physician might warn that excessive ingestion of comfrey (*Symphytum officinale*) can potentially lead to hepatotoxicity because of the amount of pyrrolizidine alkaloids, a constituent within the plant. A traditional healer might recommend that a particular healing plant be harvested only in a special area.

Nurse-herbalists must be aware of the wise and safe use of the types of plants that grow in their area. Many plant medicines have been used traditionally within the ritual practices of a particular society for centuries. The cautions related to the use of the plant may change as the information about the medicinal use of a particular plant is transmitted across cultures. Because plants and their specific cautionary issues vary greatly from place to place, the cautions presented here are general guidelines related to the use of plant therapies. Safety cannot be completely ensured even under the best of circumstances. Children of responsible parents still run out in the road, campfires get out of control, and, despite safety strategies put in place by communities and the good intentions of well-meaning people, properly-prescribed medicines still cause illness and death.

People and practitioners who partner with plants responsibly must be aware of safety considerations and the benefits and risks associated with an herb. The regulation of tobacco (*Nicotiana tobaccum*) products is just one example of why we must not rely solely upon external safety standards, guidelines, and agencies to direct health care decisions. Biomedicine may have evidence of a particular plant substance being helpful in laboratory studies, but this does not mean that an individual will benefit from the use of that plant. The response of a person to any healing intervention or modality, such as herbs, is unique. Laboratory and clinical studies provide general information, but the practitioner and the client must always be mindful of the potential for a unique response to an herbal application. Nurse-herbalists and their clients who are cautious with healing plants access their inner wisdom, insight, and common sense in choosing to partner with plants.

As a healing modality, plant therapies have been shown through scientific study and hundreds of years of traditional use to be quite safe. "Based on published reports, side effects or toxic reactions associated with herbal medicines in any form are rare. ...Clearly, then, herbal medicines do not present any more of a problem with respect to acting as potential allergenic agents following human ingestion than any other class of widely used foods or drugs."[16] Herb safety is related, however, to the use of the plant and the knowledge base of the user. Potential risks are associated with using plants as ornaments, let alone as foods and medicines. If someone were walking in the woods and thought stinging nettle were perfect for an arrangement of wild flowers, they would be surprised when they touched the leaf. The plant causes, just as its common name implies, a stinging sensation to the skin when touched.

---

16 Norman Farnsworth, "Relative Safety of Herbal Medicines," *Herbalgram*, no. 29 (1993).

Although traditionally, people have not been known to pick nettle for ornamental reasons, there is a possibility it could happen. The concern, and sometimes the conflict, between the scientists and the people is how safe use with nettle or any herb is addressed. How extensive should the controls on a plant be? Should all stinging nettle be exterminated because of its potential to sting a hiker in the woods? How do communities and governments make decisions to protect the public from the potential harm from plants, and how great is the risk from plants, really? It is the responsibility of every individual using a plant as medicine and therapy to exercise prudent care. This includes using a commonsense approach to taking herbs and understanding that the complexity of whole plants is a safety feature of herbalism.

Whole-herb applications also have a history of few to no adverse effects when used according to tradition. Herbs can also have significantly better outcomes when applied holistically in the right client, at the right time, in the right way. This is determined by assessment and pattern recognition. For example, I recently had a client who had a wound resulting from multiple surgeries that would not heal. Her surgeons were at a loss as to how to heal the wound that was weeping and causing her to be anemic. She used an herbal salve that we determined through assessment, counseling, and imagery work was best for her. After one week, the wound, which she had for more than one year, was healed. She was elated not only at the disappearance of the wound but because of the fullness of understanding of her body's healing wisdom she had received in the process of holistic nursing care.

The purpose of legal regulation is to promote the safest use of the substance as possible. It has been proposed that the safety of a medicinal plant not be judged based on information from one source. "Safety or efficacy of a particular drug can rarely be based upon the results of a single study. In contrast, a combination of information indicating that a specific plant has been used in a local health care system for centuries, together with efficacy and toxicity data can help in deciding whether it should be considered acceptable for medicinal use."[17] The World Health Organization (WHO) recommends that member states adopt some

---

17 Norman Farnsworth and others, "Medicinal Plants in Therapy," *Bulletin of the World Health Organization* 63, no. 6 (1985): 965.

form of regulation of herbal medicines to address issues of quality, safety, and efficacy. Regulation does not have to be for purposes of control of behavior of people; it also can be established for educational purposes.

Nurses often educate clients about safety issues in the home. Each year, several poisonings in which children have ingested the leaves of a house plant are reported to poison control centers; yet, there are no regulations banning people from acquiring house plants. Instead, pediatric health practitioners inform parents of the potential safety issues with house plants so that they are more aware and can put the plants out of the reach of little explorers.

Some of the guidelines presented by WHO regarding the regulation of herbal medicines have to do with assessment of use of herbs and herbal products, evaluation of manufacturing procedures and product labeling, assessment and evaluation of toxic plant materials, and the establishment of a government agency to keep records on herbal medicines in use.[18] The regulation of herbal medicines varies from country to country. Some countries exempt herbal and traditional medicines from regulatory requirements; some are subject to all requirements. Some countries exempt herbal medicines regarding registration and marketing authorization and some require registration.[19] Canada, for instance, has a system whereby the Health Protection Branch of Health Canada regulates plant medicines under its Food and Drug protectorates. It assigns drug identification numbers to an herb based on the therapeutic claims. Nurses should contact their regulatory agencies to learn more about their countries' laws regarding the safe use of herbs.

Some areas in nursing, for instance, surgical nursing, have been especially concerned about the safety and control of herbal medicines. Nurses who work in preanesthesia and postanesthesia units are particularly concerned about the interactions of herbal medicines and anesthetic drugs. This is not a new concern. In 1998, a report published in the *British Medical Journal* stated that solanaceous glycoalkaloids found in potatoes, tomatoes, and aubergines [eggplant] may slow the metabolism of muscle relaxants and anesthetic agents such as suxamethonium and

18 World Health Organization, "Guidelines for the Appropriate Use of Herbal Medicines," in *WHO Regional Publications* (Geneva 1998).
19 ———, "Regulatory Situation of Herbal Medicine," (Geneva 1998).

cocaine.[20] Thus the client may take five to ten hours recovering from anesthesia rather than the expected forty to ninety minutes. These are foods, but there is a similar concern with herbal medicines.

While nurses and other perioperative health care team members have begun to ask about the herbs that clients may be taking before surgery, what nurses and health care team members should do with the information they gather is not clear. If a client is taking an herbal formula prescribed by a traditional healer, does the nurse tell the client to stop taking the herbs, and if so, what effect might that have on the outcome of the surgery? Should clients be told to stop taking their herbal remedies used in self-care two weeks before surgery? Will that take care of the potential problem? These kinds of questions present nurses and perioperative team members with an opportunity to use an integrative approach. From an integrative perspective, the practitioner would not simply tell a client to stop taking an herb. The herb may have significant meaning to the client's health and well-being.

The benefits and risks and the timing of all interventions, surgery, and herbs need to be discussed with the individual client. They must be informed that their caregivers do not have all the answers about potential anesthetic drug and herb or food interactions. In light of the statistics on adverse reactions and deaths related to properly prescribed and administered drugs in hospitals, health team members must address the herb-drug interaction carefully, considerately, and integratively.

Is Herbalism Nursing Practice?

It is the premise of this book that herbalism *is* nursing. It is the science and art of nursing. Herbalism is not a complementary therapy to nursing. Partnering with plants holds the same status as touch in nursing care. While Therapeutic Touch or Shiatsu may be complementary therapies used by nurses in practice, touch is nursing practice. Aromatherapy, the application of essential oils—a plant constituent— may be a complementary therapy, but herbalism, particularly whole-plant herbalism, is nursing practice. Applying herbs in the care and

---

20 Janice Tanne, "Food and Drugs Alter Response to Anesthesia," *BMJ: British Medical Journal* 317, no. 7166 (1998).

comfort of clients is nursing practice that has endured over the centuries. Contemporary nurse-herbalist practice is not unlike the practice of the eighteenth-century Daughters of Charity nurses. The nurses who also held the role of "pharmacists" made their own herbal medicines for use in clients with health problems from colds to cancer.[21] They made sure that the herbal remedies were from reputable sources, prepared correctly, and administered to the proper client in the correct way. In other words, the early nurses adhered to "the five rights." The early French Daughters of Charity typically chose the right herbs to apply in the care of their clients under the tutelage of knowledgeable caregivers such as the foundress Louise de Marillac, whose spiritual writings contain numerous herbal prescriptions used by the nurses.[22] Practice was defined by those who held the knowledge in community.

Today, nursing practice is defined by a governing body. In the United States, each state's Board of Registered Nurses (BRN) is charged with the protection of public safety. The National Council of State Boards of Nursing's (NCSBN) stated mission is to provide "education, service, and research through collaborative leadership to promote evidence-based regulatory excellence for patient safety and public protection."[23] Boards of Nursing protect the public and maintain professional standards. To do so, they are authorized by state statute to conduct disciplinary procedures to establish if a nurse or advanced practice nurse has violated the documented standards of practice known as the Nurse Practice Act (NPA). The NPA is a statute approved by each state and written by the BRN. It is used to guide practice. This statute is law and each nurse is required by that law to abide by it for the safety of the public. Each state has its own NPA. The standards of care documented in the NPA are derived from many sources. Standards of professional care are gleaned from professional organizations such as the American Nurses Association, the nursing literature, testimonies and court decisions, and professional

---

21 Martha Libster and Betty Ann McNeil, *Enlightened Charity: The Holistic Nursing Care, Education and Advices Concerning the Sick of Sister Matilda Coskery, (1799-1870).* (Farmville, NC: Golden Apple Publications, 2009).

22 Louise Sullivan, *Spiritual Writings of Louise de Marillac: Correspondence and Thoughts.* (New York: New City Press, ed. and trans. 1991).

23 https://www.ncsbn.org/182.htm

recognitions of expertise in nursing practice, education, and research.

Some nurses complain about the vagueness of the NPA. Many have commented to me over the years that they wish that the NPA would be more specific in addressing herbalism. States sometimes make reference to dietary supplements, herbs, and other specific nursing interventions by name in their NPA, published white papers, or other guiding documents. But the NPA is often purposely written as a broader guide for professional practice that allows for nurses to exercise their professional judgment in the care of the unique client, family, or community. This is best for nurse-herbalism. In most NPAs, the nurse is required to have proper education and training for applying a specific intervention in practice. The nurse is also held to the standards of other specialists in similar situations. The nurse-herbalist, therefore, would be expected to abide by the foundational standards of nursing practice, have education in the application of herbs, and provide care that is consistent with others in the specialty of herbalism as defined by the experts in that field. This is reasonable.

In addition to being aware of the current state of professional scope of practice, nurse-herbalists should also be well informed as to their country's policies on herbs and herbal remedies. Many countries now have guidelines or position statements on the use of complementary therapies by the public as well as by professional practitioners. Some consider herbal remedies a "complementary therapy." In Australia, for example, the Royal College of Nursing and the Australian Nursing Federation have policies and several state nursing boards have guidelines for the integration of complementary therapies in nursing practice. All of the policies state that nurses must be appropriately qualified in a therapy when using it as a nursing intervention. Nurses in the United Kingdom must ensure that no nursing action is "detrimental to the interests, condition, or safety of clients."[24] Canadian studies have found that 71 percent of the public use "Natural Health Products" (NHPs include herbs) extensively in self-care practices[25] and therefore encourage nurses who work with clients using complementary therapies (CTs) and NHPs

---

24 As cited in Linda Nazarko, "The Therapeutic Uses of Cranberry Juice," *Nursing Standard* 9, no. 34 (1995): 34.

25 College & Association of Registered Nurses of Alberta, "Complementary and/or Alternative Therapy and Natural Health Products: Standards for Registered Nurses," (Edmonton, Alberta 2011).

to know their scope of practice, the policies of an employer regarding the CT or NHP, have competence to provide any CT in a safe and ethical manner and in the application of NHPs and CTs, and use their judgment to identify risks and expected outcomes.[26]

American reports often state that the U.S. Food and Drug Administration (FDA) does not regulate or approve dietary supplements such as herbs. The FDA does not regulate supplements *as drugs* but it is simply false that supplements and herbs are not regulated. Unfortunately, state boards often make their rules from the biomedical perspective alone—that herbs are drugs. Regulation issues will be discussed further in this chapter. Of greater concern is that some states have actually discussed and passed judgment on whether or not nurses can administer an herb prescribed by someone else.[27] The concern here is that herbs are nursing practice and therefore should not need to be prescribed. The practice of nurse-herbalism becomes distorted and complicated when ill-informed policy makers insist on treating the application of herbs as medical practice alone when in fact it is, by centuries of evidence, nursing practice as well. The remainder of this chapter addresses many of the issues associated with the five rights of nurse-herbalism that must be considered by a nurse anywhere in the world today who will deal with those who view nursing practice solely in terms of development of medical policy as separate from its historical context and current research base in nursing.

The information in this book does not replace the reader's own research into these issues of professional practice and standards. There are many arenas in which nursing is discussed as being at risk for dissolving into paraprofessional status. For nurse-herbalism to thrive, I highly recommend that nurses embrace the importance of upholding a standard of care through higher education and nursing research within their own specialty areas of practice. The role of the BRN is to protect the public; therefore, in creating a nurse-herbalist practice, consider how you can participate with your BRN in protecting the public. I recommend working closely with leadership in professional organizations both in nursing and in public groups that cultivate health freedoms and

---

26 Ibid., 4.
27 Mike Kelly and Becky Taylor, "Legislative Report: Other States' Policies Regarding Nurses Administering Prescribed Dietary Supplements," (Juneau, Alaska 2006).

pluralism, complementary therapies, and promotion of natural health care solutions. Going to a BRN by oneself is probably not the best strategy given the current level of knowledge about herbs in some states. I testified before a BRN, but that was a number of years ago.

On Oct. 13, 1993, I formally presented my "Proposal for the Integration of Traditional Chinese Herbal Science and Nursing Practice" to the BRN in Helena, Montana. I argued that herbalism was part of nursing practice and had been for centuries. I described the similarities in nursing and herbalist assessment by comparing and contrasting the Roy Model of Nursing assessment and an assessment sheet used in Traditional Chinese Herbal Medicine practice. I also demonstrated that the herbs used in nursing practice had LD_{50}'s[28] significantly higher than the caffeine in coffee that is commonly administered by nurses in hospital practice. The outcome was that I was asked why I "hadn't become a naturopath," at which point I reiterated that herbalism was nursing practice. I was also referred to the Director of the Naturopathic Board of the State who told me that what I was doing was fine. There was no interest, however, by the BRN in expanding knowledge and practice for a vital part of the profession. This event and others propelled me to write my first book on nurse-herbalism and also to conduct my doctoral research published as *Herbal Diplomats* on the history of American nurse-herbalism.

After nursing education moved into the hospital setting under the guidance of physicians and hospital administrators around 1873, the use of herbal remedies in nursing care began to dwindle. Part of the reason for this may be related to the fact that nurses, modeling their profession after medicine, desired to be paid more for their services than they had in the past. The use of herbs was often equated with self-care and domestic remedies and therefore it was harder to distinguish oneself as an "expert" who deserved to be paid as such. Physicians used fewer herbs in practice over time and nurses who worked in the biomedically dominant hospital sphere followed. There are remnants of nurse-herbalist practice in hospitals such as the use of the distillate of witch hazel (*Hamamelis viginiana*) on post-partum units for perineal swelling. More recently, documentation on nurse-herbalism can more

---

28 LD_{50} refers to Median Lethal Dose. For further information, see section in this chapter on Right Dose.

typically be found in the literature on nurse-midwifery practice.[29]

Nurses who wish to continue the herbal tradition in nursing should evaluate and document their cases thoroughly, publish outcomes and knowledge development in professional journals, and participate in education and textbook development as much as possible. Nursing textbooks that include content on herbalism are often not written by nurse-herbalists and are typically written only about herbal supplements rather than the whole-herb applications that represent the full scope of nurse-herbalist practice. Books on herbalism aimed at the nursing audience may never mention the topical applications of herbs in the care of clients that have been used for centuries. Nurses also must have an understanding of the laws regarding the use of various healing plants in their countries. Some medicinal plants are protected because they are at risk for extinction. Plants can become endangered because their habitats are threatened or because they are overused. This is especially a problem when the root or bark of the plant is the medicinal part sought.

Taking Orders

Historically, nurses have not asked permission to use herbs in their care of clients. They have known the right herb to use. It is well documented that it was common practice for nurses to use herbs in practice in all areas of nursing care and midwifery at least until approximately 1955.[30] The concept of "taking orders" from other health practitioners is a cultural construction. In the nineteenth century, the Shaker nurses, for example, took orders from physicians in their communities, but they also took orders from each other and from Shaker Elders. Sister Matilda Coskery wrote her orders for other nurses that she called "Advices" in the 1840s, documenting her professional expertise in nursing care of the mentally

---

29 Cindy Belew, "Herbs and the Childbearing Woman. Guidelines for Midwives," *Journal of Nurse-Midwifery* 44, no. 3 (1999); Barbara McFarlin and others, "A National Survey of Herbal Preparation Use by Nurse-Midwives for Labor Stimulation.," *Journal of Nurse-Midwifery* 44, no. 3 (1999); Kathleen Bunce, "The Use of Herbs in Midwifery," *Journal of Nurse-Midwifery* 32, no. 4 (1987); Eileen Ehudin-Pagano and others, "The Use of Herbs in Nurse-Midwifery Practice," *Journal of Nurse-Midwifery* 32, no. 4 (1987).

30 Martha Libster, *Herbal Diplomats: The Contribution of Early American Nurses (1830-1860) to Nineteenth- Century Health Care Reform and the Botanical Medical Movement* (Thornton, CO: Golden Apple Publications, 2004). Bertha Harmer and Virginia Henderson, *Textbook of the Principles and Practice of Nursing* (New York: Macmillan Co., 1955).

ill often with the support of herbs.[31] Nurses' practices of "taking orders" (verbal or written) and delegation are defined by the NPA. Typically, as NPAs are written broadly to allow for the professional autonomy of the registered nurse, the issues of order taking and delegation are written broadly. However, a few years ago in the state of Washington, which houses one of the largest and most prestigious naturopathic medical schools in the nation, the Washington NPA was amended to allow nurses to "take orders" from naturopathic physicians. Given the centuries-old history of the autonomous use of herbs in nursing practice, legislating taking orders for herbal remedies from a naturopath could be perceived within the context of nursing history as a significant backward step for nurse-herbalism.

Changing the NPA in Washington might be helpful in some cases, such as in a clinic where naturopathic physicians treat specific diseases and nursing care is needed. However, in the overall plan for formal integration of plant therapies in nursing practice, properly educated nurses are capable of independent application of plant therapies. When nurses pursue taking orders for herbs from naturopaths or other herbal practitioners rather than pursue their own plant therapies education and the protection of herbalism as scope of practice, a precedent is established that is not exactly congruent with nursing's heritage of healing. My preference is that nurses consider their important role in providing communities with access to consumer models of nurse-herbalist care at the very least and, at the very most, educate themselves in at least one plant that they can grow and know very well and partner with in the care and comfort of clients. One right plant remedy given at the right time in the right amount to the right person in the right way is often all that is needed in providing care for a whole list of health concerns.

Right Route

The second right—right route—has to do with the discernment of proper type of herbal application discussed in Chapter 5. The choice of application has to do with speed and specificity. Herbs are catalysts for

---

31 Libster and McNeil, *Enlightened Charity: The Holistic Nursing Care, Education and Advices Concerning the Sick of Sister Matilda Coskery, (1799-1870).* 158.

change. Ask yourself how quickly you want the herb to catalyze change and where you want the change to occur. I consider all applications equally from sublingual drops of alcohol extract (rapid catalyst) to footbaths (holographic absorption discussed further in Chapter 7). People generally discuss herbs as if they *should* be taken orally. In culinary use, this is true but not for medicinal purposes. As noted in Chapter 5, there are many effective ways of introducing the body to the healing action of a plant.

The reason so many nurses and other clinicians discuss oral application of herbs is because that is what they see on the market. The American herb industry produces oral remedies for the most part. There are a few inhalants and ear oils. One company sells castor oil with the pack materials to apply the remedy as an oil compress; but, for the most part, the industry sells capsules, pills, and liquid extracts. Part of this has to do with the influence of patent law on production choices. It also has to do with the fact that Americans as well as other industrialized societies prefer herbs in pill form like pharmaceutical drugs. Many people *want* herbs to be alternatives to pharmaceutical drugs. Therefore, thinking of herbal remedies as simply herbal remedies or what I refer to as "Gentle Medicine" does not always address the psychological need to have a substitute for drugs that will achieve the same result as a drug, look like a drug, and yet not have the adverse effects of the drug. As discussed previously, applying a remedy improperly can, over time, lead to adverse effects not unlike pharmaceutical drugs. A case in point is the improper use of ephedra (*Ephedra sinensis*).

Ephedra is a plant that has been in the Chinese *Materia Medica* for centuries. It is called Má Huáng and is classified as an herb that "releases the exterior." When a person has asthma symptoms, for example, they are unable to exhale. Ephedra opens the pores, releases the exterior, and facilitates the movement of the lung qi, allowing for the breath to descend. The person can exhale with the assistance of ephedra. However, ephedra is rarely, if ever, used as a simple or single herb in Chinese herbal medicine tradition. It is decocted with the other herbs in formulation. We have been informed through the media that there have been adverse effects from ephedra. But none of these reports that I have heard over the years has ever been about the proper, traditional use of ephedra as a tea for exterior wind pattern. They have been about the use of ephedra in weight loss or energy supplements. In some cases that I have looked more closely into, the herbal dietary supplements taken did not have whole-plant ephedra in them at all even though that was what was reported as being the "culprit." The supplement contained ephedrine, a constituent of the plant known to cause certain disturbing adverse effects as well as the speeding up of metabolism, which is the reason manufacturers have put the herb in their weight loss products. Few people have any idea of ephedra's important traditional use. But the media and the public called for its removal from the market, stating that the plant was "unsafe" when it was the people's applications that were unsafe. They were not using the right route.

Nurses understand the importance of identifying the risk and benefit ratio related to the route chosen for drug administration. Those same principles apply in herbalism. Oral doses of a plant are more "invasive" and therefore carry a greater potential for risk to client safety. Herbs that are applied topically are, for the most part, slower acting because they must enter the dermal barriers and therefore are typically not considered as great a risk. However, technology over the past few years has led to the invention of chemical and energetic means of creating "windows" in the skin that allow for more rapid uptake of drugs. Some of this topical application technology has been trickling into the supplement industry. I have spoken with R&D scientists who are creating botanical medicine "patches" for herbal weight loss products. When I was working in the group practice in Montana, I worked with electromagnetic devices to create a window in the skin so as to better treat conditions such as muscle tension with sound wave. I also developed a number of protocols for using the same technology to deliver topical herbal remedies.

The most important safety question for the nurse-herbalist is this: "Can I achieve the result the client and I seek through least invasive means?" Even within the category of oral remedies, there are some that carry more risk. A tea poses less risk than does a standardized extract in a capsule for two reasons. First, the tea is tasted. Often teas prepared for medicinal applications do not taste like beverage teas. They are often more bitter, sour, pungent, and just downright strange for a client when they try to compare their formulated tea with the teas sold in restaurants and food stores. There is an adage in Chinese herbal medicine that if the tea formula for a person is correct, they will actually crave that formula despite its repugnant taste. In more than 20 years of practice, I have witnessed this to be exactly the case. Tea application is one of the safety features of traditional herbal medicine practice. If a person does not like the taste, they will be more inclined to question the herbs they are ingesting and seek the guidance of a knowledgeable practitioner.

The question of least invasive means is also an ethical question related to the practice principle of doing no harm. While herbs are often gentler remedies than pharmaceutical drugs, there are still risks related to their improper use. Oral herbal applications, because of their predominance in society, can frequently be a mindless choice. Common sense dictates that the right route be considered.

Common Sense and Complexity

Having common sense is a very important component of one's ability to be cautious. Common sense is defined as "sound and prudent but often unsophisticated judgment."[32] Nurse-herbalists and the public do not need extensive formal herbal education to be able to reason about the right route for an herbal application. Common sense, if it is not repressed, can be helpful in determining the right herb, the right route, and the right dose. Common sense is demonstrated as an intuition or insight related to a particular experience. For example, if someone decided to eat cayenne pepper *(Capsicum frutescens)* to improve circulation, but they took it in capsule form, they could block one way that commonly has been used to measure dose—taste. Taste and other sensory experiences can activate one's common sense. If a person eats whole cayenne peppers and experiences the hot spicy taste of the herb, they would, at some point, say: "I think I've had enough."

Another example can be gleaned from the reports of the use of chaparral *(Larrea tridentata)*. I should mention here that I have never been formally introduced to this herb and do not use it in practice. I am referring to it here because of the reports in the literature. Chaparral has a very unpleasant taste. And yet the three people reported to experience

---

32 Merriam-Webster, *Merriam-Webster's Collegiate Dictionary.*

symptoms of liver toxicity related to chaparral ingestion took high doses of the herb in tablet or capsule form.[33] One could wonder what would have happened if the people had taken chaparral in tea form. Might they have not had the liver toxicity problems because they could have better regulated their intake based upon toleration of the taste of the herb? There is one clinical study of clients with terminal cancer who received 16 to 24 ounces of chaparral tea *(Larrea divericata)* per day and the participants who drank the tea did not show any signs of liver toxicity.[34] The difference in responses between the situations may have been due to the difference in route, tea versus powdered herb, or the dose. Common sense works best when the plant is experienced fully by the senses. Taste, smell, vision, and tactile sensation are all important to the proper identification of an herb and its safe use. Common sense is our own personal regulatory agency.

Complexity is one reason that herbal remedies applied through traditional routes such as teas and topicals have had such a long history of safe use. Plants have many different biochemical constituents. Used in whole form, whether decocted as tea or used as an extract or salve, the plant's action is more complex. Most of the chemical constituents occur in very small amounts. When we apply herbs, we are using small doses of particular substances. These substances are in a natural, not synthetic, state and are in formulation as they occur in nature. Many herbal remedies have been taken in their natural complex form over a lengthy period of time without toxicity or unhealthy effects. Safe use of a plant does not necessarily mean that it is effective, however. Safety and efficacy are separate issues.

Effectiveness is evaluated in relationship to the goals established by the client and their nurse-herbalist. The outcome of the application of the right herb according to a chosen route is evaluated by establishing whether or not a goal was achieved, and whether partially or fully. Continuing to apply an herb in a particular route when it is not effective

---

33 Dafna Gordon and others, "Chaparral Ingestion. The Broadening Spectrum of Liver Injury Caused by Herbal Medications," *JAMA : The Journal of the American Medical Association* 273, no. 6 (1995); "Chaparral-Induced Toxic Hepatitis--California and Texas, 1992," *MMWR. Morbidity and Mortality Weekly Report* 41, no. 43 (1992).

34 Charles Smart, "Clinical Experience with Nordihydroguaiaretic Acid: "Chaparral Tea" in the Treatment of Cancer," *Rocky Mountain Medical Journal* 67, no. 11 (1970).

is a waste of plant resources as well as a risk to the client in general. Effectiveness is evaluated over time. Evaluation begins with reviewing the right time for an herbal application.

Right Time

After assessing a client, the nurse-herbalist identifies while making a plan of care what the timing of herbal remedies should be. Establishing the time for an herbal intervention depends upon the herb and its constituents and the client's health patterns. A simple example of the importance of timing an herbal intervention is coffee (*Coffea arabica*) decoction. Coffee is a stimulant for most people so many people drink the decoction of the beans in the morning. Some people drink it anytime. My grandparents drank coffee with milk in the evening after dinner and slept better for it. Every client is different; but, initially, the nurse-herbalist assigns the herbal application to a specific time based upon their knowledge of the herb and the client. After the client tries the remedy, the nurse-herbalist evaluates the effect of the remedy in the context of time. Some herbal simples and formulas are taken with food and others are not. Some are applied before bed; others upon awakening. I have a bay leaf (*Laurus nobilis*) cordial extract I have made for clients that is taken before bed to inspire dreams. The timing of a remedy is part of the recipe for catalyzing change.

Timing is also important to consider during evaluation. Some remedies will be observed to be more or less effective at certain times than others. The nurse-herbalist, therefore, must have some understanding of the client's daily routine, diet, and health regime so that s/he can make proper recommendations for the timing of herbal interventions throughout the day. Herbal remedies must be introduced in a way that is harmonious with the client's lifestyle. For example, I often recommend a decoction of a formula of whole herbs. Many of my clients are working people and they rarely have a block of two to four hours when they can cook their teas. So I recommend that they soak their herbs Friday or Saturday night and cook on Saturday or Sunday morning. I also break with tradition slightly by having them cook enough tea for five to six days instead of three days. The teas in my experience are OK if kept in the refrigerator. I have my clients drink their teas on an empty stomach, two to three times a day so that I can better observe for potential adverse effects. All herbs effect change in the body. All foods effect change in the body. The environment in which the client lives effects change in and around their body. Therefore, to focus only on herbal interactions with any drugs a person is taking is not best practice.

Interaction and Reaction

Herbs interact with everything. Therefore, the most inclusive nurse-herbalist question related to the evaluation of right time either before or after the herbal intervention is, "*How* does this herb or formulation interact with the drugs, foods, environment. and lifestyle of the client?" I encourage the nurse-herbalist to view the client in context, what Hall and Allan have described as "Self-in-Relation."[35] Many clients use herbs and drugs in conjunction or simultaneously. However, when examining their herb use, we find that the majority of herb use is that which typically occurs in small amounts when cooking or drinking beverages. Risk related to herb use rises when the client begins to use medicinal amounts of herbs over a longer period of time. Nurses are often in excellent positions to assist clients in evaluating the effects of all interventions in a plan of care and manipulating the interventions to ensure that they do not interfere but perhaps potentiate the effectiveness of the total plan of care.

For centuries, nurses' expertise has included the ability to make judicious decisions about the "right time" for applying interventions such as drugs and herbs. For example, Sister Matilda Coskery's Advices book states:

After the Dr has named the kind, quantity and frequency of the opiates & stimulants, there is still much depending on the attendants, as in many cases these remedies increase excitement & shd therefore be discontinued until the Dr. comes again, & telling why these were not given—Hop tea is a good substitute as opiate

---

35 Beverly Hall and Janet Allan, "Self in Relation: A Prolegomenon for Holistic Nursing," *Nursing Outlook* 42, no. 3 (1994).

& tonic; & often serves better than opiates or spirits.[36] (Emphasis in original.)

Hops (*Humulus lupulus*) is best known as the flowering vine that is used in the making of beer. American nurses have historically used the flowering top in poultices applied to the chest to relieve congestion during pneumonia and to the abdomen to allay distention post-operatively. It has also been used to heal infected wounds. The knowledge of the use of hops tea and poultices is all but lost as nurses and physicians began to rely more on pharmaceutical drugs; but, the plant continues to grow and is available today for those who would learn of its healing benefits.

Some herbs such as hops can be applied as simples. Others must be used in combination with other herbs. Plants and their constituents have been shown throughout history to have a synergistic effect, an ability for the total effect to be greater than the sum of the individual effects. In TCM, for instance, certain herbs, such as dong guai (*Angelica sinensis*) and bai shao (*Peoniae lactiflora),* are almost always used in formulation together because of their synergistic effect. Sections of the Chinese *Materia Medica* explain which herbs can best be used together and which herbs should not be used together. This information from China of herb-herb interactions is the result of hundreds of years of use and scientific observation of the right time for herbs.

Knowledge of herb-herb timing and interaction is often held by traditional herbal healers. Knowing which herbs can and cannot be used together is part of the cautionary information associated with medicinal plant use. There are herbs for which this information may not exist. What can be frustrating to the biomedical practitioner is the paucity of clinical research on the interaction of herbs and pharmaceutical drugs. I find that biomedical practitioners often assume that there is a great risk of a person using both drugs and herbs. There are numerous sources of information that state that anyone under biomedical care should not use herbs because of the risk of herb-drug interactions. However, this is *potential* risk. In reality, we all know that clients have always used herbs and drugs during the same illness or about the same time. I remember

---

36 Matilda Coskery, *Advices Concerning the Sick*, Emmetsburg, MD: Archives of Daughters of Charity, St. Joseph Provincial House (n.d. c. 1840).

when the research on grapefruit juice (*Citrus paradisi*) came out stating that it "interacted" with drugs such as felodipine, nifedipine, verapamil, cyclosporin, and triazolam. Human studies have shown that the plant psoralens and possibly the flavonoid naringenin in grapefruit diminish the first-pass metabolism of the drugs by suppressing a cytochrome P-450 enzyme in the small intestine and thereby increasing drug concentrations.[37] How many years did doctors prescribe and nurses administer these drugs with grapefruit juice, never mentioning the potential effect on drug metabolism? I never remember hearing or reading of terrible results from the drugs. In fact, they have been on the market because they have been effective despite the fact that grapefruit juice is also on the market. There just seems to be an inordinate amount of fear about drug-herb interactions and little expression of scientific interest in herb-drug synergy or in developing best practices of timing client care in which both drugs and herbs are applied.

When I was at the University of Colorado Cancer Center, I worked with physicians who respected the fact that clients, particularly Asian clients, were ingesting and applying their traditional herbal remedies often on a daily basis. I consulted on a number of cases in which we determined what herbs the client was taking that had helped and made plans of care that were inclusive of those remedies. For example, the pharmacists knew the half-life of the chemotherapeutic agents and we worked the plan of care to be mindful of the client's need for the highest benefit of the drugs. We might suggest that the client stop their herbs for forty-eight to seventy-two hours while taking chemo. Often, because the client was taking the herbs every day, they were fine with stopping the herbs for a few days so that clinicians could have a clear understanding of their body's response to treatment and also to better ensure that the drug would enter the liver pathways without interference. Nurse-herbalists need to study and stay abreast of the literature on the metabolic effects of plant constituents on the liver in particular.

Cytochrome P-450 is the major member of the class of enzymes primarily localized in the liver that is involved in the metabolism of many

---

37 Uwe Fuhr, "Drug Interactions with Grapefruit Juice. Extent, Probable Mechanism and Clinical Relevance," *Drug Safety : An International Journal of Medical Toxicology and Drug Experience* 18, no. 4 (1998).

medications. Certain drugs and substances, such as cigarette smoke and estrogens, can *induce* the P-450 system and therefore detoxify chemical substances. Certain drugs, such as cimetidine and acute alcohol ingestion, *inhibit* cytochrome P-450 and therefore may potentiate other chemical substances, including drugs.[38] The individuality of the client also exists on the molecular level in the cytochrome P-450 system. The range of responses to drugs and herbs is wide. Factors that influence individual expression of the cytochrome P-450 system include gender, age, race, genetics, and hepatic condition. Just because an herb is shown in in vitro studies to affect P-450 in some way does not necessarily mean that the herb will affect all people in the same way at all times.

It is also interesting to find that although plants, such as St. John's Wort (*Hypericum perforatum*), may *induce* the P-450 system (inducing CYP3A4 in hepatocyte cells), many plants, including St. John's Wort, also contain the bioflavonoid quercetin, which is a 3A4 *inhibitor* (personal communication, Dr. Jim Duke, April 2001). What happens in the body when both inhibitors and inducers enter the body at the same time because they are both present in the same herb? Dosage, environmental, and individual factors must be taken into account. Because of the complexity of plant remedies, it is possible that there may be no clinical sequelae in taking herbs with certain drugs. However, it may also be possible that certain herbs and drugs should not be taken simultaneously by the same individual. It may also be possible that the body has the ability to sort out all the chemical interactions and produce the response it needs for greater health.

It is not possible for a drug in clinical trials to be tested against every food and herb there is, so there will be gaps in drug-food and drug-herb interaction information. From a traditional Chinese medicine perspective, all drugs, herbs, and foods are potentially interactive and/or synergistic. Drugs, herbs, and foods are evaluated from an energetic perspective when helping a client heal and find greater balance. For example, clients I have seen over the years who are on thyroid medication have a certain pulse profile, a characteristic about their pulse found on pulse diagnosis that often indicates excess heat in the body. Because I

---

38 Jonathan Treasure, "Herbal Pharmacokinetics," *Journal of the American Herbalist Guild* 1, no. 1 (2000).

have found through observation that the thyroid medication may be part of the reason for the excess heat, I consider the energetic qualities of the thyroid medication when formulating the proper tea. A client and their caregiver must decide if the herb will be used or not and, if so, when.

Some biomedical practitioners would have a client believe that there is no choice regarding the integrative use of medications and herbs or foods that may interact— the client must have their medication and therefore should avoid a specific food or herb. This really does not work. People want information and choice. Some clients, upon hearing from a biomedical practitioner that they have no choice, such as, "You are on this medication now, so do not take any herbal medicines," opt not to take pharmaceutical drugs at all, which can be life threatening. Some clients choose to take herbs and foods because they have a longer record of safe use.

An integrative paradigm of care does not mean that every person should apply herbs for health and illness; some people have absolutely no interest in working with plant remedies. It really comes down to a matter of personal choice. I have applied herbal remedies in clients at all stages of life, health, and illness and there are herbal remedies for every time. Following an integrative paradigm of care moves us toward a system of health care that acknowledges that people do use herbal medicines and sometimes prefer them over pharmaceutical drugs for very important reasons—timing being one of those reasons. I have had clients say to me that their doctors told them that their cancer was very slow growing. They weigh the benefits and risks of herbal versus chemotherapeutic remedies and choose to start their care with herbs because they often hold less risk and are known to be effective. They hold the question as to whether or not the herbal remedies will be effective in their case but when they look at timing, and realize that they do not have to go with the stronger medication right away, they may choose herbs first. This is just one example of many cases in which timing drives decision making.

Ancient health care systems such as TCM and the Ayurvedic system in India have had centuries to evaluate timing of herbal applications such as what time of day is best to take a particular herb for a particular condition and in a particular form. These systems of medicine are just two examples of the extent of the art involved in creating a health care system. The study of drug-herb-food interactions is part of the new frontier of creating an integrative health care system that includes the understanding of science and tradition. Practitioners, both traditional and biomedical, need to be very aware that it is no longer sufficient to tell a client to follow only their biomedical regimen or only take traditional remedies. People typically use both traditional and biomedical therapies, and they need practitioners who have accepted that both will be considered when health care choices must be made.

Right Dose

Some people and caregivers may believe that because a plant remedy is natural that it is safe to use, but even the most natural of elements, water, can be toxic when taken in the wrong dose. Nurses often discuss the benefits and risks of a particular intervention with a client. There are benefits and risks associated with every plant use, especially when one considers that each client is an individual. The benefits of herbs are best received when the right dose for the client is used. Paracelsus is quoted as having said that "the only difference between medicine and poison is the dose."

The word "toxic" is taken from the Greek word "toxikon," meaning "poison for arrows."[39] Many cultures have described the use of plants as poison, and not just from the tips of arrows. Socrates (469–399 B.C.E.), after being convicted of corrupting youth and interfering with the religion of the city of Athens, drank poison hemlock (*Conium maculatum*) and died. Although some plants can be deadly, a plant is not labeled toxic or poisonous just because it contains a specific toxic constituent. Botanist John M. Kingsbury writes:

> In order for a plant to be functionally poisonous, however, it must not only contain a toxic secondary compound but also possess effective means of presenting that compound to an animal in sufficient concentration, and the secondary compound must be capable of overcoming whatever physiological or biochemical defenses the animal may possess against it. Thus the presence of a known poison

39 John Mann, *Murder, Magic, and Medicine* (Oxford, New York: Oxford University Press, 1992).

principle, even in toxicologically significant amounts, in a plant does not automatically mean that either man or a given species of animal will ever be effectively poisoned by that plant.[40]

Establishing toxicity is not a simple matter. The toxicology of any substance is based on a number of variables, such as the chemistry of the substance, the dose, and the biochemical nature of the person applying the substance. Like timing, right dose and toxicity are best determined in context. To put toxicity in perspective, in 1998 in America, "about 100 people died after ingesting common, ordinary nuts. In the same period, fewer than 100 Americans died after consuming an herb in some form, and more than 90% of these people were intentionally abusing certain of the more potent members of our herbal pharmacy."[41]

One way to determine the toxicity of a chemical constituent of a plant is by studying the amount (mg/kg) of the substance needed to kill 50 percent of the mice in a particular population. The result of the study is stated as the median lethal dose (LD_{50}). These numbers are not given to complex substances such as those found in whole plants, so they are often not helpful in herbal medicine. But, to establish perspective about the toxicity of plant substances, it is often helpful to know that the LD_{50} of caffeine, a substance many people take into their bodies every day, is 192 mg/kg and the LD_{50} of carotatoxin (a substance found in garden carrot *Daucus carota*) is 100 mg/kg (Duke, 2011, www.ars-grin.gov/duke/dosage.html). For a 50-kg person to be poisoned from the caffeine in a cup of coffee containing 48 mg of caffeine, the person would need to drink 200 cups of coffee. The LD_{50} of 192 or 100 is quite low. Many plant constituents found in medicinal plants have significantly higher median lethal doses. To clarify, a higher LD_{50} means that it takes more of the substance to become toxic and a lower LD_{50} means that it takes less of the substance to become toxic. Many people ingest caffeine-containing beverages all the time, and although it may not be the healthiest practice, no deaths have resulted.

Another source of toxicity data is the list that botanists and the

40 John Kingsbury, "The Problem of Poisonous Plants," in *Toxic Plants*, ed. A. Douglas Kinghorn (New York: Columbia University Press, 1979), 2.
41 James Duke, *Dr. Duke's Essential Herbs* (Emmaus, PA: Rodale, Inc., 1999), 3.

FDA use of those plants that are generally recognized as safe (GRAS), generally recognized as food (GRAF), and generally recognized as poison (GRAP). There are certain limitations to the usefulness of this classification system. A plant may have constituents that are each classified differently. "There are probably carcinogens, mutagens, and poisons, as well as anticarcinogens, antimutagens, and antidotes in all GRAF, GRAP, and GRAS species. ... Apples are GRAF, and their extracts are GRAS but the cyanide in the seeds are GRAP."[42] Because of the complexity of plants, this system may not really be helpful to people making regulatory decisions based on a specific classification system.

Establishing toxicity of all medicinal plants used by humans is not a simple matter, scientifically speaking. Numerous specialists including botanists and clinical toxicologists would be needed to accomplish the task. Practically speaking, it is debatable whether establishing toxicity of plants is very helpful data anyway. A plant may contain a certain toxin that does not cause any problem to a human when ingested. "Toxicity is rarely an all-or-none phenomenon. Species of plants vary in their content of toxic compounds owing to unpredictable extrinsic and genetic factors. Vertebrate species and individual animals vary in susceptibility."[43] Toxicity often comes down to a matter of right dose, right use, and common sense.

So often practitioners write that herbs are horribly understudied, completely unregulated, and have serious potential for toxicity. This is just not the case. The track records of herbal medicines have been evaluated by leading botanical scientists quoted here, such as Dr. Norman Farnsworth, who have had long distinguished careers, and have been found to "not present a major problem with regard to toxicity. ... In fact, of all classes of substances reported to cause toxicities of sufficient magnitude to be reported in the United States, plants are the least problematic."[44] There is a huge body of literature on medicinal plants as well as centuries of use in health care systems. Herbs also are regulated in many countries; however, *they may not be regulated in the same way as pharmaceutical drugs.*

Although many health practitioners in the biomedical paradigm may

42 ———, *Handbook of Phytochemical Constituents of Gras Herbs and Other Economic Plants* (Boca Raton, FL: CRC Press, 1992), ii.
43 Kingsbury, "The Problem of Poisonous Plants," 5.
44 Norman Farnsworth, "Relative Safety of Herbal Medicines.," *Herbalgram* 29(1993): 36H.

believe that the system of pharmaceutical drug regulation is the gold standard in ensuring safety with herbal products, the literature does not support this. In the United States where pharmaceutical drugs are highly regulated, researched, and monitored for safe use, a meta-analysis of the incidence of adverse drug reactions in hospitalized clients reported that in 1994, 106,000 clients died from adverse drug reactions and 2,216,000 had serious adverse drug reactions. Adverse drug reactions to *drugs that are properly prescribed and administered* were the fourth to sixth leading cause of death in the country.[45] The researchers have noted that the adverse drug reaction problem is much the same worldwide and that the incidence has remained stable over the last 30 years. In Hong Kong, for example, where herbal medicines are used quite often, it was reported that 0.2 percent of general hospital admissions were due to adverse reactions to Chinese herbal medicines as compared with 4.4 percent of admissions due to adverse reactions to Western drugs.[46]

In addition, rigorous drug standards and controls also have not had much impact on the potential toxic effects of the common, over-the-counter medication, acetaminophen. One study published in the *New England Journal of Medicine* revealed that in one urban hospital alone from 1992 to 1995, 50 clients were reported to have taken acetaminophen during suicide attempts and 21 people accidentally poisoned themselves while attempting to relieve pain.[47] Although some claim that herbs are under-regulated in the United States and therefore potentially unsafe, the FDA and the herb and supplement industry have been very active in promoting the proper marketing and regulation of herbs. What are the FDA and biomedical practitioners doing about the excessive number of deaths related to properly prescribed and administered drugs in hospitals?

One of the roles of the FDA is to evaluate reports of adverse reactions to foods, drugs, and herbs along with other products marketed for human consumption. Some have suggested that adverse reactions to herbs are underreported. Therefore, the FDA has set up a telephone hotline

---

45 Jason Lazarou, Bruce Pomeranz, and Paul Corey, "Incidence of Adverse Drug Reactions in Hospitalized Patients: A Meta-Analysis of Prospective Studies.," *JAMA* 279, no. 15 (1998).

46 Tyk Chan, Ayw Chan, and Jajh Critchley, "Hospital Admissions Due to Adverse Reactions to Chinese Herbal Medicines," *The Journal of Tropical Medicine and Hygiene* 95, no. 4 (1992).

47 Frank Schiodt and others, "Acetaminophen Toxicity in an Urban County Hospital," *The New England Journal of Medicine* 337, no. 16 (1997): 1112.

to facilitate reporting. This is a public reporting site, and the detail and accuracy needed to conduct scientific analysis have not been present. The data collected and used by the FDA have been called unreliable and unsubstantiated by the U.S. General Accounting Office.

Any nurse who has ever worked on a hotline service, such as at a poison control center, learns that when someone calls in to report an adverse reaction to a substance that a scientific line of inquiry is set in motion as a result of the report. The professional who takes the report does not immediately identify or target the substance suggested by the caller as the cause of the reaction. Linking a reaction to a specific substance is not always as easy as it appears.

In order to establish causality, certain criteria must be met. Most importantly with drugs and herbs, the substance taken by an individual must be clearly identified. For example, if a client sees a practitioner because of a rash they incurred when playing in the woods, and they say that they started to see the rash after rubbing a plant on their skin, the first responsibility of the practitioner is to identify the plant the person rubbed on their skin. If the practitioner does not clearly identify the plant, they might say to the client that it is possible that the plant caused the rash, but a definitive statement should not be made without proper scientific evaluation.

In one example, there were seven cases of anticholinergic poisoning in New York City in 1994 thought by the clients to be due to drinking Paraguay tea or maté *(Ilex paraguariensis)*. When the emergency room staff obtained samples of the tea and it was analyzed by the police department, it was found that the tea was adulterated with belladonna alkaloids, atropine, scopolamine, and hyoscyamine, substances that are not part of the plant.[48] The adulterants, not the maté, were the cause of the poisoning reaction.

Standardization of Herbal Products and Practitioners

Studying the dosages of herbal supplements (i.e. pills and capsules) alone is not sufficient knowledge for the establishment of best practice in

---

48 "Anticholinergic Poisoning Associated with Herbal Tea - New York City," *MMWR. Morbidity and Mortality Weekly Report* 44, no. 11 (1995).

nurse-herbalism. Supplements are only a small part of the vast science of nurse-herbalism. As mentioned previously, there are many herbs applied historically in nursing care that have not been taken in pill form. When these herbs are crushed and placed in capsules for oral ingestion and are not applied as they have been for centuries, such as in tea form or placed on the skin for absorption, the record of safety is altered. Supplements, standardized extracts in particular, are a subset of herbal care that nurse-herbalists may or may not include in practice. Herbal supplement information may be the only information included in nursing textbooks, courses, and licensure exams, but that does not make it best practice. To associate nurse-herbalism solely with herbal supplements is not evidence-based or best practice. However, if prepared herbal supplements are used, the nurse-herbalist must know the difference between whole-plant supplements and standardized extracts.

A standardized extract is a plant preparation in which the "active constituent," if identified, has been standardized or made uniform from individual product to individual product. This is seen as beneficial by those practitioners working from a biomedical paradigm because of the perceived control over dose and quality. The belief is that the active constituents in a plant can be identified, extracted, purified, and standardized, making the remedy more like a pharmaceutical drug than any other plant preparation. Having the plant remedy standardized means that the practitioner can prescribe a specific dose of a "known" active constituent with the benefit of the constituent being in a "natural" form, as compared to synthetic drugs. It should be noted that specific dosages for whole-plant herbal remedies are also calculated specifically for clients.

The ability to produce a standardized herbal medicine rests upon the ability of researchers to identify the active constituent of a plant. In some plants such as senna *(Cassia senna L.),* a plant that has been traditionally applied in the care of the client with constipation, an "active constituent" has been identified. In senna, the active constituent that seems to have a bowel irritant or stimulant effect is identified as "sennasides." Standardization of sennasides means for the consumer that taking a certain amount of herbal product should have a laxative effect. Because the sennasides are identifiable, the sennaside constituents can be researched in much the same way a pharmaceutical drug would be. The controversy is that the history of relatively safe use of senna has to do with the traditional use of the whole leaf, not sennasides.

It is also a concern that in many plants, the goal of identifying a single constituent is not possible and that the standardization of a plant medicine to a single constituent is therefore misleading in regard to efficacy and safety. One plant researcher writes, "As there are normally more than one (or one type of) active component in a natural product, standardization based on one particular type of chemical component is not representative of the total activity of the product. Consequently, these arbitrarily selected components can only be useful as a 'marker' of product quality. And these 'markers' are only valid for extracts that are total extractions of the herbs concerned."[49]

Standardization can be helpful to identify the quality of a particular herb. Plants grown even in the same field can vary in potency of certain active constituents. Quality markers can help growers identify potential potency of the whole medicinal plant. Whole plants are, in general, less potent than an individual plant constituent. For comparison, take the apple. Most people who have eaten an apple remember the strong outer skin and the crunching sound when biting into the fruit for the first time. There is a lot of pectin and fiber in the apple skin. Now recall eating the fleshy part of the apple. Although some apples are more tart than others, they are basically a sweet fruit. The sugars in fruits are known as fructose. When extracted from fruit and processed, fructose looks much the same as the white crystallized cane sugar you might eat. Think about what it might be like to eat a spoonful of fructose sugar. How might your body respond? Sugars are known to give the body an energy boost. Does your body get the identical energy boost from an apple as it does from a spoonful of fructose? Common sense tells us that extracted (standardized) fructose is not the same as an apple and it does not have the same total effect on the body, either.

One example of when I have found that a standardized extract is very helpful is in liver damage due to toxic substance exposure from acetaminophen, environmental pollutants, or mushroom poisoning.

---

49 Albert Leung and Steven Foster, *Encyclopedia of Common Natural Ingredients Used in Food, Drugs, and Cosmetics*, 2nd ed. (New York: John Wiley & Sons, 1996), xv.

Milk thistle seed (*Silybum marianum*) has been used traditionally for more than 2,000 years for illness related to the liver. Milk thistle products are standardized to silymarin, a hepatoprotective and antioxidant constituent. According to research, a therapeutic level of silymarin cannot be achieved by taking teas or simple alcohol extracts of the milk thistle seed because silymarin cannot survive the breakdown by digestive juices and enter the bloodstream via the intestinal wall. Because silymarin is not very soluble in water and is poorly absorbed from the gastrointestinal tract, a concentrated, standardized extract or injectable form of the plant is used to fully provide the desired effects.[50] Herbalists and traditional healers may disagree that standardization is necessary for the client to receive a health benefit from milk thistle. Some herbalists have found that clients with chemical sensitivities have a negative response to standardized products because of the chemical residue in the product from the standardization process. More research is needed to fully determine the benefits and risks of using standardized herbal products.

Standardization is just one example of manufacturing or processing that goes into the production of herbal supplements. Good manufacturing practices have been identified by many, including WHO,[51] as a target for the improvement of herbal products on the market. Herbalists and traditional healers who use whole herbs have always known the importance of making a proper identification of the plant and finding a pure source for the plant. Plants that have been sprayed with herbicides and pesticides would not be used. For instance, an herbalist would not harvest mullein (*Verbascum officinale*) leaf and flowers from plants growing by a busy highway. It is important that the plant is grown in a pollutant-free environment.

Plants targeted for medicinal use, be they whole dried plant or one of the numerous products on the market, are subject to contamination and deterioration. Just as with buying a vegetable in the supermarket, the medicinal plant must be "ripe" and not decomposing to make a

---

50 Mark Blumenthal, Bundesinstitut für Arzneimittel und Medizinprodukte (Germany), and Commission E, *Herbal Medicine: Expanded Commission E Monographs* (Newton, MA: Integrative Medicine Communications, 2000).

51 World Health Organization, "Good Manufacturing Practices," in *WHO Technical Report Series Number 863* (Geneva 1996).

good product. Shelf life is different for different herbs, often based on their constituents. Storage of herbal products is very important. Whole dried herbs, for example, need to be open to the air and therefore are best kept in protective bags that have an opening. Many herbs and herb products lose their potency when exposed to heat, humidity, and/or light and therefore are kept in special areas where the storage climate can be controlled. Herbs are stored separately, sometimes in separate rooms, because of the potency of certain constituents. For example, at the Celestial Seasonings Tea Company in Boulder, Colorado, the peppermint (*Mentha piperita*) is kept in its own special vault. On public tours, the tour guides encourage participants to enter the vault where they receive a literal blast of menthol, the volatile oil that permeates any room it is stored in. For this reason, the peppermint stands alone.

Herb production facilities must be clean, and measures must be taken to prevent cross contamination between products. All products should be labeled and documented with the botanical name of all ingredients; date of harvest and/or date of process; plant source; results of screening for herbicide, pesticide, or other contaminants; the drying system used, if dried; and the results of tests for microbial and aflatoxin contamination. All processing records are kept up to date.

Although standardized herbal extracts may be very similar to pharmaceutical drugs in appearance, most plant medicines are not. Some practitioners mistakenly tell clients that herbs are "drugs" and should be used cautiously. Although the message about using caution is correct, it is not best practice to teach the public that herbs are drugs. For years, biomedical practitioners have wrestled with client noncompliance to pharmaceutical drug regimens. Clients clearly believe that they can and should regulate whether they take a drug or not. They may be quite familiar with self-medication with over-the-counter drugs. By telling people that herbs are drugs, practitioners may be inadvertently telling people that what they know about over-the-counter and prescription drugs can be applied to herbs. This can potentially lead to greater risk, mainly that the client may not seek understanding about an herb. Nurse-herbalists play an important role in community health in that they can provide education about herbs as well as care so that the record of safe use we have enjoyed for so long can continue.

Right Person

In hospital care, right person, refers to a safety measure to check and make sure that the nurse administers the drug to the right client in the room. The nurse checks the wrist band and then administers the drug. Right person in nurse-herbalism refers to the question of personal choice. Each client reserves the right to choose any nursing intervention at any time. The nurse-herbalist must not assume that all clients want herbal remedies. There are many who do but there are also many who do not. A client may perceive herbal remedies as lesser care in relation to biomedical care; they may be perceived as something significantly less than best practice.

While the nurse-herbalist educates and cares for their community with herbs, s/he must also be sensitive to the cultural beliefs and potential opposition, particularly in industrialized societies against nurses' partnership with plants. There are also many nurses who oppose the application of herbs in nursing care. My stance is that laws protect the right of nurse-herbalists to make the professional decision to apply herbs in the care and comfort of clients and that clients' rights to use herbs in self-care should also be protected. People should have the right to choose plant remedies. It would be a tragedy if any law came between the relationship of people and plants.

Each country has its own way of seeking to protect the public safety in regard to herbs and herbal supplements. The government document regulating herbs and supplements in the United States is called the Dietary Supplement Health and Education Act (DSHEA). It is not lengthy and therefore it is most beneficial for the nurse-herbalist to become very familiar with the language of this document, especially since it is often misquoted by the media, government officials, health officials, practitioners, science editors, and educators. The law can be read online at the following URL: http://www.fda.gov/opacom/laws/dshea.html The following URL is a link to the department within the FDA that implements the law: http://www.fda.gov/food/dietarysupplements/default.htm

DSHEA is an education act first implemented to ensure public access to dietary supplements in the United States. It is the opinion of the herb industry that DSHEA has adequate authority to deal with any problems in the industry. Physicians have often petitioned in their journals for greater control over herbs, including requirements that herbal supplements be registered with the FDA and pre-market approval of evidence be obtained showing that the supplement poses no risk of injury to the public.[52] However, they are essentially calling for greater controls over substances that have documented lesser risk when they have yet to find solutions to the problems in their own house caused by drugs that have a known risk to health and that are already regulated by the FDA.

There are certainly herb companies that do not produce the best products. I remember finding an herb product in 1989, prior to DSHEA, that was labeled "Echinacea" but was in fact, according to the small print, *Parthenium integrifolium*. It was clear to me that I was responsible for ensuring that my clients did not receive adulterated products. At that time, I was in the process of harvesting echinacea (*Echinacea purpurea*) root that had been in the ground for five years. One dried root yielded 0.16 grams of herb. It is not easy to grow herbs for industry-level production. I learned this first hand. It is the best safe practice for each family and nurse-herbalist to cultivate and harvest their own herbal medicines when possible. When using prepared herbal products, the nurse-herbalist should research some basics about the herb company's:

1. Commitment to their country's Good Manufacturing Practices;
2. Sources for whole herbs used in products;
3. Designation as Organic;
4. Attention to traditional use and preparations that contribute to a strong record of safety.

Herb Sales

While nurse-herbalists and midwives have traditionally grown herbs in their own gardens for use in their practice, selling herbal supplements in practice that are grown and made by someone else adds an additional

52 Loren Israelson and Thomas Aarts, "Industry Needs to Re-Think DSHEA," *Herbalgram* 58(2003).

dimension to safe and effective best practice in nurse-herbalism. As a general rule, I recommend that nurse-herbalists:

1. Cultivate and wildcraft the herbs that they partner with in practice.
2. Buy in whole-plant form herbs that are purchased for practice. Purchasing herbs in whole form allows for the inspection and verification of the proper product.
3. Learn the art and science of formulation rather than purchasing formulations. This holds true for essential oil products such as massage oils. The nurse-herbalist should purchase single essential oils and blend them according to the specific need of the client rather than purchasing someone else's formulations.
4. Know state or country regulations about selling herbal products. Preferably develop a relationship with a local pharmacy or health food store and refer clients there to purchase herbs. Very few local stores stock whole herbs. Whole herbs used in teas and topical applications can be stocked by the nurse-herbalist.

These practices lead to greater opportunity for safe and responsible practice.

The legal and safety issues surrounding the applications of plant remedies in practice are not insurmountable but they do require vigilance in the current social climate. In summary, nurse-herbalists should be able to answer the following questions related to their practice:

1. What education is required in my country/state to include the use of herbal remedies in my practice?
2. Are there any legal requirements of my country, state, and/or nursing regulatory board or agency regarding the use of herbs in caring for clients? Are those requirements specific to any particular use of herbs in practice such as oral remedies?
3. What are the legal or ethical ramifications of *not* knowing

anything about herbal remedies and *not* providing assistance to clients who are making decisions about the use of herbal remedies in self-care?

4. Are my qualifications and educational preparation adequate to address the particular need of an individual client for whom I am caring with herbal therapies? Or are there other practitioners who are better qualified to address the needs of this particular client?

5. Am I using holistic nursing process to the fullest extent in my herbal practice? Am I "practicing medicine" with herbs by becoming prescriptive, directive, and using disease-focused, medical diagnostic language?

6. Do I have sufficient understanding of the laws regarding the use of various healing plants in my country? Do I have a list of local medicinal plants that are protected because they are at risk for extinction? Do I know the wildcrafting history of the plants in my geographic location? Am I developing relationships with indigenous healers in my area?

7. When using herbal formulations, such as patent formulas or herbal supplements, am I knowledgeable about the individual plants in the formula and of the interaction and/or synergy of the herbs in formulation?

8. Do I have a conflict of interest in my practice because of the way I am selling herbal products to clients?

Plants are ready partners in teaching and healing. Their natures determine the actual expression of the five rights in nurse-herbalism. How and where they grow, their role in the larger environment and ecosystem, their medicinal constituents and fragrance, and their beauty inspire the soul, stimulate the mind, and catalyze physical changes that lead to healing and cures. Yet with all the power they hold, they go about their "work" quietly, subtly, and often gently. They move so slowly that they are easily trampled. They are highly subject to human will and consumption and therefore need a nurse's conscious protection if they are to continue to be a ready source for healing remedies.

FIRE – INTEGRATIVE INSIGHT –
BEYOND FEAR AND INTO THE FLAME
OF CONSCIOUSNESS

There is so much discussion in the media about the concerns with herbal remedies that I am often afraid that people are forgetting their roots. Our medicines are and were botanicals for centuries. I love being with plants and making medicines that I know will help people. Growing and making medicine makes my heart sing! When my heart sings, I feel no fear at all. How do we explain to people the safety that can come from really knowing the joy of healing plants? It seems that we spend so much effort on seeking to assure that the plant will not harm us that we miss the delight and the promise of healing that comes when entering the green world. Would we "ooh" and "ah" over herbs used in culinary treats, but then suspect the worst from herbs that would heal us through and through? The role of the nurse-herbalist in healing culture is not only to provide care anchored in best practice but to introduce people to the joy of healing plants and making their own medicines. It is in making medicine that we engage the fire element.

It is the fire that transforms the herb into a remedy. Fire heats water to create an infusion. The fire of the sun gently warms the herbs in a jar of oil to extract the medicinal constituents of the plants. We turn up the fire on the stove to reduce the juice of berries into syrup. Into the infusion, oil, and syrup, we also add our consciousness as we cook. We imbue each remedy with our thoughts, feelings, and beliefs about healing. The act of making medicine is a loving one. It accesses the heart's desire for healing and creates the chalice for the wisdom of the inner healer to manifest. Are we afraid of making medicine and really healing through and through? I have often wondered this when I hear or read of such suspicion of the safety of herbal remedies. My science mind just can't absorb what I perceive as such inordinate fear over the safety of plant medicine when I have partnered with plants my whole life and have benefited so much from the experiences in my own healing work and that of my clients. Perhaps there is so much concern because plants are life forms. They even demonstrate consciousness.[53] Plants are of the same elements of matter as we are—they are air, water, earth, and fire. Helena Roerich wrote of the fiery world, "The approaching fiery waves are extremely terrifying if one does not know about them and does not assimilate them with the fires of one's own heart. ... Fire is the highest element, and the approach to it must be by way of the higher consciousness. One can understand and learn to love Fire only through this higher consciousness."[54] Nurse-herbalism is an adventure in higher consciousness. I can say this because I have first-hand experience that it is so. Meditation on the beauty of the plants alone can raise our spirit and consciousness and when we taste the herbs we are transported into a different dimension all together. Herbs are not synthetic drugs; they are life forms from which we can connect to nature and the Creator in new ways every day. Medicine making is an essential element of nurse-herbalism. That is why the final chapter of this book on integrative insights for holistic practice is dedicated to the etheric aspects of making medicine.

53 Peter Tompkins and Christopher Bird, *The Secret Life of Plants* (New York: Harper & Row, 1973).54 Roerich, Fiery World 1: 12-13.
54 Roerich, *Fiery World* 1: 12-13.

Herbal Experiment: Making Medicine

Onion (*Allium cepa*) is often easy to grow. Here is a simple but powerful remedy that can be made with clients or taught to them to make in their own homes.

Onion Syrup

Slice 1 to 2 large yellow or white onions thinly. (Experience the onion's effects on your tear ducts!) Measure ¾ to 1 cup (180 to 360 ml) of honey (or any sugar). In a large container, alternately layer the onion slices and then the honey. Let it stand for three days in a dark corner of the kitchen and then strain the syrup into a colored glass bottle. Store in the refrigerator. The syrup can be taken in spoonfuls just like any cough syrup or can be added to a tea. Rest well after taking.

REFERENCES

Alberta, College & Association of Registered Nurses of. "Complementary and/or Alternative Therapy and Natural Health Products: Standards for Registered Nurses." Edmonton, Alberta, 2011.

"Anticholinergic Poisoning Associated with Herbal Tea - New York City." *MMWR. Morbidity and Mortality Weekly Report* 44, no. 11 (1995): 193-95.

Baba, Shigeaki, Olayiwola Akerele, and Yuji Kawaguchi. "Natural Resources and Human Health: Plants of Medicinal and Nutritional Value. Proceedings of the 1st WHO Symposium on Plants and Health for All: Scientific Advancement, Kobe, Japan. August 1991." Amsterdam: Elsevier, 1992.

Balick, Michael and Paul Alan Cox. *Plants, People, and Culture the Science of Ethnobotany*. New York: Scientific American Library, 1996.

Belew, Cindy. "Herbs and the Childbearing Woman: Guidelines for Midwives." *Journal of Nurse-Midwifery* 44, no. 3 (1999): 231-52.

Blumenthal, Mark. Bundesinstitut für Arzneimittel und Medizinprodukte (Germany), and Commission E. *Herbal Medicine: Expanded Commission E Monographs*. Newton, MA: Integrative Medicine Communications, 2000.

Bunce, Kathleen. "The Use of Herbs in Midwifery." *Journal of Nurse-Midwifery* 32, no. 4 (1987): 255-9.

Chan, Tyk, Ayw Chan, and Jajh Critchley. "Hospital Admissions Due to Adverse Reactions to Chinese Herbal Medicines." *The Journal of Tropical Medicine and Hygiene* 95, no. 4 (1992): 296-8.

"Chaparral-Induced Toxic Hepatitis--California and Texas, 1992." *MMWR. Morbidity and Mortality Weekly Report* 41, no. 43 (1992): 812-4.

Coskery, Sister Matilda. *Advices Concerning the Sick*. Emmitsburg, MD: Archives of Daughters of Charity, St. Joseph's Provincial House, n.d. c. 1840.

Duke, James. *Dr. Duke's Essential Herbs*. Emmaus, PA: Rodale, Inc., 1999.

———. *Handbook of Phytochemical Constituents of Gras Herbs and Other Economic Plants*. Boca Raton, FL: CRC Press, 1992.

Ehudin-Pagano, Eileen, Patricia Paluzzi, Loretta Ivory, and Marian McCartney. "The Use of Herbs in Nurse-Midwifery Practice." *Journal of Nurse-Midwifery* 32, no. 4 (1987): 260-2.

Farnsworth, Norman. "Relative Safety of Herbal Medicines." *Herbalgram*, no. 29 (1993): 36A-H.

———. "Preclinical Assessment of Medicinal Plants." In Shigeaki Baba, Olayiwola Akerele, and Yuji Kawaguchi, "Natural Resources and Human Health: Plants of Medicinal and Nutritional Value. Proceedings of the 1st WHO Symposium on Plants and Health for All: Scientific Advancement, Kobe, Japan. August 1991," (Amsterdam: Elsevier, 1992), 87.

Farnsworth, Norman, Olayiwola Akerele, Audrey Bingel, Djaja Soejarto, and Zhengang Guo. "Medicinal Plants in Therapy." *Bulletin of the World Health Organization* 63, no. 6 (1985): 965-81.

Felter, Harvey Wickes and John Uri Lloyd. *King's American Dispensatory*. 18th ed., 3d rev ed. Sandy, OR: Eclectic Medical Publications, 1983.

Fuhr, Uwe. "Drug Interactions with Grapefruit Juice. Extent, Probable Mechanism and Clinical Relevance." *Drug Safety : An International Journal of Medical Toxicology and Drug Experience* 18, no. 4 (1998): 251-72.

Gordon, Dafna, Gayle Rosenthal, John Hart, Ronald Sirota, and Alfred Baker. "Chaparral Ingestion. The Broadening Spectrum of Liver Injury Caused by Herbal Medications." *JAMA : The Journal of the American Medical Association* 273, no. 6 (1995): 489-90.

Hall, Beverly and Janet Allan. "Self in Relation: A Prolegomenon for Holistic Nursing." *Nursing Outlook* 42, no. 3 (1994): 110-16.

Harmer, Bertha. *Text-Book of the Principles and Practice of Nursing*. New York: Macmillan Co., 1924.

Harmer, Bertha and Virginia Henderson. *Textbook of the Principles and Practice of Nursing*. New York: Macmillan Co., 1955.

Israelson, Loren and Thomas Aarts. "Industry Needs to Re-Think Dshea." *Herbalgram* 58 (2003): 59-61.

Kelly, Mike and Becky Taylor. "Legislative Report: Other States' Policies Regarding Nurses Administering Prescribed Dietary Supplements." Juneau, AK, 2006.

Kingsbury, John. "The Problem of Poisonous Plants." In *Toxic Plants*, edited by A. Douglas Kinghorn. New York: Columbia University Press, 1979.

Lazarou, Jason, Bruce Pomeranz, and Paul Corey. "Incidence of Adverse Drug Reactions in Hospitalized Patients: A Meta-Analysis of Prospective Studies." *JAMA* 279, no. 15 (1998): 1200-5.

Leung, Albert and Steven Foster. *Encyclopedia of Common Natural Ingredients Used in Food, Drugs, and Cosmetics*. 2nd ed. New York: John Wiley & Sons, 1996.

Levin, Lowell S. and Ellen L. Idler. *The Hidden Health Care System*. Farmville, NC: Golden Apple Publications, 2010.

Libster, Martha and Betty Ann McNeil. *Enlightened Charity: The Holistic Nursing Care, Education and Advices Concerning the Sick of Sister Matilda Coskery, (1799-1870)*. Farmville, NC: Golden Apple Publications, 2009.

Libster, Martha. *Herbal Diplomats: The Contribution of Early American Nurses (1830-1860) to Nineteenth-Century Health Care Reform and the Botanical Medical Movement*. Thornton, CO: Golden Apple Publications, 2004.

Mann, John. *Murder, Magic, and Medicine*. Oxford, New York: Oxford University Press, 1992.

McFarlin, Barbara, Mary Gibson, Jann O'Rear, and Patsy Harman. "A National Survey of Herbal Preparation Use by Nurse-Midwives for Labor Stimulation." *Journal of Nurse-Midwifery* 44, no. 3 (1999): 205-16.

Merriam-Webster. *Merriam-Webster's Collegiate Dictionary*. 10th ed. Springfield, MA: Merriam-Webster, 1999.

Nazarko, Linda. "The Therapeutic Uses of Cranberry Juice." *Nursing Standard* 9, no. 34 (1995): 33-35.

O'Connor, Bonnie. *Healing Traditions: Alternative Medicine and the Health Professions*. Philadelphia: University of Pennsylvania Press, 1995.

Roerich, Helena. *Fiery World 1*. New York: Agni Yoga Society, http://www.agniyoga.org/ay_frame.html?app_id=FW1, 1933.

Schiodt, Frank, Fedja Rochling, Donna Casey, and William Lee. "Acetaminophen Toxicity in an Urban County Hospital." *The New England Journal of Medicine* 337, no. 16 (1997): 1112-7.

Smart, Charles. "Clinical Experience with Nordihydroguaiaretic Acid: "Chaparral Tea" in the Treatment of Cancer." *Rocky Mountain Medical Journal* 67, no. 11 (1970): 39-43.

Sullivan, Louise. *Spiritual Writings of Louise de Marillac: Correspondence and Thoughts*. New York: New City Press, ed. and trans. 1991.

Tanne, Janice. "Food and Drugs Alter Response to Anesthesia." *BMJ: British Medical Journal* 317, no. 7166 (1998): 1102.

Tompkins, Peter and Christopher Bird. *The Secret Life of Plants*. New York: Harper & Row, 1973.

Treasure, Jonathan. "Herbal Pharmacokinetics." *Journal of the American Herbalist Guild* 1, no. 1 (2000): 2-11.

Tyler, Varro. *The Honest Herbal*. New York: Haworth Press, 1993.

Vogel, Morris and Charles Rosenberg. *The Therapeutic Revolution: Essays in the Social History of American Medicine*. Philadelphia: University of Pennsylvania Press, 1979.

World Health Organization. "Good Manufacturing Practices." In *WHO Technical Report Series Number 863*, 178-84. Geneva, 1996.

———. "Guidelines for the Appropriate Use of Herbal Medicines." In *WHO Regional Publications*. Geneva, 1998.

———. "Regulatory Situation of Herbal Medicine." Geneva, 1998.

Zevin, Igor. *A Russian Herbal: Traditional Remedies for Health and Healing*. Rochester, VT: Healing Arts Press, 1997.

the Ether Element

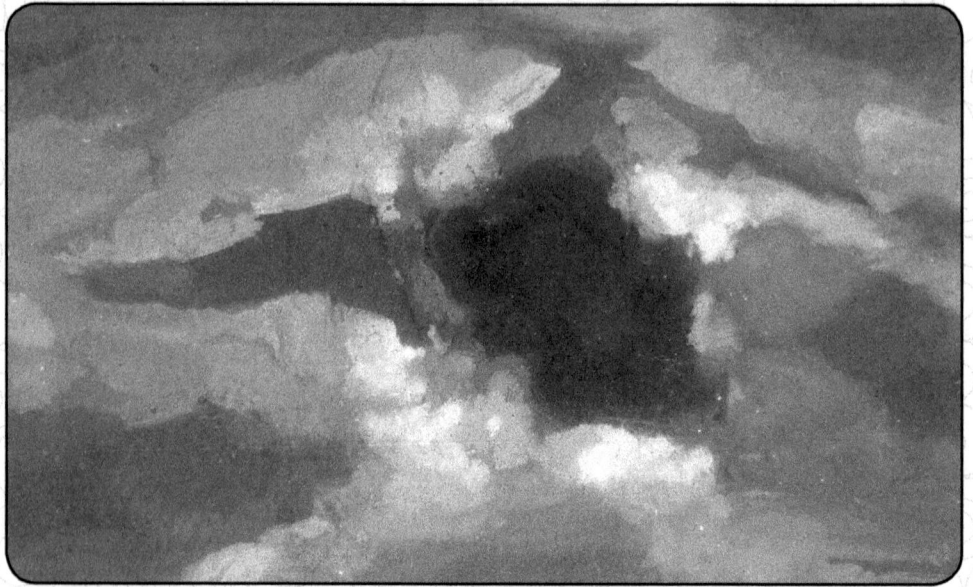

Study of Clouds
Nicholas Roerich, 1936-1942

CHAPTER SEVEN

Effecting the Ether Element

There are many facets to creating a holistic practice in nurse-herbalism. The first six chapters detail my recommendations, which are the result of years of choices that I have made in practice, education, and research. If you begin a practice following these chapters, I am confident that you will be prepared to care for people in partnership with plants. There is, however, another dimension, another gear if you will, to nurse-herbalism that I would like to introduce you to. It is the more esoteric dimension associated with the element ether and consciousness—the transformation of Self (capital S-elf refers to the true nature), which I refer to as "effecting the ether element," and the development of Self as medicine. I have spent many months wondering if I should write this chapter on a subject that has been as much a part of my herbal practice as the content in the other six—perhaps more so. Esoteric subjects, when written down on a two- dimensional page, run the risk of sounding hokey. I have already told stories of the plants such as St. John's Wort that have introduced me to the consciousness of plants and given me opportunities for spiritual experiences within the human-plant connection. This chapter contains suggestions for putting that awareness of plant consciousness and connection into action.

Nurse-herbalism is a dynamic platform for the evolution of nursing practice as a healing art and science. It is also a natural chalice for nursing as a spiritual path of Self-discovery. Partnership with plants is a special invitation to learning about the Creator and the creation, which is us, animals, the green world, and the cosmos. In partnership with plants, we become the students of Mother Nature, the powerful life force for creativity on the planet. The focus of our study is making medicine. In my heart of hearts, I know that the best medicine makers are those who perpetually stand in awe of the power of nature. They see that power as well as the wisdom and love in the heart of nature everywhere. Medicine is that healing energy we carry within us. It is our nature connected in harmony with the elements of Mother Nature. Medicine is also the remedies and interventions that we create to contain the healing energy we have to share with others. These remedies are the materialization of the elements fire, air, water, earth, and ether.

In the healing arts and in science in general, there is often greater focus on the basic four elements: earth, water, air, and fire. The fifth element ether[1] is quite elusive and therefore challenging to discuss. It has been called "infinite substance"[2] in esoteric texts on the ancient wisdom traditions. Ether is essence or life force, also referred to in alchemy as quintessence, that which binds together the four other elements. Ether is essential in healing work. It is an essence discoverable and observable through alchemical process in which the *effect* of herbal interventions is the transformation of substances in the material plane and of consciousness. The verb *effect* means to "bring into being often by surmounting obstacles."[3] There are many obstacles within and without that oppose any creative process, including transformation of matter and spirit.

One obstacle to surmount in nurse-herbalism as in all other healing art forms is what to discuss. The healing process—creating and maintaining balance—is often quite delicate. You have heard the expression that "life hangs by a thread." From my experience as a nurse, I can witness the truth of this statement. I have also seen people's healing process thwarted in the twinkling of an eye by unkind words, improper lifestyle choices, and sudden injury or trauma. Studying health patterns so closely in people provides easy viewing of the powerful effects on someone's healing

---

1   Ether, as it is used here, is not to be confused with the substance used as an anesthetic agent.

2   Helena Blavatsky, *The Secret Doctrine: The Synthesis of Science, Religion, and Philosophy* (London: The Theosophical Publishing Co., 1888), 671.

3   Merriam-Webster, *Merriam-Webster's Collegiate Dictionary*, 10th ed. (Springfield, MA: Merriam-Webster, 1999).

process, body, mind, emotion, spirit, or consciousness. The healers I have trained with have all taught me by example and verbally to keep still and not talk too freely about people's healing process. In nursing, there are laws protecting client confidentiality; but, in nurse-herbalism and the healing arts, keeping still is important to protecting the delicate presence of the ether element.

Along the same lines, I am also careful about when, where, and how I discuss herbal remedies. Nurse-herbalists have historically shared herbal recipes in the spirit of community healing and building knowledge. Many of the receipt books I have reviewed in historical collections contain recipes for herbal simples. Appendix A in this book continues the healing tradition in nursing of sharing recipes for simples. There are some aspects of herbalism that are not typically discussed in a public forum such as a book. Many healers in indigenous cultures will never write down their herbal recipes and remedies. Some say it is because they do not want the information stolen or the plant populations harmed by too many users. But another important reason is that manifesting the ether element dimension of herbalism is a spiritual experience and therefore sacred. I am referring primarily to the human-plant connection that people and herbalists alike make.

I made the decision to share some of my thoughts and stories about the sacred ether element of nurse-herbalism when that field of St. John's Wort appeared behind the hospital. I do so because I know that the experiences I have had with the consciousness of plants are a gift from the Creator. Those gifts are meant to be shared. Those who have ears will hear. The integrative insights for holistic practice in this ether chapter are important for the binding or weaving together of all parts of nurse-herbalist practice so that it becomes a cohesive offering in the healing art: alchemy, spagyrics, formulation, the wisdom of elders, diplomacy, peacemaking, and invocation. Please know that if you choose not to read this chapter, I fully understand. It may really be a bit presumptuous of me to try to give words to the formless and that which should in essence remain formless. But I have made my decision to give this ether chapter to you for consideration. I am right with my Creator. The choice and the response will be yours. We begin with alchemy and the possibilities for Self-transformation available to those who practice and receive nurse-herbalism.

ALCHEMY

Alchemy is an important term from ancient history for anyone to know about who is interested in the deeper study of herbalism as a healing art that leads to the transformation of Self. Alchemy is not a typical subject in conventional nursing, but herbalism has a strong history that includes alchemy. Alchemy is a form of chemistry and a philosophy that was practiced in the and during Renaissance. Outwardly alchemical methods were discussed in terms of refining the process of transmuting baser metals into finding a universal solvent and the ultimate panacea or elixir of life. One of the most renowned alchemists was Paracelsus.

Paracelsus applied alchemical and hermetic principles in the development of a practice of medicine that stressed the importance of clients' thoughts and emotions. He applied the Hermetic philosophy of *The Emerald Tablet* of the connection of mind and matter in the holistic care of people. Hermes Trismegistus, also known as Balinas, whom the Greeks considered a messenger of the Gods, was the third (Trismegistus) incarnation of Hermes who translated the ancient philosophy known as *The Emerald Tablet*. Hermetic texts, the oldest spiritual tradition in the West, have inspired Judaism, Christianity, Islam, Paganism, and Gnosticism. Fundamental to Hermeticism is the emphasis on Self-knowledge and the understanding of Self and all matter as the manifestation of the elements of creation.

Although today Paracelsus might be revered as a holistic physician, during his time, he— like many creative scientists and alchemists— was persecuted. Through a current cultural lens, Paracelsus' actions would be in accordance with best practice in infectious disease control. For example, he insisted that physicians stop dressing wounds with dung and instead prevent wound infections while allowing the wound to heal itself. He also "declared that diseases of miners were caused by dust particles and not by the mountain spirits upset by their mining and insisted that poisons were really chemical compounds and introduced the notion of proper dosages."[4] Paracelsus and many other scientists who have studied the ancient scientific writings such as *The Emerald Tablet*

---

4   Dennis Hauck, *The Emerald Tablet: Alchemy for Personal Transformation* (New York: Penguin Putnam Inc., 1999), 297.

are like nurses who have historically been known to be keen observers of human behavior. They know that life is not only substance but also spirit or essence. Nature, too, is also essence and substance. The Hermetic teachings applied in alchemy describe the concept this way: "That which is above, is as that which is below; And that which is below, is as that which is above." Spirit infuses all matter and matter becomes spirit.

It was easy for me to become interested in alchemy and Self-transformation in my twenties because as a professional dancer I was having experiences such as that which happened with breath and the fan dance that I described in Chapter 4. Through these dance experiences. I knew the truth of the possibility of Self-transformation according to Hermetic principle. Actively engaging this principle, we realize that there is a strong connection between the health of the body and consciousness. People talk about the body-mind connection but body-consciousness is more than body-mind. Consciousness is quintessence, that which binds or integrates all elements together in the process of Self-transformation as above so below and as below so above. The mind does not do that. Mind is the air element. It is represented in thought, belief, and reflection. Meditation and prayer can also be conducted from the level of the mind. Consciousness is ether and quintessence. According to Hermes Trismegistus, ether essence, which the Greeks referred to as "pneuma," is the "instrument or medium by which all is produced."[5] It is always present where life is, but it is intangible. Hildegard von Bingen, a twelfth-century nurse philosopher, referred to life force as "viriditas," translated as greenness, the principle of life transmitted from God into plants, animals, and gems.[6] This life force, essence, and greenness are what the great alchemists attempt to harness in their healing elixirs.

Herbalists often hold that the true medicine of any plant is in its essence, life force, or greenness. It is the plant's essence that catalyzes a certain type of change and transformation in humans. That essence might also be described as the plant's consciousness. I have also found this underlying philosophy demonstrated most clearly by traditional and indigenous peoples who have a deep respect for all life forms,

---

5 Blavatsky, *The Secret Doctrine: The Synthesis of Science, Religion, and Philosophy*: 672.
6 Hildegard von Bingen and Bruce Hozeski, *Hildegard von Bingen's Mystical Visions* (Santa Fe: Bear & Company, 1986), xxvii.

including plants. They assign names to plants as a way of conveying their understanding of the consciousness of a plant and our connection with it. For example, herbalists among the Delaware people refer to tobacco (*Nicotiana tabacum*), a sacred plant, in their medicine gathering prayer as "Grandfather."[7]

Many cultures have records of accessing the consciousness of plants. In recent times, however, these records most often have to do with the experiences that occur in relationship to the psychoactive principles of plants, a relationship often described as magical or shamanistic rather than natural or scientific. The crossover between science and spirit worlds is often blurred by certain spiritual and health beliefs or the lack thereof. Scientist and healers, such as Hildegard von Bingen, have identified numerous ways in which plants affect consciousness. Their natural beauty, their fragrance, their action in the body lift our spirits, change our perceptions, and heal us. Yet, some plants are also capable of altering our state of consciousness to the degree that Self-awareness becomes lost. While I respect the choices of those who engage in such plant relationships, I want to be clear as I was earlier in this book when I discussed the negative and positive psychic states that the practices in plant-partnership of which I write stem from a relationship with plants that is fully conscious and aware, amazing but not necessarily magical. The spiritual connection with plants leads to greater insight into their nature that can also be discovered, explained, and integrated by a human partner who is willing to delve into a study that creates a parallel and balanced evolution in botanical understanding. Botanical study takes many forms.

One of my first lessons in effecting ether in herbal medicine making came from my mother. This is not surprising because, as I mentioned earlier, my Cornish Celtic roots through my mother and her father have been the source of plant inspiration throughout my life. Every year, at the Christmas holiday in December, my mother made "Lemon Bread." Lemon Bread is actually a delicious cake that is baked in a loaf pan like bread. For those who have tasted pound cake, it is similar to a pound cake in consistency but those who have tasted pound cake quickly recognize

---

7   Gladys Tantaquidgeon, *Folk Medicine of the Delaware and Related Algonkian Indians* (Harrisburg: Pennsylvania Historical and Museum Commission, 1972), 13.

that it is not a pound cake. Lemon Bread is exquisitely delicious and in a class all by itself. In fact, it is so special that it is a family secret recipe. I watched my mother make it every year for seventeen years and on my eighteenth birthday received a recipe card with the instructions printed out by my mother. She swore me to secrecy that auspicious day and threatened "terrible things" would happen should I ever leak the recipe to a non-family member!

What makes Lemon Bread so delicious is its taste and consistency. What makes it so special is that the recipe should not work, from the perspective of culinary science. I find it most interesting to watch the transformation of the batter while I prepare it carefully according to the recipe. I am not typically a cook who follows recipes to the letter because I have enough experience to know how to achieve in the kitchen what I envision. But Lemon Bread is different. I follow the recipe. When making Lemon Bread, adding the ingredients in a particular order is part of the alchemy that ensures the transformation of the batter. You see, when the lemon (*Citrus limon*) is added to the batter, it changes consistency before my eyes. The whole process of learning to make Lemon Bread and now continuing the tradition is an experience in alchemy. My mother never told me about alchemy. She simply told me that the recipe was a secret passed down through family tradition from my great-great grandmother from New Brunswick, Canada, and Europe before that. But every year, when I begin the ritual of making Lemon Bread I am aware of the transformation that has occurred in the batter as well as within and around me.

Herbs like lemon are catalysts for change. Many of those changes that occur in nature are yet to be fully understood. Lemon has a powerful effect in the Lemon Bread recipe. Healing plants each have an effect. They catalyze changes in the environment, in the body, and in medicines that we make—sometimes in ways that may be observed but not always explained. Such is the case with our family Lemon Bread. So it remains a secret recipe for which my siblings, cousins, and I are stewards. Some who would try to coerce us to tell the recipe have said we are not stewards but controllers. But the name calling that occurs is just playful banter. In my experience, people enjoy a good game; they love the challenge of seeking to discover nature's secrets. Life, like Lemon Bread, is full of secrets. Opportunity for alchemy is everywhere; that is, the opportunity for transformation and transmutation is everywhere.

Experiences and observations in people, plants, and nature beginning with my childhood interactions with lemon and the secret recipe Lemon Bread laid the perfect foundation for inquiry beyond the substance or chemical constituents of medicinal plants and into their essence. Essence is a word often used to describe the fifth element, ether, that is rarely discussed. The essence of lemon creates Lemon Bread. Oranges (*Citrus sinensis*) do not. I know because I have tried. Each plant, like each human and animal, has its essence. That essence is important to making plant medicines that are more than just plant concoctions or constituents. The ancient science of making medicines with plants that transform and transmute includes the ancient knowledge of drawing upon the essence of plants in simples and in formulations.

PLANT ALCHEMY

Spagyrics is the term that refers to plant alchemy. The word spagyria is derived from two Greek words meaning to draw out and to bind together. Paracelsus wrote, "Therefore, learn Alchimiam, otherwise called Spagyria, which teaches you to separate the false from the true."[8] Plant alchemists expand upon the basic science of extraction to remove the essence or philosophical principles of plants through separation, then purification, and finally recombination. "In the Spagyrists view these actions lead to an increase and a release of certain curative powers in the initial species."[9] The spagyric preparation "opens the plant" to liberate stronger curative power.[10] Spagyric preparations always contain the salts obtained through incineration and calcination of the plant residue. Albrecht von Herzeele, a nineteenth-century scientist who wrote *The Origin of Inorganic Substances*, showed that living plants are continuously *creating* matter in that they "transmute phosphorus into sulfur, calcium into phosphorus, magnesium into calcium, carbonic

---

8 Manfred Junius, *Practical Handbook of Plant Alchemy* (New York: Inner Traditions, 1985), 1.
9 Ibid.
10 Ibid., 3.

acid into magnesium, and nitrogen into potassium.[11] Animals also create matter in their bodies. Louis Kervan began preparing for his career as a scientist when he noticed as a young boy that chickens ate mica in their yard but no trace of mica could be found in them when they were slaughtered. However, the chickens produced eggs with calcareous shells even though they had not ingested calcium from land lacking in limestone. He realized later that the birds were transmuting one element into another. Antoine Laurent Lavoisier, the father of modern chemistry, stated the principle that in the universe, "nothing is lost, nothing is created, everything is transformed."[12] Spanish moss is able to grow on copper wire without soil, and seaweeds (*Laminaria spp.*) manufacture iodine. It is this etheric power that accounts for the fact that some plants germinate only in spring regardless of the amount of heat and water applied to them at other times of year.

Like plants, the human body has a way of transmuting elements. Kervan noticed that laborers sweat potassium even though they had eaten salt. Kervan also did not give calcium supplements to those needing calcium. He knew that to increase calcium in the body, one would provide organic (not mineral) silicic acid such as is found in plants rich in silicon. The body did the transformation of silicic acid to calcium. One plant used in silicic-calcium alchemy is Horsetail (*Equisetum arvense*). Herbalists can often readily apply alchemical principles like this in practice because they work with plant rather than single chemical constituents as is the case with pharmaceutical drugs. By introducing the etheric and alchemical dimensions to nurse-herbalism, we open up a realm of possibilities for medicine making and healing not only in humans but also the worn out and damaged soils of the earth environment as well.

Scientific analysis is an important way of knowing. Learning about the constituents of medicinal plants is one of many perspectives that form integrative insight. But ultimately the goal of scientific exploration of anything in nature, in our case healing plants, is to understand the whole, which is greater than the sum of the parts. Scientist Johann Wolfgang von

---

11 Peter Tompkins and Christopher Bird, *The Secret Life of Plants* (New York: Harper & Row, 1973), 278.
12 As cited in ibid., 275.

Goethe, whose focus was our actual experience and perception of the living world and its spiritual as well as material basis, wrote:

> In observing objects of Nature, especially those that are alive, we often think the best way of gaining insight into the relationship between their inner nature and the effects they produce is to divide them into their constitutional parts. Such an approach may, in fact, bring us a long way toward our goal. In a word, those familiar with science can recall what chemistry and anatomy have contributed toward an understanding and overview of Nature. But these attempts at division also produce many adverse effects when carried to an extreme. ...Thus observation of Nature is limitless, whether we make distinctions among the least particles or pursue the whole by following the trail far and wide.[13]

Nurses are often focused on outcomes and effects. I have in this book contributed to that focus by applying the nursing process to nurse-herbalism. There is, however, another dimension to nurse-herbalism that is greater than the sum of its parts or its effects. In partnering with people and plants with a conscious awareness of effecting ether, nurse-herbalists manifest new life, as above so below. A metaphor for this holistic impression and synthesis of nurse-herbalism is the midwife delivering a baby and rubbing its back as it takes its first breath as it creates a new pattern of extra-uterine life. As the touch of the midwife stimulates breath and life, so, too, do the hands of the nurse-herbalist and the client who touch the plants in making medicine that they hope will create healing transformation and transmutation.

Touching Plants

All material and spiritual action for healing in nurse-herbalism begins with touching plants. Plants come in contact with the body through the senses: tasting through the tongue, touching through the skin, and smelling through the nose. The person preparing a remedy effects the

---

13 Johann Wolfgang Goethe and Jeremy Naydler, *Goethe on Science* (Edinburgh: Floris Books, 1996), 36,49.

medicine or essence within that remedy. Many cultures know this and therefore have specific rules about the preparation of remedies so that the medicine of the plant is conveyed as fully as possible to the person in need. For example, in some European cultures, plants are harvested by hand only when specific planets are in certain positions in the sky. In the Mohawk tradition, medicine women, for example, are not allowed to prepare remedies when they are menstruating because it is known that the healing energy of the plants will drain into their own bodies rather than stay within the remedy being prepared.

When we touch plants with our hands, we can deliver a wholeness current from our heart—alpha to omega—just like we do when we work with the bodies of our clients. That current infuses into the remedy an energy that can be experienced by the client when they take the remedy to Self. This flow of energy is initiated in the heart as an expression of power, wisdom, and love and then flows out through the hands. The heart is situated in the nexus of the energy centers in the body where matter and spirit meet. Spirit and matter are not opposites; they are in polarity. At the center of polarity is unity. The material universe is the negative polarity and the spiritual the positive polarity. Matter (*mater*) is mother or yin. Matter (yin energy) provides the chalice for the anchoring and evolution of spiritual (yang) energy in the physical plane. Embracing the energy of the spiral of cosmic return, mater returns to spirit. This cycle of cosmic creation, known in Sanskrit as the Maha Kalpa, is the path of wholeness in which we realize all matter as spiritual essence. Through the nexus of the heart, we find the power wisdom and love to unify science, art, and spirituality in the creation of the healing garden where nurse-herbalists and their clients can touch plants on a daily basis.

The Healing Garden

Throughout history, nurses and midwives have had their herb and vegetable gardens as their laboratories for plant alchemy. Observing and touching nature effects many changes in body, mind, emotion, and spirit. A stroll through a meadow, a walk in the woods, and gardening can decrease stress levels, affect attitude, and cultivate a positive outlook on life. Gardens and gardening provide a connection with the earth, the soil, and the life that springs forth from it. Watching a plant grow gives a sense of the continuation of life. Watching a flower fade and "go by" or a tree lose its leaves before the cold season can reassure us that all life, not just human life, is impermanent and follows a rhythm or cycle. When people are sick, they often feel isolated and afraid. Being part of nature can reconnect people with the larger processes and cycles present in nature of which they are a part. Reestablishing a connection with nature and the Creator during illness can be comforting and healing.

Many healing institutions have employed landscape architects and artists to create gardens where clients have the opportunity to interact with nature. When I was at the University of Colorado, we created a rooftop garden outside the chemotherapy infusion center where cancer patients could actually see some of the plants such as the *Vincas* that inspired the drugs they were taking for healing. My favorite plant in that garden was a rose species known as the Joseph's Coat that was named after the biblical figure. That rose produced different color roses all on the same plant at the same time. It served as a great living metaphor that resonated with many of the clients who knew that their cancer was not the same as someone else's even when the doctors gave it the same name. Their path to healing cancer was as unique as the different color roses that grew on the same bush.

That rooftop garden at the Cancer Center was an interdisciplinary project to create a healing environment utilizing principles of horticultural therapy. Horticultural therapy has been described as one of the oldest healing art forms that is probably so helpful because people view the plant world as nonthreatening. The horticultural therapist is concerned with how people interact in the environment, how people behave and feel when working with plants, and how people react to passive involvement with plants. In a therapy session, people may be given an opportunity to pot plants or seeds individually with the purpose of improving hand-eye coordination or attention skills. They may also work with others to improve socialization skills. One leader in the field wrote that, "The essence of horticulture is action. ... A person works with plants doing things with them or to them to modify and enhance their growth. ... One explanation for the positive response that man has to working with plants may be because it deals with life cycles and most people make a ready translation between the life cycle of plants and their own human life cycle."[14] Tending plant life can be engaging and Self-transformative especially when communing with the plant that will produce the medicines for simples and formulations applied in caring practice.

Power and Prescription

Nurse-herbalists can effect great changes and healing with application of herbal simples in a uniquely designed plan of holistic care with the comfort and balance of clients at heart. Formulating herbal remedies that involve multiple plants rather than simples is another dimension of practice that evolves with increasing experience and study of individual plants, botanical science, and the wisdom tradition (including alchemy) surrounding medicine making. Formulation is a specific skill often under-represented in the herbal marketplace. True formulation is not "everything but the kitchen sink" mentality. Some product formulators demonstrate their lack of botanical knowledge by putting every herb with a specific known action into a product, ergo the kitchen sink. Instead, formulations are a synergistic combination of herbs that represent different but complementary contributions of the energetic, biological, chemical, and spiritual aspects of the plants that will move the client toward a more balanced state. Formulations typically refer to the herbal remedy designed for a specific client. In nurse-herbalist practice, the formulation is most typically a whole-herb tea. The formulator also takes into account the spirit (energetics) and matter of all client Self-care and prescribed health promotion activities from the nurse-herbalist as well as other caregivers. The client's environment is also considered during the process of formulation. The healing transformative action of the entire formulation is greater than the sum of the parts—the herbs and health promotion activities as they would be applied individually.

Manifesting the power of prescription in formulation does require additional education and mastery in health pattern recognition and botanical knowledge. The foundation for formulation is knowledge of

---

14 Diane Relf, "Dynamics of Horticultural Therapy," http://www.hort.vt.edu/HUMAN/ht1. html.

the character as well as the chemistry of a plant. By plant character, I mean the botany and energetics of the plant, its history, and growth patterns. Getting to know a plant's character is similar to getting to know a client. The better a nurse knows the client, the more likely s/he is to provide care that meets the individual needs of that client. For example, in an emergency department, the nurse is more likely to follow an established best-practice protocol for care that addresses the greatest risk to client safety if the nurse does not know the client. Risk management companies teach health practitioners that risk is considerably less when the client and practitioner have a relationship. Nurse-herbalists can increase their relationships with healing plants through tea tastings, herb walks, visits to botanical gardens, gardening, and visually inspecting whole herbs used in formulation.

Secondly, formulation is attempted only after a full assessment and clear identification of health patterns. If the client situation does not allow for the time to do a full assessment of the health history, tongue and pulse diagnosis, then give simples to start. Many of the simples discussed throughout this book support the lifestyle and dietary changes that should, according to many traditions including nursing, be the first interventions introduced to bring about tremendous levels of healing transformation, leaving the application of formulas to very specific circumstances.

Many traditions such as TCM have books on established formulations that have been used for centuries. I was taught, however, to create my own formulations for clients according to TCM principles and have been doing so since 1992. Being able to prepare formulations for clients at a specific time and place is best practice in herbalism. When using an established formula, do so mindfully. Always adjust the recipe to meet the needs of the specific client. There are certain herbs that are synergistic together as there are herbs that have been found to not work together well in formulation. I pay attention to this traditional wisdom just as I follow the Lemon Bread recipe. Each formulation is applied in the care of clients according to the five rights just as is done with simples.

One of the observations that I as well as many of my herbal–teacher colleagues have made for a number of years now is that while we used to formulate regularly, we seem to now be able to effect the desired result with the least invasive means. This means that we don't seem to need to apply as many herbs in care. Focusing even more specifically on the ancient tradition of suggesting lifestyle and diet changes first with the support of simple herbal remedies, we have found formulations less necessary. There is rarely a need to rush to formulation when the benefits of working with the client and developing their connection with the plant world over the course of a few weeks or months prior to formulation is more than evident case after case.

Working according to tradition this way allows for the clearest recognition of the moment in time when an herbal formulation is needed. That clear moment emerges as an understanding of the client's overall health pattern as a combination of patterns that are best treated simultaneously so that the energy is transmuted rather than displaced. Often with herbal simples, healing is effected by moving or displacing energy that is stuck or stagnant. Nature then effects the cure because energy is in motion. But with more serious or chronic health concerns, patterns become more interwoven and the imbalances in body, mind, emotion, and/or spirit more deeply entrenched. These are the times when energy must be moved in multiple directions at one time that a formula is called for. That formula must be specific.

Each formula has a leader, an herb that provides the focus and structure for the actions of the other herbs. It is in the assignment of the herb that will take the lead position and the herbs that will support it that the nurse-herbalist's advanced knowledge of physiology as well as plant energetic characteristics become essential. As noted earlier, I have found the TCM system to be the most complementary to nursing practice. It is the most exacting in terms of identifying and delineating plants' energetic characteristics and therefore makes it easier to create balanced formulations that address the client's total need. I use the language of TCM herbalism to describe the characteristic actions of the herbs I use in formulation. Like flower arranging, an odd number of herbs is typically assigned to a formula; however, some of the client's health promotion activities are so powerfully represented in a client's life that they may occupy a prominent place in formulation and the number of herbs used would resort to an even number when the activity or drug is factored in to the overall recipe for healing.

Herbal teas made from dried or fresh whole herbs, or cut pieces in some cases such as roots and barks, allow the client and nurse-herbalist the greatest access to alchemical complementation of the client pattern. My clients love to learn to recognize each herb in their tea formula that addresses the health pattern they have been observing in their lives before receiving the herbal formula. They often comment that they "see themselves" in the formula much the way a person looking at a work of art might say the same. A personalized tea formulation is a work of art that the client then creatively engages with in the act of cooking and tasting. Some herbalists do not use whole-plant formulations, but I find their application according to the five rights after working with simple-supported lifestyle and dietary changes rapid and effective, requiring less plant material than if given immediately after first assessment.

Some clients have described the effect of formulations as magical when, in fact, following traditional science and nursing process outcomes is predictable. However, none of the outcomes are fully reproducible because formulation must be individualized for plant alchemy to occur. People, both clients and nurse-herbalists, must in my experience have a connection with the plant world and a desire to partner with plants for healing transformation to occur. The work is creative. It is inspired by health patterns and a deep desire for healing and change. To those who know medicine only as an act that is done by one person to another rather than a participatory process engaging the elements of creation, nurse-herbalism in this ether dimension of care would seem like magic from the realm of the paranormal. But for those who truly partner with plants and love them as grandfather, grandmother, father, mother, sister, or brother, there is no other normal way of healing than this. Biomedicine often seems somewhat lifeless in comparison. Nurse-herbalists have the power to infuse biomedical culture and care with life force through integrative herbal care.

Over the centuries, some have deemed the transformative power of herbal prescription "witchcraft" simply because it deviated from the status quo of orthodox medicine, religion, and science. Herbalism was a cloistered practice during the time of Hildegard von Bingen. Most nurses I have spoken with are unaware that it was women community healers, specifically herbalists and midwives, who were the stated focus of the *Malleus Malleficarum,* the document that guided the leaders of the Inquisition for 550 years from the 1300s until about 1850. So often this mass murder of peoples is discussed in regard to other histories that lasted for less than a decade, but the killing of innocent people—mostly women who were herbal healers in their communities, crossing national, political, and economic boundaries—has been paid little attention in recent years. The memory, however, still stands evident in the language, writing, and practices in which nurses and physicians within the biomedical culture and outside of it still fear marginalization as witches or some other term simply for expressing interest in the healing power of plants. Herbalism is often dubbed "unscientific" practice and the remedies "crude" by those who hold strong affiliation with the dominant biomedical culture. As Thomas Edison is often quoted as saying, "Until man duplicates a blade of grass, nature can laugh at his so-called scientific knowledge." Herbalists, traditional healers, physicians, nurses, and many others continue their scientific work with healing plants because there is much to learn and many clients seeking healing who may benefit from herbal remedies.

Fear has the ability to stifle creative expression in science. Science is exploration! When we presume to know all there is to know about the body, the mind, the spirit, and consciousness of people, animals, and plants, we may become energetically stuck. Stagnant energy becomes illness by ancient definition. Science starts with wonder! It is a process that begins with questions about life and nature that is everywhere. Some of the best life scientists are the elders in community. In the herbal tradition of many cultures, elders are knowledge holders about partnerships with plants and about life. It is the wisdom of community elders that typically guides scientific exploration of plant knowledge and the application of plants in healing. I include the elders of the biomedical community who work with plants in this statement as well. Elders such as Dr. Jim Duke and Dr. Norm Farnsworth (deceased) graciously informed my practice for decades with their plant wisdom directed at biomedical research and translation into application.

THE WISDOM OF ELDERS

The dictionary definition of wisdom is "accumulated philosophic or scientific learning; ability to discern inner qualities and relationships; insight."[15] Our insights as nurses and scientists are built on experience, observation, and study. Over time, those insights accumulate and are formed into wisdom under the guidance of our elders. Nurse-herbalism has a rich tradition in healing wisdom that can be tapped by those seeking insight. Hildegard von Bingen wrote that wisdom was less about thinking than about tasting. In Latin, the words wisdom (sapientia) and taste (sapere) come from the same root word. Nurse-herbalists and their clients know herbal remedies often by their taste as well as through the other senses. Wisdom and the ability to gain insight into the plant world are acquired through the experiences of the senses.

Wisdom for Hildegard von Bingen was an "awakening to life and to cosmic beauty."[16] Wisdom, she wrote, "resides in all creative works."[17] Nurse-herbalism is creative as well as scientific action. Nurse-herbalism involves growing, handling, harvesting, washing, and cooking plants. We have a wisdom tradition as well as knowledge of healing plants that has evolved over time and has been passed down from generation to generation. It includes ladling out bowls of healing soups to the poor, massaging herbal infused oils into painful bodies, anointing the dying with sacred herbal oil, serving a cup of tea to the stressed, bathing the sick with floral waters, and dressing the wounds of the weary. The history can continue. It is our choice to do so.

With the expansion of technology-based care, particularly in highly-industrialized nations, there has been significantly less interest and investment in continuing nurse-herbalism. I have not formally researched the current state of the science, but it is quite clear that the focus on nature, creating a healing environment, and the practice of nurse-herbalism is waning in comparison to previous times. My hypothesis for why this has been occurring is due to memory loss of the ability referred to by Cherokee elder Dhyani Ywahoo as the "turtle mind." In the elder's own words:

---

15 Merriam-Webster, *Merriam-Webster's Collegiate Dictionary.*
16 Von Bingen and Hozeski, *Hildegard von Bingen's Mystical Visions*: xx.
17 Ibid.

It's just thought regenerating, bringing together the left, right and the middle brain. We call that snake or turtle mind. That's very important. That is the balance of our whole nature. In the creation process, we say it's the emptiness that everything comes from, and it manifests through three fires. One is will. One is wisdom. The other is active intelligence. [It] is for the human being to rebuild—the rebuilding of the rainbow bridges to make the connection between those hemispheres of the brain. ... It is the seat of survival."[18]

Might it do nursing well to be more inclusive and embrace the potential of the turtle mind? Wisdom is described by elders as deep understanding and the integration of the spheres of the brain. The subsequent integrative insight that can come from activities such as nurse-herbalism heals not only the persons involved in the caring relationship. Integrative insight affects the survival of human life as a species. Some who have studied the human brain know that the hemispheres of the brain have very different functions but together they work as an integrated whole organ, which some scientists describe as holographic in nature in that it has a dimension of functionality yet is virtually unexplored. That dimension is where integration occurs as the conjunction of seemingly opposing forces. Ancient Hermetic as well as twenty-first-century Mayan tradition suggest that enlightenment is the result of that conjunction or integration of opposing forces or thought. If this is the case, as the wisdom of the elders suggest, then the integration or conjunction of technology and tradition or nature could affect the healing and survival of the planet and her inhabitants. Nurse-herbalists who pursue the integration of herbalism and contemporary nursing in a technological world may not be so much nostalgic as they are novel. Within this greater historical context, nurse-herbalism is an enduring healing tradition with the potential to promote healing and reform health care systems in the twenty-first- century global community.

Hildegard von Bingen described the essential task of personhood and citizenship as the "building of the house of wisdom in ourselves as

---

18 Bobette Perrone, H. Henrietta Stockel, and Victoria Krueger, *Medicine Women, Curanderas, and Women Doctors*, 1st ed. (Norman, OK: University of Oklahoma Press, 1989), 75.

individuals and in community with other humans and all other creatures of our earth."[19] Community building based in wisdom of beauty and viriditas was the foundation for the cultivation of justice and holiness that led to the possibility of peacemaking and peacekeeping. Given the nature of their work, nurse-herbalists are well positioned in communities to become diplomats who promote plant-like gentleness as the ethical foundation for the cultivation of healing and peace.

A LIVING ETHIC
FOR HERBAL DIPLOMACY

It is interesting to me that the words ethic and ether are so similar. This is because I have noticed the need for greater attention to ethics when involved in exploration of the ether element. Plants do not speak, they barely move, and they are highly visible. This suggests that they are in general a potentially vulnerable population. Certain species of plants are documented as vulnerable populations and legal protections are put in place to protect them. Therefore, nurse-herbalists who would work with the ether element of plant healing must have an awareness of this vulnerability and cultivate an ethic in practice that supports healing plant populations that are part of the global community.

Nurses are taught to care for individuals, families, and communities. My historical research shows that community has not only been the platform for the provision of nursing services but has also been the support base for the development of the science of the discipline.[20] Building caring community is nursing. Healing plants are part of caring community. Plants bring people together. They are a common denominator that can promote unity between cultures in that plants and the quest for healing remedies are a shared experience. They are also typically present in the exchanges that occur between peoples when sharing their cultures.

---

19 Ibid., xxi.
20 Martha Libster and Betty Ann McNeil, *Enlightened Charity: The Holistic Nursing Care, Education and Advices Concerning the Sick of Sister Matilda Coskery, (1799-1870).* (Farmville, NC: Golden Apple Publications, 2009); Martha Libster, *Herbal Diplomats: The Contribution of Early American Nurses (1830-1860) to Nineteenth-Century Health Care Reform and the Botanical Medical Movement* (Thornton, CO: Golden Apple Publications, 2004).

Yet with the increasing emphasis and the choice for more technology, people may identify less and less in consciousness with the plants that have historically unified us. Some people have no awareness that the pizza sauce they are eating is made from living plants—herbs and tomatoes, such as that high school student who was eating broccoli, not realizing it was a plant food. Some children have no connection with the plant world and even fear it. "Nature deficit disorder" is a popular term adopted to describe this social phenomenon.[21] Societal value of plant-based foods and medicines is not what it used to be. There is a growing need for an ethic for nurse-herbalist practice that can guide the development and maintenance of plant-human partnerships. The ethical framework I suggest is an active or living ethic that is grounded in cultural diplomacy that I call "herbal diplomacy."

My understanding of herbal diplomacy began with my research in 2000 of early American nurse-herbalists' healing work in community. Though they were not referred to as "nurse-herbalists" at the time, it was clear from many diaries, journals, and community and other public records that nurses of the period acted as diplomats. They shared cultural knowledge about healing and herbal remedies with peoples from other cultures.[22] Nurses such as in the Shaker communities had strong connections with the plant world. Some diary accounts of European-American women indicate that the women shared their healing knowledge with others outside their immediate communities in a spirit of "gentleness and fairness."[23] Cherokee elders report that their botanical healing knowledge was shared in the belief that "all are in communion with the universe and that every part of life is related."[24] A spirit of unity led to cultural diplomacy demonstrated in community building through the sharing of recipes for healing with herbs.

I have taught and written about cultural diplomacy in nursing ever since I learned about our professional heritage. For the last two decades, the concepts of cultural competence, cultural sensitivity, and cultural

---

21 Richard Louv, *Last Child in the Woods : Saving Our Children from Nature-Deficit Disorder* (Chapel Hill: Algonquin Books of Chapel Hill, 2005).

22 Libster, *Herbal Diplomats: The Contribution of Early American Nurses (1830-1860) to Nineteenth-Century Health Care Reform and the Botanical Medical Movement*: 256.

23 Ibid.

24 Ibid.

awareness have been explored extensively as they relate to nursing practice and education. Cultural diplomacy is the *active* expression of these concepts of cultural awareness, sensitivity, and educational competence. Cultural diplomacy is demonstrated in certain skills through which the nurse's caring ethic is demonstrated. Diplomacy is the highly refined communication skill used in developing and maintaining relationships between different cultures. It is an antidote to the culture clashes between nations and peoples that lead to frustration, power struggle, anger, argument, and violence.

The goal of cultural diplomacy in general is to build long-term relationships that can lead to an increasingly peaceful global community. The purpose of cultural diplomacy in health care is improving communication and understanding between peoples who hold different health beliefs so that there is a possibility for exchange of health care knowledge and resources as is appropriate for building a caring peaceful community. Culture clash is the greatest obstacle to building a global health care community. At the center of culture clash in any community or nation, including the health care community, is the fear of loss of control and the subsequent need to dominate others and convert them to one's own cultural beliefs and practices. Psychologist M. Scott Peck wrote that the purpose of community building is peacemaking. He also stated that as long as people try to "convert and heal" others and attempt to turn them toward their own paradigm of the world, true community is not possible.[25] The diplomat does not seek to convert and heal; s/he uses the skill of tactful negotiation to maintain open communication and diminish any hostility between parties. The cultural diplomat in health care inspires an ideal of a peaceful global health care community working together toward a plan of health care for all that is inclusive of all health beliefs, practices, and systems.

Nurse-herbalists are uniquely situated for the bridging work of the cultural diplomat because they are educated and experienced in the biomedical, traditional, and Self-care paradigms and because healing plants are common to all paradigms. Nurse-herbalists also walk between the plant and human worlds, acknowledging the importance

---

25 M. Scott Peck, *The Different Drum: Community Making and Peace* (New York: Touchstone, 1987).

of the relationship between the two. The living ethic of forging diplomatic relations between people and plants and also among health care cultures evolves naturally out of the responsibilities of the nurse-herbalist. Herbal diplomacy begins with dialog and discussion about plants.

Herbal Experiment: Power Object

This is actually an experiment in Herbal Diplomacy.

1. Choose an object that represents your personal power. Study it carefully and write down how you came to choose the object.
2. Make a list of the qualities of your personal power object.
3. Make a list of the qualities of a nurse-herbalist that represent power to you.
4. Compare and contrast the lists. Now make a separate list of what power qualities you hold that are your strengths. Make another list of the qualities of power you need to fulfill your role as a nurse-herbalist.
5. Go to your safe place and ask the question, "What is the first step I can take to develop the qualities of power that I need for herbal diplomacy?"

Understanding your beliefs and perceptions about power in general and your own personal power is foundational preparation for herbal diplomacy work.

The following is a list of suggestions for developing communication skills in cultural and herbal diplomacy:

1. Differentiate advocacy from diplomacy. Dialog should be inclusive and inviting. Nurses are taught in education programs to advocate for clients. Then they become employees and have to learn to juggle the switch to diplomacy in which they honor the needs of clients as well as the needs of their employer. The biomedical culture often

demands of nurses that they serve as advocates for those who are incapacitated in some way and therefore cannot speak or act in their own interest. Diplomacy typically involves more than one party and the nurse's role in diplomacy is to represent all parties' interests in negotiation rather than advocate for or champion one party or one view. Advocacy implies polarization of some kind whereas diplomacy suggests neutralization. I recommend striving for diplomacy in nurse-herbalism as informed consent is more possible within a context of diplomacy. For consent to be "informed," three criteria must be met:

    a. The risks and the benefits as well as potential alternative interventions must be discussed with the client. In herbal diplomacy, the benefits and risks of herbal intervention are clearly delineated and alternatives to herbal care discussed.

    b. The client must give their consent freely. There can be no coercion. Applying techniques discussed earlier in the book such as Modeling and Role Modeling help the nurse-herbalist establish and maintain stronger boundaries with Self and clients so that diplomacy is a possible approach to care. I have met nurses who advocate so strongly for herbalism with their clients that they sound and act coercive.

    c. The client must be competent to make a rational choice for herbalism.

2. <u>Create a mutual frame of reference</u>. It is helpful to parties with different beliefs and ideas if the diplomat suggests a frame of reference that all parties can relate to. That frame of reference may be a mutual goal for the outcome of the meeting, for example. The mutual frame of reference is helpful when one or both parties become disturbed and the risk of communication breakdown becomes apparent. The mutual frame of reference can be used to re-focus discussion.

3. <u>Question your approach</u>. Ask yourself what questions you have about a client, an herb, or anything that you study. If you have no questions at all (which I often hear students say though they rarely actually mean it), and you think you already have all the answers, you are most likely in a state of mindlessness. It is best to cultivate a combination of confidence and uncertainty. This state, according to Ellen Langer, researcher and author of the book *Mindfulness*, leads to an ability for creativity.[26] Diplomacy requires a person to be nimble, mindful, and highly creative.

4. <u>Engage with culture of others</u>. Prepare for diplomacy work. Modeling the client's culture is part of modeling their worldview. Read the writings of another's culture. Learn the language. Visit their museums and study their art. Learn their medicine and nursing practice. This is a big task so it is best to follow the lead of your hosts, guests, clients, or students.

5. <u>Take care of yourself</u>. Respectful relationship with the Self is fundamental practice for diplomacy work with others. One Buddhist Lama writes, "We could not have gotten sick in the first place without some kind of loss of interest and attention. Whether we were run down by a car or we caught a cold, there was some gap in which we did not take care of ourselves—an empty moment in which we ceased to relate to things properly…disease is a direct message to develop a proper attitude of mindfulness…a sense of composure."[27] In addition to taking care of your body, mind, and spirit, it is important to cultivate the health of the emotional body. Emotion is energy-in-motion. In health diplomacy negotiations, as in all aspects of nursing care, emotions run high. The nurse-herbalist can reduce the amount of the effect of emotional strain and drain with visualization. See emotions as liquid—water. Visualize the emotional body

---

26 Ellen Langer, *Mindfulness* (Reading, MA: Perseus Books, 1989), 143.
27 Chogyam Trungpa, "Healing & the Reality of Death," *Shambhala Sun*, no. March (1994).

as a tank or chalice holding water. Leaks in the vessel lead to stress, strain, and fatigue. Strong vessels emote by releasing energy into motion by choice rather than having the energy leak out. Many diplomats are emotionally passionate about such concepts as the desire for freedom and creating policy and practice that will unify and raise people up. Diplomats, like psychotherapists, develop emotional mastery as well as communication skills that help others channel emotional energy tied to beliefs, thoughts, and practices into constructive change that creates caring community and peace.

6. <u>Cultivate respect as an innate quality of one who would carry medicine.</u> Respect is a value that is part of the nursing heritage. The French Daughters and American Sisters of Charity nurses, for example, highly valued the demonstration of respect for others. They even cultivated respect for those who persecuted them and the religious beliefs that guided their ability to nurse the sick, wounded, and dying in times of plague and war when others in community would not. Respect is an internalized state of being that enables one to be in the presence of others who differ greatly from oneself. Respect is extended not only to people but also to the diplomatic process in which the people are engaged. Respect for the diplomatic process often guides the choices the herbal diplomat makes regarding initial actions, communications, and negotiations. Numerous scientific experiments and anecdotes suggest the sentience of plant life.[28] Therefore, respect for plants is also fundamental to herbal diplomacy.

7. <u>Seek cooperation not co-optation.</u> Some of the best diplomats I have met are members of indigenous communities. They have a respect and reverence for life that is palpable and that extends to all life forms, including plants. I suggest that this reverence for life is a core value

---

28 Tompkins and Bird, *The Secret Life of Plants.*

of the herbal diplomat who would seek to heal the planet as well as human beings and create a culture of peace. Here is one example of the spirit of diplomacy that I have experienced in relationship with indigenous elders:

Witch hazel (*Hamamelis virginiana*) was dropped from the National Formulary in the United States in 1955 because it was believed to be without any medicinal virtues. The formulary states that witch hazel water is an "embrocation which appeals to the psychic influence of faith."[29] Traditional evidence must not be overlooked. Witch hazel has a history in North American Indian medicine as a powerful healing herb. I have been to Zezi's house after she has harvested witch hazel and watched her strip the bark. She would not do all that work for nothing! I have partnered with witch hazel in skin care for decades because it helps, not because of faith. Experience and learning from a wise elder are hardly the psychic influence of faith. Not long after I had taught this plant medicine to nursing students a few years ago, I was invited to assist at a small medical museum with an herb garden. Standing majestically in the corner was a witch hazel. The docents talked about the little garden plants but not the tree even though it was labeled. The day I was there, the docents had been lovingly weeding and beautifying the garden. In the corner by the tree was a huge pile of witch hazel twigs and small branches that had been trimmed from the tree. I asked what they planned to do with the pile and was told that it was going to the trash. How do I express my horror at such human mindlessness and ignorance? There is so much of it related to plants and, therefore, I have compassion to a degree. But from my perspective and experience, that pile of twigs destined for the trash was a pile of gold. The people knew it was medicinal but in talking with them I found out that they did not know

---

29 *The Dispensatory of the United States of America*, ed. Arthur Osol and George Farrar, 24th ed. (Philadelphia: J.B. Lippincott, 1947), 529.

how to make medicine from the tree. What concerned me most was that after I told them about the important medicine in the tree bark, they showed no remorse or attempt to retrieve that pile. They did not ask me what to do next. They did not care that they were wasting a very large amount of medicine. Ignorance became negligence at that moment in time. What happens to a planet when humans exhibit such negligence? The indigenous peoples have legends about that. Herbal Diplomats® warn about the importance of listening to the plants, tradition, and indigenous peoples who are the stewards of their place. I listened as Zezi taught me, a plant-lovin' herbal diplomat who grew up on the Mohawk Trail in New England, about her ways. When the time came, I tried to pass on the wisdom of the witch hazel, a mighty teacher indeed. No one there would receive it. I do not know what happened to that particular garden but I have seen what happens when the plant healer is rejected. Healing energy and the plant withdraw peacefully as if bowing to human power and will and Earth changes as a result.

Peace is promoted through cultural expression and exchange. The healing arts are a vital part of peaceful culture. As people heal, they often experience peace and as they seek peace, people experience healing. It is important to protect the possibility of peace through culture. Nursing, herbalism, and all expressions of healing should experience the same freedom of expression in culture as do all forms of music, dance, and visual arts. Plant healing should not be censored nor should it be relegated to the controls of a particular group of individuals. Plants, their power and prescription, belong to everyone. The science, art, and spirituality of herbalism are cultural constructions. It is up to people to protect herbalism within their communities. Nurse-herbalists have a legacy of protecting and promoting herbalism. Perhaps it is time once again for nurses to bring herbal diplomacy to the forefront as the need for accessible, inexpensive, and effective care that is represented in integrative herbal care grows exponentially nation by nation.

Peace and Planet Healing

Herbal diplomacy is like a forest of redwood trees. The redwoods' roots are very shallow but they grow into some of the largest trees on the planet because of their power in community connection. Redwoods rely on each other for growth. Herbal diplomacy is practiced within community. It also promotes the building of connection in a caring community. The diplomat's vision for the purpose of a meeting often extends beyond the people at the negotiation table. They take on the difficult task of negotiation in the first place because they know that their efforts in the resolution of one cultural dilemma will, like the redwood community, potentially affect others.

Trees stand peacefully and exude a presence in a given space. They also serve as symbols for life force and power in nature. That quest for understanding the power innate in trees and nature is expressed in the writings of philosopher H.P. Blavatsky: "If thou wouldst believe in the Power which acts within the root of a plant, or imagine the root concealed under the soil, thou hast to think of its stalk or trunk and of its leaves and flowers. Thou canst not imagine that Power independently of these objects. Life can only be known by the Tree of Life. ...The roots, the trunk and its many branches are three distinct objects, yet they are one tree."[30]

Trees as well as plants often hold revered positions in indigenous peoples' creation stories and legends of healing. One of the most famous in America is the story of the Tree of Peace of the Peacemaker and Hiawatha. The Peacemaker and his spokesman Hiawatha effectively stopped the warring between the tribes of the Six Nations that ultimately became the Iroquois Confederacy: the Oneidas, Mohawks, Senecas, Onondagas, Cayugas, and Tuscaroras. They did this by establishing the Longhouse (Kannonsionni) where peace was law and sacred endeavor. In the thoughts of the people of the Iroquois Confederacy to this day, "peace is inseparable from the life of man. ...Peace is a way of life, characterized by wisdom and graciousness."[31] The Tree of Peace was given to the people of the Six Nations by The Peacemaker as the symbol that

---

30 Blavatsky, *The Secret Doctrine: The Synthesis of Science, Religion, and Philosophy*: 58-59.
31 Paul Wallace, *The White Roots of Peace* (Philadelphia: University of Pennsylvania Press, 1946), 7.

represented the shelter under which the people of Six Nations gathered together in peace and the wisdom that emerged since the establishment of the Longhouse.

Just as nurses describe health as more than the mere absence of disease, peace for the people of Six Nations is more than the absence of conflict and war. Peace as the law is righteousness in action. Right action is ethic. The Peacemaker helped the warring tribes of the Iroquois Nation find their ethic in unity. They realized their strength in unity was grounded not in the notion of *E Pluribus Unum* but in *Ex Uno Pluria*,[32] defined as the strength of the whole made safe through the individuality of the members. The fires of each of the individual nations burn under the canopy of the Longhouse. The Peacemaker gave the Six Nations the symbol of fire, around which they sat together, as well as the Tree of Peace. He also gave Hiawatha and the Nations the symbol of the bundle of five arrows, a symbol of strength through union.[33] He taught them that while a single arrow can be broken, in unity, as in a bundle, it cannot. The purpose of the union in the Longhouse was to "provide a strength that casts out fear."[34] The Peacemaker established peace through an alchemy in community using all five elements to transform war. Within this legend of the Six Nations, we find a simple model for righteous action or ethic guiding the actions of the herbal diplomat who facilitates the peace and negotiation process:

1. Begin with a prayer of thanksgiving to the Creator.
2. Chiefs (leaders) need to have courage, patience, and honesty most of all.
3. Think not so much of the present advantage as of the future welfare of the people.
4. Each separate group discusses (delegation) issues within their group and then one person speaks to others with one voice.
5. Next, the tribes on each of the two sides of the fire compare with their brother so that each side of the fire speaks with one voice in the Longhouse.

---

32 Ibid., 31.
33 Ibid., 34.
34 Ibid., 31.

6. In the Longhouse, all people are represented. Each tribe passes its decision to the Atotarho,[35] or leader, of Six Nations.

This model represents both practical and spiritual aspects to diplomacy. It suggests ideas for structuring dialog so that all are heard and represented before the fire of transformation. Skilled communication and dialog are fundamental to community building. Herbal diplomacy and building caring community are the future of nurse-herbalism in which nurses and traditional healers can expand their work together with the plant world to bring hope for healing and peace to individuals, families, communities, and the planet.

35 Ibid.

ETHER – INTEGRATIVE INSIGHT–
OUR UNDER-STANDING OF ALCHEMY

One of the experiments I like to recommend for those interested in nurse-herbalism and herbal diplomacy is administering an herbal footbath. The herbal footbath is one of the simplest healing interventions that I have used over the years. It is also an intervention in which all of the qualities of herbal diplomacy are activated in the promotion of healing and peace. The herbal footbath is also very alchemical in that it is a spiritual and practical act that can be transformative for the client. Footbaths are portable, accessible, inexpensive, and effective.

Bathing the feet is a time-old hygienic practice. Every nurse is taught in nursing school to put a patient's feet in a bucket of water as part of a body bath. But the herbal footbath that I speak of here adds a different dimension. It is a footbath that supports the expression of the ether element in that it includes ablution and anointing, two ancient healing traditions. I learned the basic herbal footbath from Oma in 1984 and have been practicing and developing it since. During the herbal footbath, the nurse-herbalist bathes the client's feet. Feet represent the client's "under-standing."

Holographic science suggests that every bodily organ, system, structure, and energy field is represented in the feet. The two feet together are a holographic representation of the entirety of the Self. When we hold the two feet in our hands, we are holding the entirety of the person and their under-standing. The patterns of energy flow in the feet tell many stories about a person. When described to a person, these patterns and stories often cause the person to pause and reflect. Time and again I have witnessed the client's experience of pattern analysis in the feet improving their understanding of their health, illness, and lifestyle patterns and choices. This understanding is the beginning of the healing process and is why I include the herbal footbath as part of nurse-herbalist practice and preparation for herbal diplomacy work.

Reading the patterns and stories of the feet, however, is not a simple task. I apply the same nurse-herbalist principles. First, create a healing environment. Do this by inviting the client to partner with me and healing plants in creating an herbal footbath. To do this, present a selection of herbal bath infusions to the client for them to choose from. Use a dishpan-size, rectangular bucket placed length-wise and filled with very warm water. The client puts their feet in the water. The nurse-herbalist kneels before the person. I have used the footbath many times in my healing work with families as a peace-promoting exercise. It is very difficult to remain angry or hostile with someone who kneels before you and bathes your feet.

The warm water opens the pores of the soles of the feet, which are the largest in the body's integumentary system. Through these pores, the person absorbs the physical healing properties of the plant infusion. I also float specially-chosen flowers (such as rose petals) or herbs (such as rosemary or bay leaf) in the bath water so that the energetic vibration of the plant can surround the entirety of the feet and the person's under-standing. Often clients will mention that their "feet are dirty." It is a great opportunity to teach the difference between herbal interventions that address hygiene such as wiping the body or space with vinegar versus the herbal footbath offered to energetically weed out all blocks to under-standing.

The first purpose of the footbath is to strip the energy fields of the feet through ablution. Ablution is a term used to denote ritual washing and purification. When a person walks the earth, their feet pick up on the energies lodged in the places they walk. Some of those energies are discharged throughout the day but not all. The herbal footbath catalyzes the changes in the energy patterns around the feet. Then the nurse-herbalist, kneeling before the client, performs an ablution to the client's feet and ankles. The nurse-herbalist uses her/his hands like swords to strip the accumulated energies from the feet. This is done by bringing the water up above the ankles with cupped hands and then, with two hands to one leg, gently stripping or pulling the energy toward the toes and into the water. The action is repeated if the hands jump off the ankles or feet at any point during the stripping action.

After both feet are stripped, the water is thrown down the toilet. Do not underestimate the energetic pollutants in that water! Oma always told the story that when she started practicing as a reflexologist and doing the foot washings, she would throw the herbal bath water into the garden, thinking that she was being helpful to the environment by preserving water. But what happened to the garden is important to our energetic understanding of the power of ablution. In the places where she routinely tossed the bath water, these gnarly plants emerged that did not look healthy at all. Please toss the water into the toilet with a prayer for the transmutation of that energy extracted by water and herbs. This is part of the alchemy of the herbal footbath in which energy is transformed and transmuted by intentions and actions of the client and the nurse-herbalist.

Alchemy begins with prayer or invocation. Invocation is the philosopher's stone—s – sacred –tone sought by ancient alchemists in their quest for Self-transformation. A good time for invocation is when the client's feet are in the herbal footbath. I always ask the client if they would like to say a prayer or invocation for healing or if they would like me to do so. The purpose of the invocation is to invite the light to enter the footbath and our bodies so that it will purify our heart's intention and increase awareness and understanding through the process. I often say very simple invocations that are respectful and inclusive of a person's religious and health beliefs. The following is an example of instruction for an invocation given by Basil Valentine, a fifteenth-century alchemist who was well known for his deep knowledge of nature:

> First invocation to God, with a certain heavenly intention, drawn from the bottom of a sincere heart and conscience, pure from all ambition, hypocrisy, and all other vices which have any affinity with these; as arrogance, boldness, pride, luxury, petulancy, oppression of the poor, and other similar evils, all of which are to be eradicated from the heart; that when a man desires to prostrate himself before the throne of grace, for obtaining health, he may do so with a conscience free from unprofitable weeds, that his body may be transmuted into a holy temple of God … [36]

After the ablution, take each foot out of the water, one by one, and wrap each in a towel straight away so that the foot does not get cold. After the feet are dry but still warm, anoint the feet with massage oil, using a rhythmical and spiraling motion around the heel and ankles and into the feet. I then like to put the client's socks on for them. Putting the socks on the client's feet for them quickly not only preserves the warmth of the client's feet but it is also a demonstration of love and caring as the ablution ritual is completed and the feet return to the socks.

The herbal footbath, ablution, and anointing are simple but powerful interventions. Clients often express the profound transformative healing experiences they have during and after the bath. As we invoke healing and call for the light to enter our bodies to transform us and others, we transmute not only the client's personal blocks to healing. The nurse-herbalist who engages in these types of ancient herbal interventions and rituals has the opportunity to transmute his or her own blocks to healing. In the alchemical tradition of "as above so below; as below so above," it is known that what happens to the one affects the all. Transmutation can take place at all levels of time and place. By turning our thoughts to creating a healing environment in partnership with plants, such as in the ritual of the herbal bathing of the feet, we embrace the potential for becoming more at peace with ourselves as human beings co-existing with nature. We can become more comfortable walking the earth and experiencing Earth's changes as we relate more to the image of the Green Woman or Green Man emerging from the leaves and flowers of the green world. In the process of figuring out how to partner with plants, we become more human. In touching plants with pure intention of making medicine in the form of baths, teas, compresses, syrups, tinctures, and floral waters, the nurse-herbalist is transformed by the radiations of a plant-like gentleness that freely invites the manifestation of new ways to help and heal humanity and create caring community.

---

36   Arthur Waite, *Alchemists Through the Ages* (New York: Rudolf Steiner Publications, 1970), 17.

REFERENCES

Blavatsky, Helena. *The Secret Doctrine: The Synthesis of Science, Religion, and Philosophy*. London: The Theosophical Publishing Co., 1888.

The Dispensatory of the United States of America. Edited by Arthur Osol and George Farrar. 24th ed. Philadelphia: J.B. Lippincott, 1947.

Goethe, Johann Wolfgang and Jeremy Naydler. *Goethe on Science*. Edinburgh: Floris Books, 1996.

Hauck, Dennis. *The Emerald Tablet: Alchemy for Personal Transformation*. New York: Penguin Putnam Inc., 1999.

Junius, Manfred. *Practical Handbook of Plant Alchemy*. New York: Inner Traditions, 1985.

Langer, Ellen. *Mindfulness*. Reading, MA: Perseus Books, 1989.

Libster, Martha. *Herbal Diplomats: The Contribution of Early American Nurses (1830-1860) to Nineteenth-Century Health Care Reform and the Botanical Medical Movement*. Thornton, CO: Golden Apple Publications, 2004.

Libster, Martha and Betty Ann McNeil. *Enlightened Charity: The Holistic Nursing Care, Education and Advices Concerning the Sick of Sister Matilda Coskery, (1799-1870)*. Farmville, NC: Golden Apple Publications, 2009.

Louv, Richard. *Last Child in the Woods : Saving Our Children from Nature-Deficit Disorder*. Chapel Hill,: Algonquin Books of Chapel Hill, 2005.

Merriam-Webster Inc. *Merriam-Webster's Collegiate Dictionary*. 10 ed. Springfield, MA: Merriam-Webster, 1999.

Peck, M. Scott. *The Different Drum: Community Making and Peace*. New York: Touchstone, 1987.

Perrone, Bobette, H. Henrietta Stockel, and Victoria Krueger. *Medicine Women, Curanderas, and Women Doctors*. 1st ed. Norman, OK: University of Oklahoma Press, 1989.

Relf, Diane. "Dynamics of Horticultural Therapy." http://www.hort.vt.edu/HUMAN/ht1.html.

Tantaquidgeon, Gladys. *Folk Medicine of the Delaware and Related Algonkian Indians*. Harrisburg: Pennsylvania Historical and Museum Commission, 1972.

Tompkins, Peter and Christopher Bird. *The Secret Life of Plants*. New York: Harper & Row, 1973.

Trungpa, Chogyam. "Healing & the Reality of Death." *Shambhala Sun*, no. March (1994): 27-31, 69.

Von Bingen, Hildegard and Bruce Hozeski. *Hildegard von Bingen's Mystical Visions*. Santa Fe: Bear & Company, 1986.

Waite, Arthur. *Alchemists through the Ages*. New York: Rudolf Steiner Publications, 1970.

Wallace, Paul. *The White Roots of Peace*. Philadelphia: University of Pennsylvania Press, 1946.

APPENDIX A
Nurse's Herbal

HOW TO USE THIS NURSE'S HERBAL

This *Nurse's Herbal* serves as a compendium of plant solutions for client care and comfort. Following nurses' historical tradition, this herbal is a recipe book of herbal simples. The recipes are a montage of evidence from my personal experience, history, in vitro studies, ethnobotanical data, and the results of human clinical trials. As per tradition, this herbal's focus is on helping the nurse-herbalist identify what and how specific herbal simples can be used in nurse-herbalist comfort and care. It does not focus on contraindications and cautions. If you have not partnered with a plant listed here, please be sure to research it before applying it in client care. Applying these plant solutions in a unique plan of care for the client in accordance with the principles of timing, type, and tuning and the five rights is the responsibility of the nurse-herbalist. The recipes in this *Nurse's Herbal* do not replace common sense or best practice in nursing.

> Note on Nurse's Self-Care: The best way to partner with healing plants and understand their healing actions is to try these remedies yourself. General Rule – do not recommend an herbal application until you have tried it yourself.

This *Nurse's Herbal* is organized by health patterns that are commonly identified in nursing practice. Within each health pattern category are a list of herbal simples and a brief description for their application. The simples are organized according to the most common herbal applications in nursing practice: <u>Oral</u> Remedies include teas, liquid (alcohol) extracts, syrups/soups, and supplements that I have applied in client care. <u>Topical</u> remedies include compresses, poultices, infused oils, and ointments. The <u>Environmental</u> applications include baths, inhalations, and steams. Details of herbal preparation and application are defined and described throughout *The Nurse-Herbalist,* particularly Chapter 5, and therefore may not be repeated here.

HEALTH PATTERNS

Pain and Fever Relief

Emotional and Hormonal Balance

Skin and Strong Boundaries

Sleep, Rest, and Peaceful Restoration

Mobility, Energy, and Transitions (ex. Pregnancy, Birth, Death)

Digestion and Elimination

Immune Response

HERBS

The herbs included in this herbal are referred to by common name. Please use this list for clarification of botanical names for the herbs. Some pin yin (Chinese) names are also included.

Aloe (*Aloe vera*)

Angelica (*Angelica archangelica/sinensis*) (*Angelica sinensis* = Dang Gui)

Arnica (*Arnica montana*)

Bilberry (*Vaccinium myrtillus*)

Black Cohosh (*Cimicifuga racemosa*) (Sheng Ma)

Calendula (*Calendula officinalis*) Note: Do not confuse with the ornamental marigold (*Tagetes spp.*)

Carrot seed (*Daucus carota*)

Cayenne (*Capsicum frutescens*)

Celandine (*Chelidonium majus*)

Chamomile – German (*Matricaria recutita*)

Chlorophyll

Cinnamon (*Cinnamomum zeylanicum*)

Coffee (*Coffea arabica*)

Cranberry (*Vaccinium macrocarpon*)

Echinacea (*Echinacea purpurea or angustifolia*)

Elder (*Sambucus nigra*)

Eleuthero (*Eleutherococcus senticosus*)

Evening Primrose (*Oenothera biennis*)

Fenugreek (*Trigonella foenum-graecum*)

Feverfew (*Tanacetum parthenium*)

Garlic (*Allium sativum*)

Ginger (*Zingiber officinale*) (Sheng Jiang)

Goldenseal (*Hydrastis canadensis*)

Hawthorn (Craetegus *monogyna*)

Hops (*Humulus lupulus*)

Horseradish (*Armoracia rusticana*)

Horsetail (*Equisetum arvense*)

Kudzu (*Pueraria lobata*) (Ge Gen)

Lavender (*Lavandula angustifolia*)

Lemon (*Citrus limon*)

Lemon Balm (*Melissa officinalis*)

Lemongrass (*Cymbopogon citratus*)

Licorice (*Glycyrrhiza glabra*) (Gan cao)

Milk Thistle (*Silybum marianum*)

Mustard (*Brassica nigra*)

Myrrh (*Commiphora spp.*)

Oat (*Avena sativa*)

Onion (*Allium cepa*)

Parsley (*Petroselinum hortense*)

Peppermint (*Mentha piperita*)

Psyllium (*Plantago psyllium*)

Red Clover (*Trifolium pratense*)

Rhubarb root (*Rheum palmatum*)

Rose (*Rosa gallica*)

Rosemary (*Rosmarinus officinalis*)

Sage (*Salvia officinalis* and *Salviae miltiorrhiza*) (*S. miltiorrhiza* = Dan Shen)

Saw Palmetto (*Serenoa repens*)

Seaweed (*Sargassum spp.* or Kelp – *Fucus vesiculosus*) (Hai Zao)

Soy (*Glycine max*)

St. John's Wort (*Hypericum perforatum*)

Stinging Nettle (*Urtica doica*)

Tea (*Camellia sinensis*)

Thyme (*Thymus vulgaris*)

Turmeric (*Curcuma longa*) (Yu Jin)

Valerian (*Valeriana officinalis*)

Watermelon (*Citrullus lanatus*)

Wild Yam (*Dioscorea villosa or opposita*) (*D. opposita* = Shan Yao)

Wintergreen (*Gaultheria procumbens*)

Witch Hazel (*Hamamelis virginiana*)

Yarrow (*Achillea millefolium*)

HERBAL GLOSSARY OF ACTIONS

Adaptogen	A substance that increases overall, nonspecific resistance to stress. Ex: Eleuthero (*Eleutherococcus senticosus*)
Alterative	A substance that gradually changes the metabolism and elimination of the body to improve general health. Often referred to as a tonic. Formerly known as blood purifiers. Ex: Red Clover (*Trifolium pratense*)
Analgesic	Reduces pain by affecting nerve signals to the brain or releasing muscle spasm. Ex: Wintergreen (*Gaultheria procumbens*)

Anti-Catarrhal   Relieves chronic inflammation and excessive mucus in the body. Ex: Ginger (*Zingiber off.*)

Antihelminthic A substance that is antiparasitic. Ex: Garlic (*Allium sativa*)

Antiseptic   Prevents the growth of microorganisms. Ex. Thyme (*Thymus vulgaris*)

Antispasmodic   Prevents or reduces muscle spasms. Ex. Chamomile (*Matricaria recutita*)

Aphrodisiac   A substance that increases sexual desire. Ex. Cayenne (*Capsicum frutescens*)

Aromatic Bitter A substance that stimulates appetite through its scent. Ex: Hops (*Humulus lupulus*)

Astringent   A substance that causes a contraction of tissue or mucous membranes and reduces the secretion of mucus often as the result of tannin constituent. Ex: Witch Hazel (*Hamamelis virginiana*)

Bitters   A substance (with a bitter taste) used to stimulate appetite and aid the liver in detoxification. Action starts in taste buds. Ex: Goldenseal (*Hydrastis canadensis*)

Blood Cleanser An older term used in herbalism referring to herbs that increase overall vitality of the body and detoxify the blood of impurities due to poor diet, overeating, constipation, improper breathing, and drinking impure water, to name a few. The term used today is alterative. Ex: Milk Thistle (*Silybum marianum*)

Carminative   A substance that stimulates peristalsis and relaxes the stomach, thereby relieving flatulence. Ex: Peppermint (*Mentha piperita*)

Cathartic   A substance that induces bowel evacuation. Ex: Rhubarb root (*Rheum palmatum*). Also known as purgative.

Counterirritant A substance that warms and stimulates circulation to a particular part of the body where the herb is applied. Ex: Cayenne (*Capsicum frutescens*) or Mustard (*Brassica nigra*). Also known as Rubefacient.

Demulcent A substance that soothes by providing a moistening, protective coating and relieving inflammation of the membranes. Ex: Kudzu (*Pueraria lobata*)

Diaphoretic A substance that promotes perspiration. Ex: Elder (*Sambucus nigra*)

Diuretics A substance that increases the excretion of fluid. Ex: Parsley (*Petroselinum hortense*) and Watermelon (*Citrullus lanatus*)

Emmenagogue Promotes flow of menses. Ex: Angelica (*Angelica archangelica/sinensis*). Some of these herbs may also be perceived as abortifacient because of their action. But not all herbs that move energy in the body so as to promote menses have a history of action or use as abortifacients—a substance that causes abortion. Herbs that cause abortion should not be used in my opinion. There are many herbs that aid conception and fertility, such as carrot seed (*Daucus carota*) and myrrh (*Commiphora spp.*), that also have been used for centuries as strong contraceptives but are not abortifacients.

Escharotic A caustic acid or base substance that causes a chemical reaction with the tissues of the body, manifesting as heat, itching, burning, and breakdown of the tissue involved. Ex: Red clover (*Trifolium pratense*) – This refers to a special preparation, not red clover tea or extract.

Expectorants A substance that expels mucus from the respiratory tract. Ex: Lobelia (*Lobelia inflata*)

Galactagogue A substance that increases the flow of breast milk. Ex: Fenugreek (*Trigonella foenum-graecum*)

Hemostatic	A substance that stops hemorrhage and internal bleeding. Ex: Yarrow (*Achillea millefolium*)
Nervine	A substance that is healing to the nervous system and relieves nervous tension. Ex: Valerian (*Valeriana officinalis*)
Rubefacient	A substance that is used externally to increase blood supply to the skin. See counterirritant.
Sedative	A substance that induces rest and calmness. Ex: Lemon Balm (*Melissa officinalis*)
Stimulants	A substance that quickens and increases the energy of the body. Ex: Rosemary (*Rosmarinus officinalis*)
Tonic	A substance that improves overall general health. Ex: Stinging Nettle (*Urtica doica*)
Vulnerary	A substance that promotes wound healing. Ex: Calendula (*Calendula officinalis*)

PAIN AND FEVER RELIEF

Oral Remedies

A tea brewed from **lavender** flowers is useful in relieving headaches caused by fatigue and exhaustion.

It is believed that the first written record of **feverfew** occurred in the *Materia Medica* by Diocorides. Since at least 78 A.D., feverfew has been used to treat headache, stomach pain, menstrual irregularities, and fever. Early Europeans believed that the herb was ruled by the planet Venus and therefore was a good herb for women. Feverfew contains compounds that act to prevent spasms of the smooth muscles in the walls of the cerebral blood vessels. It is believed that these compounds may produce the antimigraine effect similar to methysergide, a serotonin antagonist. Constituents in feverfew have been found to inhibit prostaglandin production and arachidonic acid release in vitro and in animal studies. This may account for its antiplatelet and antifebrile actions. Changes in the chemistry of platelets in human clients taking feverfew have not been detected. Extracts also inhibit secretion of serotonin from platelets and proteins from polymorphonuclear leukocytes (PMNs). The pattern of the effects of the feverfew extracts on platelets is different from that obtained with other inhibitors of platelet aggregation and the effect of PMNs is more pronounced than with high concentrations of non-steroidal, anti-inflammatory agents. For headache in children, my usual preference is to try a chamomile compress to the back and neck, followed by a gentle massage with an herbal oil such as Saint John's Wort or arnica before giving oral remedies such as bitter-tasting feverfew. While feverfew may be helpful in suppressing pain and promoting comfort, it is important for nurses to provide clients with information regarding potential underlying patterns that create and re-create pain, the body's signal of need for attention. It is also important to take time to help the client begin to identify personal and environmental triggers for their pain. Holistic evaluation of those clients with chronic pain or chronic use of plant therapies for pain reduction must be done. Note: Bees dislike feverfew. so take care when growing the plant. The suggested dosage of feverfew extract (1:5 g/ml, 25 percent ethanol) needed to prevent migraine headaches is 5 to 20 drops daily.

Cranberry juice, fruit concentrate, and tablets are helpful in the relief of urinary tract discomfort. I find "pushing" cranberry juice, or drinking as much of the juice as you can, to be the most effective in pain relief. Bacteria can enter the bladder from the urethra and result in the symptom of burning pain during urination. Additional symptoms include the desire to urinate even if the bladder is empty; urine that is cloudy, dark, or foul smelling; low back pain; fever; and chills. At first it was speculated that cranberries exert their beneficial effects by lowering urine pH, but data conflict. Cranberry's action is now thought to be due to its ability to prevent bacteria from adhering to the lining of the urinary tract. Cranberries also are used for relieving heat symptoms such as itching related to yeast infection. Because of this, one would think that it would be best not to drink sweetened cranberry juice because it would "feed" the bacteria or fungus; but, my experience is that cranberries are so incredibly astringent that the unsweetened juice can cause severe cramping in the abdomen. I have tried recommending that clients dilute unsweetened juice without success. Clients experience the pain-relieving qualities of pushing cranberry juice when the juice is lightly sweetened and diluted.

Black cohosh, in addition to its renowned status as an herb for women's discomforts, has been used extensively for muscular and rheumatic pain, headache, and eyestrain. Black cohosh is best extracted in alcohol. Dose of tincture is 15 to 30 drops in a small amount of warm water. In the early 1840s, black cohosh was a popular remedy for rheumatism and neuralgia. It was used for all kinds of muscular pain and tension, especially abdominal muscle soreness, tension in the neck and back, and internal abdominal pain. This is true today as well.

Cooling **peppermint** tea clears heat and fever in the head.

Lemon balm tea reduces fever. Lemon balm eases the pain of gout.

Wintergreen tea has been used internally as an antirheumatic, anti-inflammatory, and diuretic agent.

Fresh **turmeric** root in food or as tea helps relieve pain and swelling caused by traumatic injury.

The oil of **evening primrose** seeds contains gamma-linolenic acid, which is the precursor of linoleic acid and prostaglandin E_1. This natural, polyunsaturated fatty acid is used for the pain and discomfort associated with inflammation, diabetic neuropathy, mastalgia (and polycystic breasts), menses, and rheumatoid arthritis. The oil is typically taken as a dietary supplement. This is one supplement I have recommended in practice. Because the human body needs a balance of omega-6 and omega-3 essential fatty acids (EFAs), evening primrose oil has often been studied with fish oil, a rich source of omega-3 EFAs. Evening primrose oil is considered safer than borage oil for long-term use because borage seed oil may contain enough toxic pyrrolizidine alkaloids, as does the whole plant, that it may make long-term therapeutic use unsafe.

Parsley tea is helpful in people who are suffering from gout or kidney pain. I use flat leaf Italian parsley rather than curly parsley. Chop the leaf and pour boiled water over the leaf. Let it steep for 5-10 minutes until the water is green. Strain and sip.

Aloe is also given internally for healing gastrointestinal wounds such as ulcers. My grandfather showed me many times as a child how he would tap his aloe plants to create a drink from the leaf pulp for people he knew who had ulcers. They would drink the gel in some water and be pain free.

St. John's Wort tea and liquid extract have been used extensively to repair nerve damage. I have used it internally and/or externally with stroke and brain-injured clients. St. John's Wort has been used in the treatment of spinal cord injury, shock, and concussion. Some herbalists also use it with clients who have pain related to shingles.

Topical Remedies

Ginger is applied externally to painful joints to decrease inflammation. Fresh ginger compresses are very effective for increasing circulation of blood and body fluids in an area of the body when stagnation exists, manifesting as enduring joint pain, toothache, backache, menstrual cramps, and pain associated with passing kidney stones. I have taught teens with chronic pain how to apply fresh ginger compresses to the kidneys of their class partner. They were amazed at the relief they experienced from the compresses and that they were able to use fewer doses of over-the-counter, non-steroidal, anti-inflammatory drugs. Ginger essential oil in a carrier oil can be applied to the specific trigger point to relieve pain. Use a spiraling motion to work the warming oil into the point. It is especially helpful in headaches (apply to trigger points at the base of the skull) and back pain (apply to points along the sacroiliac joint and greater trochanter). Ginger is very hot energetically; therefore, the nurse-herbalist should recommend internal use judiciously, especially in those with symptoms of interior heat.

Wintergreen essential oil, usually about 0.5 percent to 0.8 percent from wintergreen leaves, is obtained by steam distillation of the leaves in a carefully controlled process that yields methyl salicylate. The absorption of methyl salicylates from the gastrointestinal tract is slower and more erratic than skin absorption. Wintergreen oil is not taken internally. Wintergreen essential oil is readily absorbed by the skin. It is used in the form of salves and liniments to relieve pain, rheumatism, sprains, sciatica, muscular pain, and neuralgia. Note: The wintergreen in some over-the-counter joint creams is typically a synthetic copy of the plant and may contain no salicylates.

Hops are used for the pain-relieving properties of the strobiles. Nurses historically have applied hops poultices to the chest and abdomen to relieve congestion during pneumonia and to relieve abdominal distention postoperatively; poultices also have been applied to wounds that are infected, painful, or inflamed.

Cayenne is a warm, powerful stimulant, and is recognized as a substance that increases circulation. Nurses have a long history in the use of cayenne as a counterirritant. Cayenne also has been used topically as a counterirritant or as a stimulant of blood flow to a body part or internal organ. Capsaicin (a constituent in cayenne pepper) cream can be used externally for pain, but when applied to the skin, it should not be used on or near any open sores. Cayenne tincture and the extract of capsaicin are used in topical counterirritant preparations to treat arthritis, rheumatism, fibromyalgia, neuralgia, low back pain, and mild frostbite. It also has been used to treat herpes zoster outbreaks; backache, sprains, and strains; diabetic neuropathy, especially in the feet; post-mastectomy pain; psoriasis; and cluster headaches. The cream is best applied with plastic gloves because the cream does not come off the hands easily with water. Vinegar can be used to remove cream that gets on the skin. When applied, capsaicin cream may cause a burning or tingling sensation at first. This is the normal action of the plant therapy. It is not normal for the skin to blister or cause excruciating pain during a topical application of cayenne. Studies have shown that significant pain relief may not occur for two to four weeks.

The boiled leaves of **feverfew** can be used to make hot compresses for pain due to congestion and inflammation of the lungs, stomach, and abdomen.

Warm **tea** bag compresses are often helpful for headache.

The essential oil of **lavender** flower is used for colic and chest congestion and to relieve biliary complaints and headaches. Although most essential oils have pain-relieving qualities, lavender oil is considered to be especially analgesic. The linalool and linalyl aldehyde in lavender seem to reduce the flow of nerve impulses, such as those that transmit pain. Warm, moist applications of the flower also help relieve pain associated with rheumatism and neuralgia.

External applications of **lavender** have been used for toothache, neuralgia, sprains, and rheumatism and to cleanse wounds, varicose ulcers, burns, and scalds. At one time, it was common for the French to keep a bottle of lavender essence in the home to be used for bruises, bites, aches, and pains—both internal and external.

Lemon Compress is a topical application of an herbal infusion (water extraction) of lemon using a cotton, silk, or wool material. For fever, fill a large bowl half full of tepid water. Take a fresh lemon and paring knife. Submerge the lemon under the water and cut it in half and then score each half of the lemon into star shapes. The lemon is cut under water so that the volatile oil does not escape. Using the bottom of a small cup, express the juice from the pulp and the essential oils from the skin under the water by pressing down on the lemon. Place the cloth in the infusion; wring out until cloth is not dripping. Use it to sponge the fevering client. Begin sponging by wrapping the ankles in the tepid cloth. Flip the compress as soon as the cloth draws heat from the body. The room temperature should be regulated so that the client is not chilled by drafts or by the room temperature itself. The client is covered for warmth. A woolen cloth with safety pins attached is placed on the bed in preparation for being placed around the lower legs. Place another piece of soft material on top of the wool that will fit around the legs. Then the dipping cloth is prepared. A bandage-type material that will go around the lower legs is folded to fit the legs and then rolled on both sides up to the middle. Place the bandage on another cloth that can be used to wring out the bandage. This cloth should have both ends rolled, too. Place water, temp 37.6 °C, in a bowl and, using a fork to hold a lemon submerged in the water, use a knife to cut the lemon in half into a star shape. Use the base of a glass or small bowl to press the lemon halves. Then put the cloth with the bandage on it in the lemon water, holding onto the rolled ends so that they do not get wet. The compresses are wrapped around the lower leg from the top of the metatarsals to below the kneecap while the client is reclining. The lemon compresses are left in place for 60 to 120 minutes. Blood pressure, temperature, and perspiration are observed to be sure that the client's temperature is lowered gently.

A floral water made from **elder** flower is used to take away headaches and the first symptoms of colds by bathing the head.

Rose water is very helpful in relieving headache and pain in the eyes, ears, throat, and gums. Apply the water with a spiraling motion at the temples and pressure points around the skull and mandible.

Horseradish root poultice can relieve sinus pain.

Black cohosh tincture is used as a topical application for inflammation of the nerves, spine, ovaries, and the eyes or old skin ulcers; tic douloureux; rheumatism; and stiffness in the neck, back, or side.

Environmental Remedies

Chamomile steams relieve sinusitis pain. Essential oils in the flower head are antibacterial and anti-inflammatory. Chamomile calms the throbbing in the sinus very quickly and is relaxing.

Rosemary herb and essential oil have a long history of use in comforting clients by increasing circulation and warmth, relieving joint pain, and stimulating the mind. Elderly clients often experience a warm rosemary footbath as the best remedy for helping ease the discomfort related to the generalized aches and pain and cold extremities they experience, especially when they are in an unfamiliar place such as a hospital or nursing home. The essential oil of rosemary in a carrier oil can be very helpful when massaging clients who complain of headache, stress, and pain.

Yarrow leaf and flower infusion makes an excellent sitz bath for the discomfort women have with fibroids and pelvic pain. Use 4 ounces (100 g) of yarrow in 5 gallons (20 L) of warm to hot water, or just enough to cover the hips with the knees bent up. Wrap the upper body in towels and soak for ten to twenty minutes. Rinse.

Coffee is classified as a narcotic stimulant. One cup of coffee usually contains approximately 100 mg of caffeine. Caffeine is used in many analgesic preparations because it potentiates the effect of aspirin and paracetamol. When weighing the benefits and risks of intervention, the knowledge that drinking a small amount of coffee with an over-the-counter analgesic can lessen the need for stronger prescription pain medicines may be the preferred choice. Note: Caffeine is addicting. It acts by blocking the normal action of adenosine, resulting in an overactive adenosine system, abnormal sedation, and therefore a subsequent craving for caffeine whenever the effect wears off. Adenosine is known to inhibit dopamine release. If its action is blocked, excess dopamine in the body results. Coffee infusion is also used effectively for fullness in the head (congestive headache) and pain in the back. The client sips a wine glass full of a coffee infusion as they soak their feet in a warm coffee footbath for twenty minutes. The footbath is an old nursing remedy for draining excessive energy (stuffiness and pain) from the head to the feet.

Horsetail sitz baths and tea are helpful for pain related to the passage of kidney stones.

EMOTIONAL AND HORMONAL BALANCE

Oral Remedies

Some health practitioners, including Carl Jung, have used the aroma of **lemon balm** to strengthen the memory and alleviate feelings of melancholy and sadness. This plant is also known as the scholar's herb because it helps the memory and clears the head. Lemon balm tea, hot and cold, is uplifting to mind, emotion, and spirit. Lemon balm is a great cool tea during summer months.

Eleuthero has been shown to be a very effective adaptogen herb for helping improve the body's ability to adapt to change and environmental and physical stressors. An adaptogen is a substance that has a nonspecific action and a normalizing action irrespective of the direction of the pathologic state. Its exact mechanism of action as an adaptogen is not fully understood. It has been studied and used extensively in Russia and China, where it is believed to influence the energy of the body as a *qi* tonic. The importance of the herb is now recognized in other countries. Nurses may want to consider the clinical use of eleuthero with clients with stress-related conditions, immune deficiency symptoms, altitude sickness, and generalized *qi* deficiency or weakness. Eleuthero is also helpful in preparing clients for stressful situations, such as undergoing chemotherapy and radiation treatments. Liquid extract in a small amount of water following the standard adult dose found on labels is what I typically suggest.

In Chinese medicine, 10 or more species of **angelica** are used. The most popular one, *Angelica sinensis*, also known as "dang gui," is a well-known remedy for female disorders. It has been used in China for several thousand years. TCM classifies angelica as an herb that tonifies and moves blood. It is most often used in formulation, not as a single herb. It works synergistically in combination with certain other herbs such as white peony (*Paeonia lactiflora*). *A. sinensis* is taken as a tea or in soup as a health promotion measure for maintaining a healthy reproductive system. Angelica is used for the treatment of menstrual disorders, hemorrhage, colds, gastrointestinal complaints, and many other conditions. It is believed that the plant has the ability to increase blood flow to the female reproductive organs and therefore creates balanced menstruation and acts as an aphrodisiac and a postpartum healing agent. Angelica root is traditionally cut in a way that emphasizes its three sections—the head, the body, and the tail. Sometimes only a particular section of the root is included in a formula because the different sections have different actions. The head is the uppermost part of the root and is thought to be the most tonifying, but the least effective part for moving blood. The tail, the lowest part of the root, is said to be the least tonifying but the most effective in moving blood. The body of the root is thought to be more tonifying. The Chinese have known for years that angelica's effect in women is not related to any plant hormone activity. *A. sinensis* does have an effect on the uterus, however, both stimulating and relaxing it. The volatile oil component of the plant is believed to be responsible for the relaxing effect on the uterus and a nonvolatile component seems to stimulate the uterus. Ligustilide may be the active constituent in the essential oil, which is able to inhibit the smooth muscle of the uterus. Decoct (do not boil) 3 to 9 g of the root in 500 ml of water for approximately forty-five minutes.

Traditionally, **St. John's Wort** has been used for people with mild to moderate depression. Standardized extract of St. John's Wort, 300 mg, three times a day for four weeks in combination with daily light treatment for two hours is also effective during a randomized study in relieving 20 subjects' symptoms of seasonal affective disorder. St. John's Wort tea also can be given as a sedative to children (1 teaspoon [3 to 5 g] of cut herb to 6½ oz [200 ml] water, 2 to 3 cups per day for children over 3 years; children [age 1 to 3] 1 cup per day). The dose of liquid extract for school-age child depression, 10 drops, up to three times per day; a small child, 5 drops two times per day. St. John's Wort tea can also be given at bedtime for bed-wetting.

Using the Kupperman index for evaluation (measuring menopausal symptoms such as sweating, hot flushes, irritability, insomnia, depression, vertigo, concentration, and heart palpitations), a randomized, controlled study of 60 women demonstrated that **black cohosh** ethanol extract, 80 drops per day for three months, was equal to conjugated estrogens (0.625 mg/day) and diazepam (2 mg/day) in significantly decreasing neurovegetative and psychiatric symptoms in women.

As early as the eighth century B.C., **lavender** was described in an ancient Indian medical text as useful for psychiatric disorders. Lavender is used specifically for depressive states associated with chronic digestive disturbances. In Ayurvedic medicine, lavender is called the "broom of the brain" because its use is said to sweep away sluggishness of thought, strengthen brain power, and clarify the intellect. Lavender is still used today in the form of an edible medicinal butter by Tibetan Buddhist medical practitioners for treating insanity and psychoses.

Oat (food or oatstraw tea) is used to treat neurasthenia, an emotional and physical disorder characterized by fatigue, lack of motivation, feelings of inadequacy, and psychosomatic symptoms. Oat is very calming.

Many people experience heart palpitations and high blood pressure. **Hawthorn** berry syrup can be added to the diet for those seeking a strengthening of the heart and increasing vasodilation.

Women enduring hot flashes often find some relief from drinking **peppermint** tea. The coolness of the tea rises to the head.

Lemongrass tea raises the spirits and calms anxiety. One of my favorite recipes to offer clients and families is a cup of lemongrass tea with an oatmeal cookie. The lemongrass tea raises the spirit and the oat calms the nerves...at the same time.

Red clover tea and liquid extract can be used during perimenopause. It should be taken throughout the month and amount increased if and when symptoms accentuate. Red clover contains plant constituents called isoflavones that when ingested are known to increase estrogen levels in women. The lack of estrogen produced after menopause contributes to decreased arterial compliance, leading to hypertension and increased left ventricular workload. This double-blind, placebo-controlled study found arterial compliance to be improved within weeks of ingesting isoflavones from red clover. Genistein and daidzein bind at estrogen receptor sites and tend to normalize estrogen and progesterone.

Soybean cultivation is thought to have begun in China sometime between 2967 B.C. and 2597 B.C. Soy was called one of the five sacred crops. Currently, TCM uses soybean preparations for patterns of yin deficiency, irritability, restlessness, insomnia following fevers, and for tightness in the chest. TCM practitioners believe that soy should not be given to nursing mothers because it inhibits lactation. The Chinese classify soy/tofu in general as cooling, slightly sweet, and somewhat damp. If someone were to have a condition that has qualities of cold and damp, soy or tofu would be contraindicated. An extreme dampness condition in TCM is known as "phlegm." The phlegm condition can be hot or cold and is aggravated by poor digestion. The condition of phlegm can manifest in what is called in the West, a tumor. Health care providers who are not aware of the energetics of foods, as are TCM practitioners, often recommend soy, based on its plant constituents, in extreme amounts to people with tumors in particular. I have heard well-meaning practitioners say, "Eat as much soy as you can!" From a TCM standpoint, if the cancer client has a cold phlegm condition or spleen qi deficiency, soy and tofu would not be recommended. Soy also should not be eaten when coming down with a cold when there is excess mucus with a wet, productive cough. Although there have been some inconsistencies in the data, there appears to be an effect of the phytosterols in the form of isoflavones in soy on hormone balance in humans and on the incidence of some diseases such as breast cancer and heart disease. Soy contains four main isoflavones (genistein, daidzein, genistin, and daidzin) that have phytosterol activity and are thought to act as estrogen antagonists. Genistein, the most active phytosterol, has the highest affinity for estrogen receptors. It is absorbed in the gut. In vitro studies of human breast cancer cell lines found that genistein effectively inhibits cell growth whether or not the cells express an estrogen receptor, suggesting that the mechanism of action of the isoflavones in preventing appearance of mammary tumors may not be a direct antiestrogenic effect. Animal and in vitro studies suggest that the protective effects of soy may be equally applicable to both hormone and non-hormone-related cancers. One limitation often found in the biomedical literature is that investigators do not clarify the individual soy product used in their studies. Studies have determined that fermented soy products such as miso and natto contain much higher levels of the isoflavone genistein than those that are not fermented, and that fermentation of soy increases the availability of isoflavones to the body. Some soy products have been processed in such a manner that the isoflavones have been removed. Soy protein isolates are one example. When purchasing soy products, it is important to look at the label to check the isoflavone content. Foods known to contain isoflavones are soy protein granules, roasted soy nuts, tofu, tempeh, soy beverages, soy butter, and cooked soybeans.

As early as 1785, **black cohosh** was used by the American Eclectic practitioners. In 1832, it was introduced to the medical profession and became a valuable and commonly used remedy of physicians. It is used currently in Europe most often in supplement form for its estrogen-like action and to suppress luteinizing hormone in menstrual disorders such as premenstrual syndrome, dysmenorrhea, and uterine spasms and in the treatment of symptoms related to menopause. Black cohosh is believed to tone the tissues of the female reproductive tract. This was perhaps why it has been able to relieve pelvic pain associated with menstruation and restore delayed menses. It was used for sterility and ovarian pain in women, and aching sensations of the prostate gland in men. Many of the studies that have evaluated the effects of black cohosh on symptoms related to hormone balance (e.g., menopause) have used ethanol extract of black cohosh, a standardized black cohosh product called Remifemin®. The biologic activity of black cohosh is thought to be related to the triterpene glycoside constituents—actein, cimicifugocide, deoxyacetylacteol, and 27-deoxyactein. Each 20-mg tablet of the standardized product called Remifemin® contains 1 mg of deoxyactein. Several of the studies involving Remifemin® have been conducted by the manufacturer of the product. For the liquid extract – 1:1 (g/ml): 0.04 ml daily. The German Commission E recommends that the use of black cohosh be limited to six months for human safety reasons. Black cohosh should also be used wisely so as to protect plant populations. It is considered an at-risk plant by the United Plant Savers because of high demand and overharvesting in the wild.

Seaweed, particularly kelp, is used medicinally for its ability to balance hormonal activity of the thyroid. It is often used in herbalism for the treatment of symptoms related to hypothyroidism and obesity.

When high levels of purified constituents of **garlic** are used on a regular basis, iodine uptake by the thyroid is reduced.

Topical Remedies

Rose essential oil is used as a general tonic, especially for the heart. Rose massage oil soothes the nerves. The scent of roses can increase concentration and act as a sedative and antidepressant. It is used for emotional shock, bereavement, and grief.

Lavender has been used topically as a stimulant in nervous conditions.

Angelica essential oil can be applied topically in the treatment of people suffering from shock.

Some nurses have found that giving their intubated clients a gentle hand massage with dilute **lavender** essential oil twenty minutes before extubation allows the client to relax and not struggle against the tube. The clients are able to relax in preparation for extubation, but not so deeply that they are not able to breathe on their own.

Wild yam is an inexpensive source of building blocks for human cortisones, androgens, estrogens, progestogens, and topical hormones. These drugs are used to treat menopause, dysmenorrhea, premenstrual tension, testicular deficiency, Addison's disease, allergies, dermatitis, psoriasis, impotency, prostatic hypertrophy, and many others. In addition to providing the blueprint for the development of these drugs, wild yam also serves as a source of diosgenin for "natural" hormone pharmaceutical products such as natural progesterone creams. Natural progesterone can be made from animals or plants. Some bio-identical or natural progesterone products on the market contain only wild yam. Some contain wild yam and progesterone that has been converted in a laboratory from the diosgenin extracted from the wild yam rhizome. This converted progesterone resembles human progesterone and is the most effective product. The herb, in any form other than the laboratory converted product, is poorly absorbed by the body. At this point, scientists believe that humans lack the enzyme necessary to convert diosgenin to human progesterone. Many practitioners I have worked with prescribe the cream for women with perimenopausal and menopausal symptoms. The cream is applied to the chest, inner thighs, or inner arms usually twice a day and may be absorbed at different rates, depending on the woman. While the cream can be very effective in relieving menopausal symptoms, exact dosage of progesterone received by the client is not as easily calculated as with oral pharmaceutical preparations of synthetic progesterone (progestins) and/or estrogen. Typical recommendation: Postmenopausal women use 1/4 teaspoon cream one to two times per day on days 8 to 30 or 31 of the menstrual cycle and no cream on days 1 to 7. (To determine their cycle, postmenopausal women can pick a date and call that Day 1 of their cycle, then calculate from there.) Perimenopausal women do not use the cream during menstruation. Use 1/4 teaspoon two times a day on days 8 to 21 and 1/4 to 1/2 teaspoon two times a day on days 22 to 28. The dosage range of natural progesterone creams derived from diosgenin is less than 2 mg per ounce (28 g) and up to 400 mg per ounce (28 g).

In North and Central America, wild yam is used as a relaxing treatment for menstrual cramps and ovarian pain. The inner part of the root can be made into a salve and applied topically for vaginal dryness related to menopause. In all cases of topical use, the absorption of the wild yam cream is clinicians' concern. The following company is a resource for natural progesterone cream:

Women's International Pharmacy
5708 Monona Drive
Madison, WI 53719-3152
1-800-279-5708
1-608-221-7800
Fax 1-608-221-7819
www.WomensInternational.com

Many ask if a natural hormone replacement is safer for long-term use than a synthetic hormone replacement. The use of the replacement option or model, whether applied to synthetic or natural hormone products, may be what needs to be questioned. The answer probably lies in adaptation, helping the body to *adapt* to new hormone levels. The body is highly adaptive, so nurses might ask why there are so many concerns regarding hormonal discomfort, particularly in industrialized countries. Discomfort associated with menopause in some cultures, such as the traditional Navajo, is virtually unknown.

Environmental Remedies

Lavender essential oil is used in aromatherapy for the treatment of emotional disorders, such as nervousness, irritability, insomnia, and manic depression. Old medical books document its use in "raising the spirits" and "comforting the brain." Lavender essential oil has the ability to bring balance to body and spirit because it both relaxes and stimulates. Lavender aromatherapy is effective in allaying the anxiety of women undergoing mammography screening.

Rosemary, typically applied as a bath or massage oil, is an effective nerve stimulant, helpful for memory loss, lethargy and general dullness, and improving alertness. The scent is refreshing and invigorating, has an uplifting effect on the spirit, seems to dispel confusion, and promotes mental clarity. Rosemary's antioxidants and other compounds may work to prevent oxidation and the breakdown of acetylcholine in the brain, leading to a potential prevention and/or suppression of the symptoms of Alzheimer's disease.

The essential oil of **angelica** is used for symptoms of all types of nervous debility, as a general restorative, and for those who are timid, weak, and have trouble making decisions. It is said to help those with an unbalanced nervous system.

SKIN AND STRONG BOUNDARIES

Oral Remedies

In the first century A.D., the Greeks reported that **sage** decoction stopped bleeding from wounds and cleaned ulcers and sores. The Anthroposophical approach to healing regards sage as being able to support the warmth-creating process within the body. One of the ways it does this is to stimulate perspiration in those who sweat little and to stop perspiration in those who sweat heavily.

Evening primrose oil capsules taken orally are helpful in dry skin conditions that accompany viral infections, eczema, and chronic diseases. It can be applied to the edges of wounds to facilitate the healing process.

Red clover tea and liquid extract can also be used by those with acne and other skin problems such as boils and carbuncles.

Chlorophyll water is very helpful in increasing the oxygen-carrying capacity of the blood, thereby increasing the nourishment to the skin.

Topical Remedies

Calendula is a medicinal plant with light green leaves and golden orange to yellow flowers. Each daisy-like flower has a central orange disk with numerous yellow-orange florets. Calendula flowers open in the morning and close in the afternoon. If the flowers are closed after 7 a.m., it is said that there will be rain. Many renowned physicians and healers, including Hildegard von Bingen, Abbe Kneipp, and Maria Treben, have used calendula as a remedy for symptoms related to the skin such as impetigo, bedsores, and malignant growths. The German Commission E approves the internal and topical use of calendula flowers for inflammation of the oral mucosa. It is approved for external use for poorly healing wounds, including bedsores, ulcerations, and swelling. Calendula possesses anti-inflammatory, wound-healing, and antiseptic properties. It is applied topically to cancerous tumors and ulcers. Calendula infusion with 1/2 to 1 teaspoon (1 to 2 g) dried flower petals in 5 ounces (150 ml) water is an excellent topical application to prevent gangrene, infection, and tetanus. It is used on the skin of infants to prevent or heal chafing, excoriation, and diaper rash. Preparations of calendula are used to wash abscesses, eczema, burns, and skin ulcers. It has been used postoperatively on the surgical wound to aid healing. Calendula not only improves wound and skin healing but also can help prevent scar tissue formation and has been used historically in healing wounds created by herbal escharotics in the treatment of tumors. Calendula cream is helpful in the care of a baby's sensitive skin, especially in relieving symptoms related to diaper rash. Calendula compresses can be applied to clients with decubitus ulcers and other wounds, and calendula ointment for burns, diaper rash, and wound care. For conjunctivitis, rinse both eyes three times a day with 1 to 2 ounces (30 to 60 ml) of room temperature water with 5 to 10 drops of calendula extract.

Rose water and salves are indispensable for relieving inflammation of the skin, particularly of the face. Rose ointment is helpful in the relief of radiation burns and radiodermatitis in cancer treatment.

Chamomile ointment is comparable to hydrocortisone in reducing inflammation and bacterial infection of the skin. The polysaccharides in chamomile are immune-stimulating. They activate macrophages and B lymphocytes needed for the healing of wounds.

Witch hazel leaf and bark have astringent and hemostatic properties that have been attributed to the tannins present in the shrub. The leaves contain 8 percent and the bark from 1 percent to 3 percent tannins. Tannins have strong astringent properties. When a distillate or decoction of the plant is applied topically, it causes proteins to precipitate out of cells, causing the superficial cell layers to tighten and shrink. This produces local capillary vasoconstriction or hemostyptic action. This decrease in vascular permeability results in an anti-inflammatory effect. The tightening, or astringent, action on the tissues deprives bacteria of a growth medium. Tannins also have a mild topical anesthetic action that soothes pain and itching. Witch hazel preparations help in the treatment of minor skin injuries, acne, hemorrhoids, varicose veins, and local inflammation of skin and mucous membranes as well as swellings, skin ulcers, bedsores, and external inflammation, especially of the eyes. A strong decoction 2-3 teaspoons (10 g) of witch hazel leaves or bark in 1 cup (250 ml) of water steeped for thirty minutes also has been injected into the vagina for prolapsed uterus.

Historically, **St. John's Wort** has been used for healing "hurts and bruises" inside and out. St. John's Wort has a long history of safe use in the relief of internal hurts such as depressed mood, stress, and insomnia, and external hurts or wounds. It is taken orally as a tea, tincture, liquid extract, or standardized extract and used topically in infused oil form. St. John's Wort is best known for its use in promoting the healing of wounds and bruises. It can be used topically in the form of infused oil or tincture. Midwives, including one trained in England that I used to work with, often use St. John's Wort oil to gently massage the perineum during labor in preparation for delivery, to mitigate any need for episiotomy, and to promote healing of the perineum. St. John's Wort oil can be the treatment of choice in children who have first-degree burns, such as sunburn, after the burn is cooled with water. A gauze dressing soaked in St. John's Wort oil is applied for about ten hours to help in healing the burn and preventing formation of scar tissue.

Celandine is very effective in wart removal. The outer layer of skin of the wart is gently scraped with a scalpel until the blood supply of the wart is exposed. Then the celandine oil is applied and the wart covered. I have seen warts that were still growing after medical treatments with chemotherapeutic agents and cryotherapy disappear after a few days' use of topical celandine infused oil that I made from the fresh leaf.

The antiviral constituents, rosmarinic acid and other polyphenols, have been identified in **lemon balm.** Lemon balm compresses and ointment are helpful in the treatment of skin lesions related to herpes simplex viral infection. Lemon balm was shown in studies to be significantly effective in reducing recovery time from herpetic infection from the normal ten to fourteen days to four to eight days. Lemon balm can also has been mixed with salt and applied topically to cysts in the skin. It is effective in cleansing sores.

Aloe is popularly known as the "burn," "first aid," or "medicine" plant. The fresh gel from the leaf can be immediately applied topically to burns, sunburns, insect bites, acne vulgaris, and wounds to promote healing. Aloe vera gel is used as a demulcent, wound healing agent and it has been successful in the treatment of pressure ulcers. In vitro studies have demonstrated that aloe vera in concentrations greater than 70 percent (for gram-positive bacteria) and 60 percent (for gram-negative bacteria) has an antimicrobial effect similar to silver sulfadiazine. Some studies have shown that aloe vera dressings have been better than Vaseline gauze. Midwives apply aloe vera gel to a torn perineum after birth. Because the bottled gel may contain preservatives that may irritate sensitive skin, use the fresh gel directly from the leaves. Express the gel onto a gauze pad or a menstrual pad and fix it in place. The gel is remarkably healing and cooling.

A floral water made from **elder** flowers is used topically for sunburn, freckles, and to bathe old sores and ulcers of the lower extremities to help them heal. The floral water was used as a wash to take away redness of the eyes. One traditional remedy used by midwives is an infused oil made from elder flowers and olive oil that is applied to sore nipples and breasts during lactation. This will relieve the pain and sensitivity.

Onions also are mashed and applied as a poultice to burns, and the skins can be boiled gently and applied to the skin for conditions such as scabies. The skin of onions can contain as much as 3 percent quercetin, a flavonoid that has a known skin-soothing and anti-inflammatory action.

The colloidal (gelatinous) fraction of **oatmeal** is successfully used as a bath preparation to relieve the irritation of eczema and dry skin. Oat straw tea is used to treat shingles, herpes zoster, and herpes simplex. The German Commission E limits the use of oat straw to baths for reduction of inflammation and pruritus.

The juice or tea from **Angelica** (*Angelica archangelica*) plant, or powder of the root, is applied to skin ulcers to promote new growth.

Tea bag compresses can relieve sunburned areas, swollen eyelids, and tired eyes.

Lavender essential oil is considered to be safe for all skin types and is believed to regenerate skin cells. It acts to prevent the formation of scars and stretch marks and slows the formation of wrinkles. It can be used on burns, sun-damaged skin, rashes, wounds, and skin infections.

Red clover poultices are used for cancerous growths on the skin and for symptoms related to ailments such as psoriasis or eczema.

Dressings made from a constituent in **seaweed,** calcium alginate, have been used extensively in the treatment of exuding pressure and leg ulcers. Eleven clients in one study of calcium alginate dressing use for exuding wounds reported significantly less discomfort with dressing changes, especially in those clients with lower extremity ulcerations. In addition to the increased comfort to the client, calcium alginate dressings were found to be easy to use, conforming to the wound surface, and absorptive without macerating healthy surrounding tissue.

Turmeric ointment and wash are very antiseptic in wound and skin care.

Environmental Remedies

Some experts think **rose** water's medicinal value is almost equal to rose oil. It can be used in the bath to soothe the skin. It contains acids that restore proper pH and are beneficial when applied to the skin. It is believed that these acids are responsible for its ability to soften, hydrate, and act as an anti-inflammatory on the skin. Rose water is especially good for soothing dry, delicate, and mature complexions.

SLEEP, REST, AND PEACEFUL RESTORATION

Oral Remedies

Chamomile tea and tincture are taken internally for restlessness and mild insomnia. Chamomile is a mild sedative that has no depressive effect. Children often like the taste of chamomile tea. Chamomile tea can be given before bed to help relax the child who has difficulty sleeping for reasons such as teething pain.

Lemon balm tea helps in difficulty falling asleep related to nervous conditions. It has mild vasodilating properties so it can reduce heart rate and lower blood pressure.

Oats are such a common food that they can easily be overlooked when searching for healing remedies. A tincture of the oat seed when it is in its immature, milky stage of development is used as a nervous system restorative, to help with convalescence after an illness, and to strengthen a weakened constitution. Oats extract is a nervine and is used for those suffering from nervous exhaustion and insomnia. When oat is in its earliest stage and just flowering, the green grass is rich in avenin, a constituent considered a nutrient for nerve cells. Looking at the plant, or a picture of the plant, one can sense its signature, or personality—strength and vitality as manifested in the straight stem, and gentle repose and rest as demonstrated by the arching flowers. Clinically, oats and their extract have demonstrated an ability to soothe and comfort as well as nourish. Oat is a tonic, or stimulant, for the nervous system and it also can promote restful sleep. It can stimulate the vitality of those who have suffered nervous exhaustion and calm those who are anxious. Oat seems to be able to create balance within the nervous system. Informing people about the importance of giving their nervous systems a rest from the bombardment of various environmental stimuli by having quiet time at home and including whole grain oats as a regular part of their diet can be an important addition to the health promotion program of some clients, regardless of the person's blood cholesterol level.

Valerian root is a nervine. I do not talk about the plant as a "sleep aide." Rather it is mildly sedative and relieves the agitation and imperil that may precipitate sleeplessness. Imperil is chrystallized irritability on the nerve endings throughout the body. Some plant researchers have published that the herb's sedative effects are due to valepotriates and volatile oils in the roots. However, valepotriates are highly unstable compounds that deteriorate rapidly when in solution or exposed to oxygen. They are not well absorbed by the gastrointestinal tract after ingestion; are water insoluble; and, according to some researchers, are not present in aqueous or alcohol extracts of valerian root. Many are puzzled about why the water extracts that contained no valepotriates and little volatile oils have proved to be effective in promoting sleep. Research suggests that any sleep-promoting effect may be due to an interaction of a constituent with central gamma-aminobutyric acid (GABA) receptors. The monoterpene bornyl acetate and sesquiterpene valerenic acid as well as other sesquiterpene acids in valerian have a direct action on the amygdaloid body of the brain, and valerenic acid inhibits enzyme-induced breakdown of GABA in the brain, resulting in a calming effect on body, mind, and spirit. Many people do not like the smell of dried root (dirty socks) and therefore take it in a capsule like a drug. This is a part of the reason why the responses to valerian are erratic. Some find it sedative and others stimulating. It is also quite warming and therefore I check pulse, tongue, and history before recommending this even as a simple per the consumer model. Because this herb is a special nervine, it must be tasted. Taste is where the action on the nervous system begins according to Ayurvedic tradition. I agree and know that it is best to grow it and smell its flowers, too, when establishing partnership. Biomedical science's holistic understanding of the anatomy and physiology of the nervous system is rudimentary. I recommend turning to writings of the ancient wisdom and healing traditions to develop a greater understanding of the nervous system, including psychology (ex. Tibetan tradition) and the corresponding energy system (ex. Ayurveda and TCM). As a simple tea: 1 to 5 cups per day of tea with 1 to 3 g (0.06 to 0.10 oz) of dried root per cup. Liquid extract: 20 to 30 drops two to three times a day.

Hops tea has been used in relieving insomnia, restlessness, nervous diarrhea, intestinal cramps, lack of appetite, and other nervous conditions. It is also effective for delirium tremens.

Lavender is licensed in Germany as a medicinal tea for sleep problems and for nervous stomach.

Horsetail tea is very helpful in providing silicon for the restoration and strengthening of bone.

Milk thistle has been studied extensively. Most studies have been done on the standardized extract form of milk thistle and that is why this is one herb that I apply biomedically in capsule, standardized extract form. Studies show that milk thistle can normalize liver enzyme levels and regenerate the liver while improving discomfort related to liver diseases such as cirrhosis and hepatitis. Milk thistle's antioxidant action is thought to alter the structure of the cell membranes of hepatocytes to prevent entrance of the liver toxin into the cells. It stimulates the liver's regenerative ability and the formation of new hepatocytes by stimulating protein synthesis. Silymarin, a constituent in milk thistle, has been shown to increase the glutathione content of the liver by more than 35 percent in healthy volunteers. Glutathione is the compound responsible for detoxifying a wide range of toxic chemicals, pesticides, and heavy metals, including mercury, lead, cadmium, and arsenic. Silymarin has strong free-radical scavenging (antioxidant) activity, ten times stronger than vitamin E. Children are also exposed to environmental pollutants and toxins. I recommend introducing children to the flavonoids and lignans that may be responsible for the hepatoprotective effects of milk thistle by having them eat artichokes (*Cynara cardunculus subsp. Cardunculus*). Artichokes are a relative of milk thistle. Some children really like them and can learn a lot about herbs and plants from eating them leaf by leaf. Nurses are also exposed to toxic substances and environments as well as toxic chemicals, such as disinfecting solutions, chemotherapeutic agents, and blood and body fluids that carry hepatitis. A healthy liver is very important to a long, healthy life. Nurses can take milk thistle on occasion to support the liver's natural ability to regenerate.

Red clover tea has been used for many years both internally and externally to treat and prevent cancer and to relieve symptoms related to malignant ulcers, scrofula, indolent sores, bronchial conditions, renal conditions, and sore throat. Red clover is normally used over a period of time because its therapeutic action takes time. I heard one of the most remarkable stories about red clover and cancer while at a conference on complementary therapies and cancer care. Dr. Benjamin Carson, a world-renowned professor of neurosurgery, oncology, plastic surgery, and pediatrics at Johns Hopkins University, told his remarkable story of red clover tea. He had accidently injected his own finger with VX2 carcinoma when attempting to inject the same into the brain of a rabbit while doing laboratory research. The cancer was not a human cancer and his immune system attacked it vigorously. None of the scientists at Johns Hopkins or the National Institutes of Health could save his life. He happened to come across the old American herbal by Jethro Kloss, *Back to Eden*, in which he read about red clover tea. He drank gallons of the tea and the finger cancer and the nodules in his thyroid began to disappear. He credits the victory to red clover.

Liquid **chlorophyll,** more specifically chlorophyllin, is very helpful in restoring the oxygen- carrying capacity of the blood. Some porphyrins, the ringlike structures in heme and chlorophyll, stimulate the synthesis of the protein portion of the hemoglobin molecule, enhancing the body's ability to produce globin. Liquid chlorophyll can be added to water and drunk regularly throughout the day. I prefer that my clients use chlorophyll extracted from stinging **nettle** rather than alfalfa because nettles is an agent of change. Alfalfa also potentially increases inflammation in the body whereas nettles will relieve inflammation.

Nettles tea or liquid extract also helps restore and build blood.

Bilberry supplement (standardized extract in capsules) is one herb that clearly provides support for the restoration of the microcirculation in the eye and other tissues and can be considered as a supplement in those clients who suffer repeated retinal hemorrhage or diabetic retinopathy, for example. The positive effects of bilberry on night vision and visual acuity are related to its ability to decrease the breakdown of rhodopsin (retinal purple), a light-sensitive pigment located in the rods of the retina. It also has the ability to regenerate rhodopsin.

Topical Remedies

Topically, a few drops of essence of **lavender** can be used in footbaths to alleviate fatigue.

The name "**valerian**" is derived from the Latin *valere*, meaning "to be well." Spikenard, a precious, aromatic oil used in Egyptian and Eastern civilizations in spiritual practices such as anointing, comes from a plant (*Nardostachys jatamansi*) that is a close relative of valerian. I have used valerian in making ointments and waters for those performing anointing in spiritual rituals where spikenard might have been used in the past. Valerian's fragrance and topical presence is soothing to the nervous system.

Red clover escharotic salve or ointment, enema and/or douche are used in the treatment of breast and ovarian cancer.

Celandine tincture or infused oil help eye conditions. The word "chelidon" in Greek signifies a swallow, the bird. Swallows are known to use greater celandine to apply to the eyes of their babies whose eyes get pecked. People also use celandine for the restoration of the eyes. Either the sap directly from the stem and leaf or a bright green oil made from the celandine leaf can be applied to the eyelids (not the eye) to relieve and restore aching, tired eyes. I have used the external application of celandine tincture with clients. For example, I have used the tincture when a woman client got gasoline in her eyes. Her eyes were pain and infection free by the following morning.

Environmental Remedies

The essential oil of **lavender** is used as a restorative during fainting and to treat nervous palpitations.

The **tea** ceremony in Japan is a renowned ritual of beauty and grace. It has social, aesthetic, and religious aspects, and takes practitioners much time to learn and perfect just as with any other art form. The tea ceremony has a tension-reducing effect both on practitioners and guests.

The therapeutic and sedative effects of **hops** have been observed over the years to be related to the inhalation of the aroma from the oil in the strobiles. A hops pillow can be given to adults or children to promote sleep. A small decorative cotton or linen bag can be filled with a few ounces of dried hops strobiles. The filling may be used for about seven days before the aromatic principles evaporate. A warm bath with hops bath oil or infusion might be considered to promote the inhalation of hops' aroma, which is known to have sedative effects. Hops are rarely recommended as a single herb to be taken for any medicinal purpose except in a bath to promote sleep. Consider combining hops with other relaxing herbs such as chamomile or valerian.

The essential oil of **Angelica** (*Angelica archangelica*) root may be inhaled to reduce the symptoms of postpump depression and promote sleep, and has been used by nurses to ease the transitions occurring during the postoperative period.

MOBILITY, ENERGY, AND TRANSITIONS
(Ex. Pregnancy, Birth, Death)

Oral Remedies

Arnica is not taken internally in whole herb form or preparations. Oral homeopathic preparations of arnica, because they are diluted to the point at which the molecules of arnica are chemically undetectable, are used for many conditions, such as mental and physical shock, trauma, pain and swelling, dental extraction, bone fractures, headache, and concussion.

In a national survey of 500 members of the American College of Nurse Midwives, 90 members said that they use herbs in practice to stimulate labor and of those 90 members, 45 percent use **black cohosh**. Black cohosh tincture used in doses of 10 drops under the tongue every hour is given by midwives to facilitate the softening of the cervix. It is especially helpful if labor is to be induced before the cervix has had time to ripen naturally. Black cohosh has been used during labor to produce natural intermittent uterine contractions, rather than the constant contractions produced by ergot. It has stimulated and toned the uterus to produce the normal contractions necessary for childbirth. After birth, it has been given to decrease the after-pains and relax the nervous system taxed by the exertions of labor. It was thought that a strong decoction of the recently dug roots in tablespoon doses was most effective for these conditions. Black cohosh is combined with blue cohosh and given by midwives when labor needs to be encouraged. It has been used to strengthen or restart contractions. Fetal monitoring has shown that the blue cohosh may increase the heart rate of the baby. It may also cause decreased blood pressure in the mother. One extensive source of information on the use of herbs in pregnancy, including the use of black cohosh during labor, is the writings of the Thomsonian and Eclectic physicians of the 1800s in America. Much of this literature is housed at the Lloyd Library in Cincinnati, Ohio. The Lloyd Library material is indexed online through the University of Cincinnati at www.libraries.uc.edu.

One of the first herbs I tasted as a child with my mother was **wintergreen** berry. The Mi'kmaq healers give wintergreen berry to people to eat as a heart attack preventative and to people who are recovering from heart attacks. It is used by those with blood clotting disorders and those who have had strokes. The plant is believed to thin and regulate (move) the blood, similar to the action of aspirin, thus preventing the formation of blood clots.

Cinnamon, called *gui zhi*, has a long history of use in TCM. It opens the energy channels in the body, relieves wind chill, and disperses cold in the muscles, meridians, and the exterior of the body. Cinnamon decoction warms the kidney energy system and tonifies the yang in states of decreased physical vitality. Symptoms that may indicate a yang deficiency condition include aversion to cold, cold limbs, weak back, decreased libido, impotence, and frequent urination. Cinnamon also helps in clients who are wheezing (asthma) due to the failure of the kidneys to grasp the *qi*. Cinnamon prevents symptoms of misplaced *qi* from rising in the body. Cinnamon "leads fire back to its source," meaning that it corrects upward-floating energies that should be restrained by the internal organs. It acts to redirect excess energy in the upper half of the body to revitalize deficient energy in the lower half of the body. Cinnamon does this by warming the kidneys. Cinnamon bark decoction is used for fever, headaches, inflammation caused by sinusitis, and colds. These properties also make it effective for certain types of pains in the chest and abdomen, diarrhea, and decreased function of the kidney. Cinnamon tea controls hemorrhage in the body, but it has a specific effect upon the uterus, acting to stop bleeding by causing contraction of the uterine musculature.

In TCM, it is believed that **coffee** can tonify the yang. People like the warming yang tonic effects during cold winter months. However, coffee also readily drains kidney (energy system) yang and aggravates the liver energy system. In India, coffee is thought to hasten old age and decrease longevity because it disturbs the normal metabolism. Some cultures have developed ways to deal with the stimulating effects of coffee. The Arabs serve coffee, as do Turks, in a little cup with the grounds. They roast and grind the coffee immediately before serving, add the coffee to a pot with sugar and water, and boil it. The coffee is served with the grounds in the cup because they believe that the grounds neutralize any excessively stimulating qualities associated with the caffeine in the coffee. There are nurse-herbalist applications for the stimulating effect of coffee. Coffee is effective in relieving symptoms associated with asthma because it contains xanthines, such as theobromine and theophylline, which help stop bronchospasm. If people with asthma forget their inhaler, they can drink a few cups of coffee while waiting for their medication. Asthma can be life threatening and coffee has been reported to be successfully used in potential emergencies.

Many women after vaginal delivery often like drinking **cranberry** juice. It is astringent (helpful after the loss of fluids and blood from an herbal medicine perspective) and also prevents bladder infections that are often an issue for pregnant and postpartum women. I do not recommend that the juice be drunk over ice but rather at room temperature. Cranberry is energetically cooling, which is helpful in postpartum women, who typically exhibit a yin or heat deficiency pattern, meaning that they are energetically hot and yin or fluid deficient.

If the client insists on cold food, the following is my family's recipe for cranberry sherbet, a natural alternative to popsicles.

Ingredients:
4 cups cranberries
4 cups (960 ml) water
2½ cups (566 g) sugar or sweetener
1 cup (240 ml) orange juice
4 tablespoons (60 ml) lemon juice
2 tablespoons (30 ml) rose water

Simmer berries in water for fifteen minutes until mushy. Mash and strain. Add the sugar or sweetener and stir until dissolved. Add fruit juices and freeze in the bowl until mushy. Take out of freezer and beat with electric beater on low, then medium, then high until very frothy. Add rose water. Line a cupcake pan with cupcake papers and spoon frothy sherbet into the papers and freeze until hard. Usually makes 18 servings of sherbet. Decorate with fresh flower or candied violets before serving.

Lemon balm tea or liquid extract brings comfort to the bereaved family of one who is dying. It also has been given to the person who is dying and seems to bring solace to them with its relaxing, yet uplifting, properties. The name "balm" suggests the action of the herbal remedy as a soothing extension of the caring touch and nurturing spirit of the nurse when providing comfort.

Oats are a tonic that improves the condition of the heart muscle. Clinical trials reveal that Oatmeal or oat bran intake lowers low-density lipoprotein cholesterol without affecting high-density lipoprotein cholesterol.

Tea has been shown to promote significant increases in alertness and information-processing capacity, which did not decline throughout the day, as compared with water. Green tea has significant thermogenic and fat-oxidizing properties. The tannins in tea leaf are thought to be carcinogenic; however, adding milk has been found to bind the tannins to a protein in the milk, thereby preventing any harmful effects.

Historically, **goldenseal** has been thought to stimulate the respiratory and circulatory systems, bringing tone to the arteries and increasing blood pressure in the capillaries. It is thought that this action brings more nutrition to the muscles and helps in various cases of muscular debility.

Oral **evening primrose** oil is widely used by midwives to promote cervical ripening in pregnant women.

Rose petals and leaves can be used as an astringent tea for toning the uterus and healing the perineum after the birth.

Ginger can be helpful in pregnant women with nausea and hyperemesis. Some women respond best to fresh ginger tea and others dry ginger powder in capsules.

Chamomile is useful during the latter months of pregnancy and during the birth process to decrease anxiety in the mother and family members. Hispanic women drink chamomile (Manzanilla) tea as soon as they feel labor pains. Chamomile tea stops the labor pains if the woman is in false labor and continues the labor if it is truly her time to deliver. This traditional evidence suggests that chamomile is also a thinking herb.

After the bombing of Nagasaki, Japan, in 1945, Tatsuichiro Akizuki, the medical director of internal medicine at St. Francis Hospital (located 1 mile from ground zero), fed all clients and staff who survived (most survived the initial blast) a strict macrobiotic diet of brown rice, miso (**soy**) and tamari (soy sauce) soup, wakame and other sea vegetables, Hokkaido pumpkin, and sea salt. Although many people died from radiation sickness in Nagasaki, Dr. Akizuki saved everyone in his hospital. Japanese medical researchers continue to study the effects of miso and sea vegetables, in particular for protection against radiation sickness, as well as cancer and heart disease. Miso, a salty, fermented soybean paste, is used in preparing soups and sauces. It contains enzymes that aid digestion and minerals that aid metabolism. Miso also is used to prevent allergies and tuberculosis.

Midwives recommend drinking **sage** leaf tea to help reduce excessive engorgement of breasts during lactation. Hot sage tea also is used to reduce the secretion of milk in nursing mothers who are beginning to wean their babies.

Thyme affects the rhythmic system of the body, relaxes convulsive coughing, and strengthens the nervous system. Some women sip thyme tea during childbirth to hasten delivery.

Yarrow tea or liquid extract stops excessive bleeding and hemorrhage.

From a traditional Chinese medicine viewpoint, the use of **cayenne** internally needs even more consideration because of its extremely hot nature. Cayenne would most likely be contraindicated in clients such as the elderly, who often have yin deficiency (interior heat) conditions. Although taking cayenne internally has many beneficial joint-pain relieving and gastrointestinal-protecting phytochemical activities that may be helpful for elderly clients, it also may aggravate other symptoms related to heat in the interior of the body, which can cause a dissipation of fluid, potentially leading to such symptoms as stiffness and stagnation.

Turmeric is known in Chinese as "jiang huang" (rhizome) or "yu jin." In Chinese herbal medicine, turmeric root tea is used to move the blood and *qi*, especially in the abdomen and shoulders. Often when the gallbladder is inflamed or stagnant, the shoulders and nape of the neck become sore and stiff. Traditionally turmeric has been used for both. It is used as a treatment for inflammation, dysmenorrhea, liver damage, gall bladder stagnation and stones, and jaundice to stimulate the flow of energy through the shoulders.

Topical Remedies

A compress or poultice of **yarrow** leaf or a compress with yarrow extract stops bleeding. It is best to also apply direct pressure and elevation.

Arnica has a long history of use in nursing for bodily injuries that result in limitations to mobility. Hildegard von Bingen used arnica in the twelfth century. Topical arnica applications in the form of oil, ointment, jelly, and tincture are quite common and currently are recognized by the German Commission E as antiphlogistic or anti-inflammatory for use in hematoma, sprains, bruises, contusions, rheumatic pain of muscles and joints, and for edema related to fracture. For sprains and strains, arnica used topically usually results in the subsiding of swelling or congestion after twelve to twenty-four hours. I have observed topical arnica infused oil quickly reduce pain related to sprains and injuries and help swelling and bruising disappear within two to four days. For many years, I have used topical arnica oil with lavender for clients with ankle and low back sprains, wrist and elbow pain, carpal tunnel syndrome, bruising, fractures, and joint pain. It is important to help the body stay mobile during these types of conditions because the tendency is for the body to tighten and protect the injury long after the initial insult warrants the protection. Herbal applications such as arnica oil massage encourage the stimulation of circulation and oxygen exchange in the injured area of the body. Arnica prevents stagnation and promotes healing.

Gently apply **rose** oil (infused not essential) to the skin of newborn babies. This recipe helps protect the baby's nervous system as they adjust to extra-uterine life. Rose oil and essential oil applied topically to the face, neck, and body are helpful in women who are transitioning in perimenopause. Rose oil baths and face sprays may help with discomfort related to menopause.

Nurses continue to use **witch hazel** in the care of pregnant and postpartum women. Witch hazel compresses are helpful in reducing perineal pain and swelling of tissues. Witch hazel water may be applied to varicose veins of the legs during pregnancy by spraying it on with a spray bottle or using a saturated cloth. It helps tighten the skin and reduce pain and swelling. It can also be applied to hemorrhoids during pregnancy. Witch hazel water can be used topically for care of the umbilical stump of the newborn. Applied with a cloth, it will help the stump heal and dry quickly.

With education and experience, **cayenne** can be a very helpful herb to use in topical and internal applications when there is blood and/or qi stagnation, especially of a "cold" nature. There are systems of assessment such as in Chinese medicine that help determine the thermal nature of a condition, especially as it may manifest in the joints and muscles of the body. If these assessment systems are unknown, one can also try an external application such as a poultice or ointment and, through observation of an initial trial, determine if the client benefits from the heat and counterirritant action to a particular body part. Nurses are generally familiar with recommending hot and cold applications for structural injury. There are times during the healing process when heat or cold feels better to the client. In general, cold is applied immediately after an injury to decrease inflammation, and heat is applied later to relax the muscles that have been protecting the injury. The heat in topical herb applications is not only used to stimulate joints and muscles but also to stimulate internal organs such as the lungs where thick stringy mucus may be lodged. Using a basic understanding of applying heat is fundamental to the use of cayenne. It is recommended that to get the full benefit of creams containing cayenne or capsaicin, they should be applied at least four to five times daily until relief is obtained. This process could take three to four weeks to achieve maximum pain relief. After relief is noticed, capsaicin can be applied less often.

Environmental Remedies

Midwives often recommend herbal sitz baths to aid in the healing of perineal tears or sutures after the birth. **Goldenseal** root decoction is frequently one of the ingredients included in the sitz.

Witch hazel water can be used in sitz baths after birth to soothe perineal tears, aid healing, and prevent infection.

Rosemary massage oil and footbaths can be used with clients whose memories are impaired, such as those with Alzheimer's disease or dementia, as long as the client's blood pressure is within normal limits. Rosemary shampoo, baths, and tea have been found to have an effect similar to the drugs given to clients with Alzheimer's disease because several of the plant constituents known to retard the breakdown of acetylcholine are readily absorbed through the skin and some are thought to be able to cross the blood-brain barrier.

DIGESTION AND ELIMINATION

Oral Remedies

Chamomile tea and tinctures are taken internally for gastrointestinal spasms, inflammatory conditions of the gastrointestinal tract, dyspepsia, epigastric bloating, poor digestion, and intestinal gas. Chamomile tea helps relieve abdominal pain in infants with colic. Historically nurses have added a small amount of chamomile tea to a baby's bottle to relieve colic pain. It is very helpful, especially when the parents also massage the baby's abdomen in a clockwise direction following the movement pattern of the intestines.

Kudzu is a twining, hairy perennial vine that grows quickly and can cover large areas of ground and trees. The plant is native to eastern Asia and was introduced in the United States more than 100 years ago. It proliferates in the southeastern United States. Most people I have met only know this plant as a weed. But the leaf is a good source of protein and the root is a healer. Kudzu can be used like corn starch in cooking to thicken soups, sauces, and stews. Kudzu root powder, the starch that dissolves out from the root and is then hardened, can be purchased from health food stores. To make Kuzu Pudding: One heaping teaspoon (5 g) of the powder is stirred into cold water. A cup (240 ml) of cold water is added and brought to a boil and cooked until the kudzu starch is translucent, at which time other ingredients can be added. For a salty taste, add some tamari or sea salt. For diarrhea, a salty/sour taste is preferable. Add a half a teaspoon of Japanese *ume boshi* plum paste little by little because it will just be suspended in the pudding and will not dissolve. The *ume* plum paste is more astringent and is helpful if the client is losing a lot of fluid from diarrhea. For moistening the gastrointestinal system, such as in cases of ulcer or burning pain, cook the kudzu with apple juice or pear nectar instead of water. Chopped apple or pear can be added also. I have also recommended this to clients after they have drunk the chemical-based preparatory fluids for sigmoidoscopy and other gastrointestinal tests. Those preparations are energetically scalding to sensitive mucous membranes. The lungs and large intestine are paired organs in TCM. If heat is created in the bowel from those chemical preparations, the client often begins coughing after the test. Kudzu helps moisten the intestines and thus the cough resolves.

Cranberry juice, fruit concentrate, and tablets are helpful in the relief of urinary tract discomfort. I find that drinking as much cranberry juice as you can, or "pushing" the cranberry juice, to be the most effective.

Lemon, fresh fruit or juice, increases salivary flow, the first part of the digestive process. Warm lemon water often acts as a gentle cathartic.

Peppermint tea is helpful for relieving indigestion and abdominal gas.

Chlorophyll water can significantly decrease constipation and excessive flatus.

Coffee produces therapeutic results that caffeine alone does not. An infusion of roasted coffee has been used as a digestive stimulant and an antiemetic. It mildly increases biliary flow and intestinal peristalsis. Coffee is used to decrease a feeling of fullness after a large meal and to regulate the bowels. Caffeinated coffee has been found to stimulate colon motor activity more than decaffeinated coffee or plain water. I recommend warm lemon juice in water for those who do not want the caffeine effects. Coffee also has a diuretic action. Nurses routinely offer coffee as a part of a clear liquid or regular diet to clients. Many of the medicinal plants used in clinical herbalism are not nearly as toxic, considering median lethal doses, as a cup of coffee, yet coffee is provided with other medications after surgery and other biomedical procedures often without question. Nurses could create clearer guidelines for providing coffee to ill and postoperative clients. Roasted dandelion root or chicory root beverages could be used in a clear liquid diet as a non-stimulant alternative to coffee.

The Chinese *Materia Medica* makes a distinction between the medicinal properties of fresh and dried **ginger**. Fresh ginger is known as "sheng jiang" and is classified as an herb that relieves wind chill (an exterior condition); dry ginger is called "gan jiang" and is classified as an herb that warms the interior. Dried ginger root is used in Traditional Chinese Medicine to warm the stomach and spleen energy systems in cases when either deficiency or excess are present. It also is used with symptoms such as epigastric pain, vomiting, dysentery, and abdominal pain with feelings of gnawing hunger. Fresh ginger root is used to release the exterior of the body and disperse cold and for symptoms of cold in the stomach and may be used in cases of vomiting, coughing, and excess sweating. Chewing ginger promotes salivation. Swallowing it stimulates digestion, increases the secretion of gastric juice, and dispels flatulence. Because of its stimulating effect on digestion, ginger may increase the bioavailability of certain pharmaceutical drugs. Whole herb ginger (fresh root and powdered root in capsules) has been studied for its anti-nausea and antiemetic effect. Ginger root is useful in motion and seasickness. Dried ginger does not work like pharmaceutical drugs for motion sickness. The positive antiemetic activity has been attributed to an effect on gastric activity rather than on central nervous system mechanisms, specifically oculomotor and vestibular systems that are characteristic of pharmaceutical anti-motion sickness drugs.

Psyllium seed has been used traditionally in the United States and Europe as a bulking laxative to treat the symptoms of chronic constipation. It is used in current herbalism for its ability to decrease bowel transit time, absorb toxins from the bowel, regulate intestinal flora, for its beneficial fiber, and its demulcent action on the digestive tract. Psyllium also is recommended for use during chronic yeast (*Candida albicans*) infections. It is believed that psyllium can absorb the byproducts of the yeast growth, thereby preventing the systemic reabsorption of the toxins. In the presence of water, a plant constituent called mucilage, found in psyllium seed and husk (primarily), swells to form a slippery mass. Psyllium exhibits adaptogen action. It can regulate the fluids in the bowel, so if a person has diarrhea, psyllium helps retain fluids. Psyllium's ability to retain fluid also helps the person with constipation because the moistening, bulking action of the herb helps the person eliminate smoothly and comfortably. Although the biomedical diagnoses of diarrhea and constipation would seem to be on opposite ends of the spectrum, psyllium can work on either health concern with a similar action. When taken into the gastrointestinal tract, psyllium swells either because of the fluid in the gut or the fluids taken in with the psyllium. When the psyllium swells, it can cause a sense of fullness in the stomach. It ultimately becomes part of the feces. It adds bulk to the stool and keeps it hydrated and soft. The resulting bulk promotes more efficient peristalsis and evacuation of the bowel. Lots of plain water must be taken with psyllium to keep the stool moist so that the colon does not become impacted. Psyllium draws fluid from the moist mucous membranes of the gastrointestinal tract if there is not extra water in it. A client I worked with years ago who had been taking a psyllium powder product as part of an intestinal "cleansing" program came into a clinic where I worked. She had abdominal pain, was admitted to the hospital, and ended up needing an appendectomy. When the surgeon opened her belly to remove the appendix, her bowel had perforated and psyllium was caked on her intestines. Part of her bowel had to be removed as well. She later admitted to not having read the label on the product and having no idea that she needed to drink lots of plain water with the psyllium. This is the only time I have seen a problem with psyllium self-care. Elderly clients, in particular, should take psyllium with caution because they are often prone to dehydration.

Saw palmetto has been shown to be an effective alternative to drug therapy for benign prostatic hyperplasia (BPH), especially in those clients who are worried about serious adverse effects of drugs such as erectile dysfunction and hypotension. Saw palmetto is typically taken as a standardized extract in capsules (160 mg twice). This is partially due to the fact that the taste of saw palmetto is highly objectionable to clients. A standardized extract is more often used than a tea or liquid extract. All of these herbal alternatives cost about $15 to $45 per month compared with $45 to $85 for pharmaceutical therapy. Men often have symptomatic relief within three months of starting to take the herb. Saw palmetto berries are used for the symptoms associated with BPH, such as hesitancy in initiation of the urinary stream, dribbling, urinary urgency, pressure over the bladder, and incomplete emptying of the bladder. Saw palmetto often is used in combination with other herbs, such as stinging nettle, for the relief of lower urinary tract discomfort. The clinical trials on the use of saw palmetto in the care of those with BPH are related to the effects of a standardized extract of the berries on the prostate and related urinary tract symptoms as well as those with mild-to-moderate symptoms of prostatic hyperplasia who fulfilled specific inclusion criteria.

Horseradish is a warm and pungent herb that carries the energy of the metal element, related to the Five Element Theory used in Chinese medicine. Poor digestion causes food to move slowly through the gastrointestinal tract and, thus, to ferment. This is especially the case with protein foods, which can be harder for some to digest. Horseradish has extensive traditional use as a digestive aid, especially in clients who have sluggish digestion. Horseradish is also an excellent addition to a regular, balanced diet when used as a condiment (i.e., in very small amounts mixed with other foods). Horseradish seems to stimulate digestion through its warming action of the digestive tract. A little horseradish goes a long way in helping those who need the benefits of protein-rich foods, such as meat and fish, but who often have trouble digesting them.

Angelica (*A. archangelica*) is used as an aromatic and bitter preparation for digestion, to stimulate the appetite, and for symptoms of digestive disturbance. It is used for symptoms related to dysfunctions of the liver, gallbladder, and gastrointestinal tract. Germany has licensed angelica for the treatment of symptoms such as bloating, flatulence, mild gastrointestinal cramps, and insufficient gastric juice.

Feverfew traditionally has been used in herbalism to relieve intestinal gas and dental pain; promote the onset of menstruation; as a mild laxative; and as a "bitter," an agent that promotes digestion.

If a client's digestive "fire" is low, consider suggesting the use of **rosemary** in food. Rosemary has been shown to exert an antispasmodic action on gall bladder passages and on the small intestines.

Several studies have been conducted on berberine, one of the active constituents in **goldenseal** root, and its effect on infection in the human body. Goldenseal contains active principles isoquinoline alkaloids, consisting mainly of hydrastine and berberine (0.5 percent to 6 percent). In one double-blind, placebo-controlled trial, men from Bangladesh with diagnosed *Escherichia coli* diarrhea infection, given berberine sulfate 400 mg orally as a single dose, experienced a 48 percent reduction in stool volume and 42 percent had stopped having watery stools within twenty-four hours as compared with 20 percent in the control group ($p < .05$).

Elder was used by American Eclectic physicians as a stimulant to increase secretion of various bodily functions. A warm infusion of elder flowers was used as a diaphoretic and a gentle stimulant. The juice of the berries prepared as syrup was used as an alterative and as a mild laxative.

Oats also are used as an easily digested food for the mother after childbirth. An easy way to make a hot oat cereal is to first purchase some Irish oats. These are not the typical rolled oats that are commonly sold in stores. Irish oats are the cut whole grain. Toast 1/4 cup (56 g) of the grain gently in a skillet. Put it into a thermos jar. Add 1 cup (240 ml) of boiling water. Let this sit overnight. Open it in the morning for a quick breakfast cereal. Add sweetener, nuts, or fruit only if the digestive system is strong. Traditional herbalists recommend that those recuperating from recent illness when the digestion has been weakened eat oats plain so that the grain does not ferment in the intestines.

Sage tea is used to aid digestion and to treat inflammation of the gallbladder and urinary bladder. It is used for flatulence.

Hops tea is used as a digestive tonic in jaundice and indigestion.

Aloe leaf yields two different medicinal substances, each from different parts of the plant. Aloe vera gel is contained in the center part of the succulent leaves. The bitter, yellow-colored latex from the plant is derived from cells that line the inner surface of the leaf skin. The latex is used as a harsh laxative and is known as the drug "aloe" or "aloes." The latex is obtained by cutting the leaves and allowing the bitter sap to drip out. It is then processed into the drug form. The gel does not have laxative properties.

The fluid extract (1.5 to 3 g of 1:1 g/ml) or tincture (1.5 g of 1:5 g/ml) of the root of **Angelica** (*A. archangelica*) can be given to children for discomfort related to gastrointestinal problems and loss of appetite.

Calendula possesses antispasmodic, diaphoretic, anti-inflammatory, wound-healing, and antiseptic properties. Calendula tea is very helpful for "stomach flu" symptoms such as nausea and abdominal cramps.

Recipe for Miso (**Soy**) Soup: Miso is a dark paste made from soybeans, sea salt, and fermented rice or barley that are aged together. Miso contains enzymes that facilitate digestion and strengthen the quality of the blood and alkalize the body. To make miso soup, purchase some dark brown miso paste. Boil 1 cup of water. Add a small amount of the boiled water to approximately 1 tablespoon (14 g) of miso. The strength of the miso broth can be adjusted to taste. After the paste is thinned with a little water, add it to the rest of the boiled water. Do not boil the miso soup. The soup can be drunk plain or a small amount of green onion can be added for flavor and color along with a few drops of brown sesame oil. This is a great home remedy when you are feeling out of balance. I like to have miso soup when traveling, especially on long, international flights. For travel purposes, dried, powdered miso is available.

Soybeans are low in saturated fat, cholesterol-free, and a good source of protein and omega-3 fatty acids. The German Commission E has approved soy *lecithin* for treating disturbances of fat metabolism, such as hypercholesterolemia in cases in which dietary management is not effective. Although Asians have eaten soy products for many centuries, people of other races often find soy to be indigestible. This may be due to the difference in digestive enzymes between races, and therefore, people who have not grown up in a culture where soy products are eaten as part of a staple diet may want to ingest soy sparingly, or perhaps not at all. Raw soybeans contain trypsin inhibitors that interfere with protein metabolism by the pancreatic enzyme trypsin. This process may damage the pancreas. Also, soybeans contain substances that can reduce the absorption of iodine by the thyroid gland. It is recommended that those with diminished thyroid function avoid eating soy to prevent further aggravation of this condition.

The **seaweed** Sargassum, or "hai zao," is classified as salty, cold, and bitter in TCM and is used to clear heat and phlegm conditions. It is used for the treatment of symptoms often related to diagnoses of both hypothyroidism and hyperthyroidism. It is used as a gentle laxative because up to 45 percent of its weight consists of a complex carbohydrate that swells in the presence of water. Kelp contains iodine, an essential trace element that is required for normal functioning of the thyroid gland. The only abundant, naturally occurring sources of iodine are in seaweeds and sea vegetables. Vegetables grown on land have very minute amounts of iodine compared to those found in the ocean. Kelp, depending upon when it is harvested, can have 100 to 500 times more iodine than shellfish. Kelp and other sea vegetables are food sources with a rich mineral content. For example, sea vegetables such as hijiki and wakame contain more than 10 times the calcium in milk, and wakame and kelp contain four times the iron in beef. People should drink plenty of water when adding sea vegetables to their diet. In TCM, medicinal amounts of seaweeds are contraindicated when using licorice root. Kelp's clathritic nature—its ability to absorb fluid and nutrients from its environment—provides a signature for its action in the body. Therefore, seaweeds and kelp powders should only be eaten if they are harvested from pollutant-free waters and processed without formaldehyde. Fresh kelp powders are green in color. If you have never eaten kelp or any sea vegetables and you would like to try some, start off slowly as it takes the body up to three to four months to adjust to the addition of marine plant polysaccharides in the digestive tract. Get some kombu (*Laminaria*) or wakame (*Undaria*), preferably whole pieces rather than powder, and soak the seaweed for a few minutes. You can add the kombu to a pot of rice you are cooking and taste it afterward. After soaking, wakame is bright green in color and can be thinly sliced and added to miso soup. You must chew the sea vegetables thoroughly or they will expand exponentially and be excreted pretty much in the same form in which they are ingested.

Topical Remedies

Thyme, in particular thymol, has an extensive history of successful use in dentistry related to its antiseptic qualities. Thymol is the main ingredient in Listerine, an over-the-counter mouthwash. In vitro studies of the effect of thyme oil on bacteria commonly found in the mouth such as *Streptococcus mutans,* one of the major etiologic agents of dental caries, and *Staphylococcus aureus,* one of the major organisms associated with dental infection, showed that thyme oil has significantly effective germicidal action against these microbes.

Hops are used as a compress to the abdomen to relieve spasms of the internal organs.

Environmental Remedies

Coffee enemas are sometimes helpful in detoxification, such as when a client is exposed to environmental pollutants or large doses of vitamins and/or medications such as occurs in cancer treatment programs. Coffee footbaths followed by a foot massage or foot reflexology treatment are helpful for promoting defecation.

Lemon essential oil blended with a carrier oil and massaged into the feet often promotes salivation and digestion.

See immune response – **elder** and **yarrow** – herbs that promote perspiration/elimination through the skin.

IMMUNE RESPONSE

Oral Remedies

Infusion of **elder** flowers or berries is taken at the first signs of a cold or flu. Tea: 1/2 to 1 teaspoon dry berries or flowers (3 to 4 g) in 5 ounces (150 ml) water. Take 1 to 2 cups several times daily as hot as can be sipped safely. Peppermint leaf can be added to the tea also to cool the heat in the head. The infusion promotes sweating, sleep, and increased bronchial secretion activity. It has demonstrated anti-inflammatory, antiviral, and diuretic activity in in vitro studies. Elder has demonstrated antiviral activity in vivo. It prevents influenza virus from entering respiratory tract cells. Elderberry extract and syrup have been shown to significantly reduce the time a person experiences flu symptoms to days rather than weeks. While there may be no "cure" for the common cold or influenza, elder has been shown to support the body in moving through the illness in a shorter period of time. The concept of moving through an illness is important in health care. People develop immunity when they experience the diseases that occur around them. Some might even say that those who live through an infectious disease can be strengthened by the experience because they then have acquired primary immunity to the disease. An infectious illness, such as a cold or flu, becomes more serious when it continues to produce symptoms that go on for weeks and even months. The viral illness gradually weakens the body and the spirit, because the person may feel exhausted just from feeling sick for so long. Bacterial illness, weakness, fatigue, and anorexia can then become complications of what was originally a viral illness. One goal of nursing care during viral illness must be to help the client maintain their strength and ability to move through the illness as quickly as possible so that the viral illness does not weaken the client and allow other complications to occur. Elder flowers assist in moving the virus through the body by opening the pores and increasing perspiration. This also helps with regulation of fever. Elder flower/berry tea should be taken hot while in bed because the diaphoretic effect is best experienced when physically warm. It also should be taken in the afternoon when the natural diurnal pattern of the body creates a rise in temperature. When taken during this time, it will produce prompt sweating.

Elderberries, although the mechanism is not exactly clear, are able to help the person move through their illness more quickly. This is considered beneficial in herbalism so that the client is not overcome by the illness and can experience it at a manageable level. Elderberries are used to promote sweating, but the berries are not as effective as the flowers in this regard. Elderberries are an excellent source of vitamin C. Although birds eat the berries raw, humans must only eat them cooked because they contain the cyanogenic glycoside, sambunigrin, the ingestion of which can cause nausea, vomiting, or severe diarrhea. I also recommend that people observe their bowel habits while taking elderberry. Some berries can be very astringent (drying) and the last thing someone with cold or flu needs is to be constipated. Although no side effects have been noticed in the studies that have been reported, I have observed some people experiencing slight constipation from taking elderberry syrup straight. Therefore, I usually recommend taking elderberry syrup in a small amount of warm water and making sure to drink plenty of fluids throughout the day. Elder blossom extract can reduce infant's fevers. Use 1 drop of tincture per pound of body weight. Put drops in small amount of water and place under the infant's tongue. Adult dose of extract is 1/2 to 1½ teaspoons (2.5 to 7.5 ml) three times daily.

Nettles liquid extract is very helpful in allergic reactions and asthma. Nettles works on the histamine response in the body. I recommend that it be used with vitamin C and/or quercetin supplements for more severe allergic response. Tea can be used in adults and children with less severe responses.

Kudzu pudding (for recipe see the digestion/elimination section) releases the tightness in muscles that occurs in the early stages of an infection, nasal allergies, colds, inner ear infection, or sinusitis. Kudzu has the ability to open certain energetic pathways in the body to allow the release of trapped, pathologic influences from tight muscles. Kudzu is also helpful for diarrhea. Puerarin, a constituent in kudzu that has 100 times the antioxidant activity of vitamin E, helps prevent cancer and heart disease, and has been shown to reduce blood pressure in animals. Kudzu pudding improves coronary circulation and decreases the heart's oxygen requirement. It relaxes the muscles in the heart and lowers the heart rate.

The **onion** bulb has been used as a food and medicine for thousands of years, especially for coughs and the common cold. The onion allicins and cepaenes, organosulfur compounds, have a wide range of therapeutic activities including antiasthmatic effects. The anti-inflammatory effects of onion are thought to be related to the cepaenes constituents. With the increase in lung disease, asthma, and tuberculosis (some report related to increases in air pollutants), the lungs are often weakened through repeated viral and bacterial infections. The risk for infection such as pneumonia is greater. Preventive care, including lifestyle and dietary changes, can be recommended, especially at the beginning of cold and flu season. Nurses may want to consider adding onion as part of their recommendations. Nurses may want to suggest that clients increase their intake of onion in foods and learn to make an onion syrup to be taken when congestion, cold, or flu begin to cause discomfort. Nurses also might consider clinical research to explore the traditional use of onion poultices applied to the feet or chest in the care of people with upper respiratory discomfort or the external application of onion skin to promote wound and skin healing. Nurses have used onion poultices applied externally to areas of inflammation, especially to the chest. Part of the onion's personality and its therapeutic effects involves causing the eyes to tear and the sinuses to run when preparing the onions for use. The nose runs when a person is coming down with a cold to help the body shed the virus. Onions help by assisting this process of keeping secretions moving and therefore are often used in breaking up mucus in the head and chest. Onion is warming, stimulating, and penetrating, and it doesn't have to be eaten to do its work. Onions are often applied externally. When used externally, their pungency can be inhaled and felt. Local heat from the onions increases the "fever" to the area, bringing with it all the benefits of localized fever in terms of controlling the spread of infection. For the immune system to do its work, it has to be able to send its messengers to the place of infection or inflammation. Onions help break up or clear mucus and other substances that block the immune system from doing its work. Pungent substances like onions gently but diligently clear the way for the immune system. Onions also introduce their own antibacterial, antiviral, or antiparasitic substances. Pharmaceutical antibiotics have only the ability to address the exact bacteria they were designed to destroy. Antibiotics, energetically speaking, are cooling and therefore may not have the ability to penetrate mucus and other secretions as do other warming pungent substances. Onions, especially fresh chopped or lightly cooked, perform multiple actions at one time; at the very least they increase heat, provide an antimicrobial action, and break up mucus. Accepting that a substance has the ability to perform multiple actions at the same time may make it difficult to understand the substance fully from a biomedical perspective, but it also makes the substance less likely to fail as a healing agent as the environment changes and bacteria and viruses mutate.

To make **Onion** Cress Soup: Two large yellow or white onions chopped into small pieces but not minced. Put in pot with 4 cups (960 ml) vegetable or onion stock. Cook the onions in the stock on medium low heat until the onions are very tender. Do not boil. Add the liquid aminos or sea salt to taste. Prepare two large bunches of watercress (*Nasturtium officinale*). The leaf is used in many countries to relieve symptoms associated with respiratory illness and catarrh. In therapeutic amounts, it is contraindicated in pregnancy. Trim the leaves from the cress stalks and before serving the soup, add the cress to the onion soup. Cook for two minutes. The cress is best if it is still green when served so only add as much as you plan to eat at one time.

To make **Onion** Syrup: In a large container, alternately layer the slices of 1-2 large yellow or white onions with 3/4 to 1½ cup (180 to 360 ml) of honey (or any sugar). Let it stand for three days in a dark corner of the kitchen and then strain the syrup into a colored glass bottle. Store in the refrigerator. The syrup can be taken on a spoon just like any cough syrup or can be added to a tea.

Valerian is an excellent cough syrup for coughs that are not productive and serve only to keep one from resting well. Valerian root is boiled with licorice root, raisins, and aniseed. This syrup is an expectorant for those who are short winded. It helps open the bronchial tubes and expectorate phlegm easily.

Sage tea has historically been used by nurse-herbalists, such as the American nurse-midwife Martha Ballard in the late 1700s and early 1800s, as a tea for the sick. Sage is antibacterial, astringent, secretion-stimulating, perspiration-inhibiting, and has the ability to stop the growth of certain viruses and fungi. The flowers and leaves of sage have been found to inhibit the growth of *S. aureus* and *Streptococcus pyogenes*. The phenolic acids, salvin and salvin monomethyl ether, have antimicrobial activities, especially against *S. aureus*. Hot sage tea is used as a gargle for sore throats in both adults and children. Use 1/2 to 1 teaspoon (1 to 3 g) dried leaf in 5 ounces (150 ml) of water, three times per day. Sage contains high levels of tannins, plant constituents that have an antimicrobial and soothing effect, which may explain its use for sore throat. Large doses of sage tea should not be taken. Sage tea gargles at the earliest feeling of the scratchy throat that accompanies a cold or flu are often helpful in healing. It is best to recommend making the gargle with sage leaf rather than essential oil. Gargling stimulates the lymphatic system in the throat and, with the antimicrobial activity of sage, supports the overall immune response in the throat and head area. Sage also helps regulate fever and perspiration of the skin during viral illness such as the common cold. Sage exhibits adaptogen activity in that it either increases or decreases the perspiration of the body, depending on the client's need. Adequate perspiration is key to the illness being resolved without the virus lodging in one area of the body and weakening any particular organ. Excessive perspiration, however, such as occurs during many days of fever, can actually weaken the body.

Thyme and its extract, thymol, are used as an antiseptic and disinfectant. The essential oil of thyme has analgesic and antiaging properties and inhibits certain bacteria, fungi, and viruses. It also can stimulate the immune system. Several species of thyme, including *Thymus vulgaris,* are used in treating cancer. The wide spectrum activity of thyme oil is thought to be due to the phenol component, thymol. Thymol can be bactericidal or bacteriostatic, depending on the concentration used. Thymol, the plant constituent that has been studied more than the whole plant, is considered quite toxic, causing nausea, vomiting, headache, dizziness, convulsions, coma, and cardiac and respiratory arrest. Therefore, I recommend the use of whole plant or whole plant essential oil. Many infections that are resistant to antibiotics can be eradicated with essential oils. This especially applies to sinus and respiratory tract infections. One in vitro study analyzed the antibacterial activity of several volatile oils and found thyme oil to have the widest spectrum of antibacterial activity. Just a few of the bacteria that thyme was most active against include *Aeromonas hydrophila, Clostridium sporogenes, Flavobacterium suaveolens, Proteus vulgaris, Salmonella pullorum,* and *S. aureus.* It was also highly active against *E. coli, Klebsiella pneumoniae,* and *Pseudomonas aeruginosa. Thymus vulgaris* aqueous extract has been shown to significantly inhibit *H. pylori* in vitro and was more effective than some antibiotics. Thyme oil is currently used in cough drops, liniments, mouthwashes, and in topical antifungal preparations. Thyme is often combined with other herbs in a tea for chest congestion, bronchitis, and whooping cough. Use 1/2 to 1 teaspoon (1 to 2 g) of herb for one cup of tea. More often I use thyme syrup made from fresh thyme from my garden and local honey. My pediatric clients like to help make the syrup and they come back each year for more, saying that it is the "best" medicine when they get sick. In the second century, Galen gave the thymus gland in the chest its name because it reminded him of a bunch of the thyme plant. The thymus gland is considered by some healers to be the seat of life energy and is therefore the first organ to be affected by stress. Thyme helps clear the chest area where the thymus gland does its work to develop the immune response in the newborn and later on develop a healthy immune system and promote the maturation of T cells. Clearing the chest also means clearing the area around the heart. The heart and lungs are vital organs of survival. Some healers use thyme to stimulate the immune response of the whole chest area, including the heart. TCM has long asserted that there is a subtle energy flow through the heart and on to the thymus gland and thus to and throughout the body's immune system. What we feel in our heart is conveyed to our immune system. Thyme reminds us to take the time to connect with our heart as the center of discernment and healing to recognize that which invades our healthy world and causes us excessive stress and inharmony. Out of that heart connection is the opportunity for a greater and more effective immune response.

Currently, **garlic** is one of the most popular herbs used to reduce certain risks associated with cardiovascular disease. Current uses of garlic include its ability to lower serum lipids and decrease blood pressure and blood sugar along with its antimicrobial activity. Garlic also is used to prevent and alleviate the symptoms associated with bacterial, parasitic, and fungal infections, and viral infections such as colds and influenza. Garlic is an excellent expectorant. Garlic with purple skin is thought to demonstrate the most effective action against microbes and amoebic infection. Garlic and its constituent allicin are effective against certain multidrug-resistant strains of bacteria. Most bacteria are unable to develop resistance to it because its mechanism of action is not like other antibiotics. The parent substance of allicin, alliin, is a sulfur-containing amino acid derivative that does not have antimicrobial activity. Alliin becomes allicin when the garlic bulb is ground and the alliin comes in contact with an enzyme in the bulb that converts the alliin to allicin. The active principles in fresh garlic are released through grinding as in chewing; however, many people do not like the after-effects of chewing fresh garlic cloves. Fresh garlic extracts with the constituent allicin also demonstrate antifungal, antiparasitic, and antiviral activity in vitro. Little *clinical* research has been conducted to address the traditional use of garlic in preventing infectious disease in humans and strengthening the immune response in some way. A 1993 metanalysis of the literature that included five studies ($N = 365$) found that garlic, in supplements approximating 1/2 to 1 clove per day, did exhibit a significant reduction in total cholesterol levels by at least 9 percent and sometimes up to 15 percent. One limitation of the metanalysis is that in three of the five studies, Kwai garlic tablets were used; in one study, spray-dried powder was used; and in the fifth study, garlic aqueous extract was used. None of the studies placed dietary restrictions on participants. As the list of resistant strains of microorganisms grows, nurses may need to deal with a public that is restless for suggestions for dealing with infection. Garlic has been shown to be capable of inhibiting viruses, fungi, and gram-negative and gram-positive bacteria, without resistance developing. The antithrombotic and significant antifungal action of garlic is related to its ajoene consitutent. Dried garlic preparations do not contain allicin or ajoene. Dried preparations do contain alliin, both allicin's and ajoene's precursor. The enzyme that converts the alliin to allicin and ajoene is very unstable in the presence of acids, such as gastric secretions. Therefore, enteric-coated, dried garlic preparations may be more effective. There are no known interactions between garlic and prescription drugs; however, garlic is known to substantially increase the anticoagulant effect of warfarin and therefore could increase bleeding times. It has been reported that blood-clotting times have doubled in clients who are taking warfarin when taking garlic *supplements*. Medicinal amounts of garlic can significantly thin the blood.

Black cohosh (*Cimicifuga racemosa*) rhizome, called "sheng ma," is classified in TCM as an herb that relieves wind heat. The species is *Cimicifuga foetida*. Chinese black cohosh root decoction is used for headaches and releases the exterior of the body so that rashes, such as measles, can erupt. Black cohosh is not used after measles have already erupted.

Echinacea is known for promoting natural powers of resistance against infectious conditions in the nose and throat, influenza, inflammatory and purulent wounds, abscesses, headaches, metabolic disturbances, and as a diaphoretic and antiseptic. Internal preparations are used to stimulate the immune system at the onset of colds and flu symptoms and for treatment of *C. albicans* infections, chronic respiratory infections, prostatitis, and rheumatoid arthritis. In one German study of 203 women with recurrent vaginal yeast infections in which all of the women were treated with the standard medication, topical econazole cream, and some of the women also took oral doses of Echinacin (*E. purpurea* leaf juice extract) for ten weeks, the women who took the echinacea had a 16.7 percent recurrence rate, whereas those that did not had a 60.5 percent recurrence rate. The dose of extract is 1:5 [g/ml], (55 percent alcohol), 30 to 60 drops three times daily. An herb teacher of mine once told me that herbs can be "irritants." This was not meant to be derogatory of herbs but was simply a descriptive statement of the action of some herbs in the human body. Echinacea is an irritant in a sense. Its prickly nature is represented in the bristles of its cone and how it tingles or prickles the tongue. It irritates the body's immune system to act against bacteria, viruses, or fungi. Biomedical evidence has some idea how the plant accomplishes its stimulating work, but as is true for several herbs, the action of echinacea cannot be ascribed to one constituent. It is probable that a synergy of constituents and activities occurs that enables echinacea to cause its response in the human immune system. It is not known exactly which constituents in echinacea have the immunologic effect but a lipophilic substance, isobutylamide, is thought to be responsible for the tingling sensation on the tongue often associated with therapeutic effect. The antiviral activity of echinacea is said to, in part, be due to caffeic acid, chicoric acid, and echinacin. Echinacea's therapeutic effects on wound healing and upper respiratory infection are thought to be related to its ability to stimulate the production of properdin, a serum protein that neutralizes viruses and bacteria, and to inhibit microbes from secreting the enzyme hyaluronidase. Dr. Varro Tyler, botanical researcher, showed that preparations of echinacea are thought to be effective because they stimulate the lymphatic tissue in the mouth and therefore initiate an immune response.

A tea made of **rose** petals is given to infants in small amounts for fever and is used to ease children's coughs.

Goldenseal root is considered a specific remedy for inflammation of the mucous membranes, especially if chronic. One exception to this was in cases of acute otitis media in which goldenseal was said to work better than in chronic cases. It has been used for gastric inflammation. It is not used in cases of acute inflammation. Goldenseal is used in cases of inflammation of the gallbladder ducts, hepatic congestion, severe diarrhea, and dysentery. It is taken internally and applied topically to hemorrhoids, anal fissures, rectal ulcers and eczema, and prolapsed rectum. Noted British infectious disease physician Edward Bach, who performed original research in bacteriology and homeopathy and eventually created the Bach flower remedies, found that gram-negative bacilli, in particular those found in the intestines that are often regarded as having no significance in relationship to disease processes, are actually associated with chronic disease. Perhaps goldenseal's effective antiseptic action on the intestines and its immune-stimulating effect should be studied further in relation to its potential to be preventive and/or healing for some chronic illnesses. Goldenseal serves as a good reminder that herbs need to be used for the right situation, at the right time, and in the right amount. Goldenseal must be used for the right condition and in the right amount because it has been overharvested, and its existence may be endangered if its populations are not conserved. Goldenseal also must be used at the right time. For example, in the case of intestinal infection, it is best used for chronic conditions. The dose of a 1:1 [g/ml] extract, 60 percent alcohol (0.3 to 1.0 ml) is three times daily. Goldenseal tincture or powder taken orally stimulates the salivary glands, the appetite, the liver, stomach, and intestinal mucosa. It is used for inflammation and sores in the mouth and in chronic conditions of the gastric mucosa such as gastritis and ulcers. Goldenseal has been reported to increase the blood supply to the spleen, and one of its constituents, berberine, is said to activate macrophages in the body. However, goldenseal does not act like an antibiotic in that it does not work systemically to scavenge and kill harmful or healthy bacteria. Nurses have partnered with this plant for a long time. Mary Ann Bickerdyke, an American nurse-herbalist who is highly regarded for her service during the Civil War, was known to dose the soldiers/clients suffering from infection with smallpox with "black root and goldenseal, sassafras tea and beet juice, and all the milk and fresh vegetables they would take," after which a large number recovered.

Seaweeds also have been used as a blood purifier and for athero-sclerosis, rheumatism, and benign and malignant tumors. It is believed to help these conditions because its mucilage content is very absorptive of toxins in the bowel. Kelp and its constituent, sodium alginate, have been shown to effectively reduce the absorption of heavy metals and radiation, such as strontium 90 and cesium, in humans. The kelp absorbs the radioactive substance or heavy metal and carries it out in the stool. In a human trial of 40 people in which 10 ingested stable strontium, sodium alginate from *Sargassum siliquastrum* (12 to 15 g of 2 percent solution in orange syrup or 6 percent in bread) was found to significantly reduce absorption of radiostrontium, a hazardous nuclide that has a half-life of twenty-nine years. A review of animal in vivo studies have shown that hot water extracts of *Laminaria* and *Sargassum* demonstrate significant tumor inhibition effects, in particular with Ehrlich ascites carcinoma and Sarcoma 180 tumors. As seaweeds have been shown to have the ability to scavenge hydroxyl radicals, *Sargassum* has demonstrated high antioxidative activity in vitro. It is best to rehydrate dried seaweeds and then cut them up in soups and foods.

Calendula possesses antispasmodic, diaphoretic, anti-inflammatory, wound-healing, and antiseptic properties. Calendula tea or extract can be used internally for sore throat and nausea.

Topical Remedies

Garlic-Mullein Flower Ear Oil: Peel and thinly slice the cloves of one garlic head. If you have access to fresh mullein flowers *(Verbascum thapsus)*, use equal parts flower and garlic. There is no need to wash the flowers as the tap water will contaminate your oil. If you do not have flowers, just make garlic oil. Put the herbs in a wide-mouthed jar and cover the herbs with olive oil. Place a piece of cheesecloth over the jar opening and secure it with a rubber band. Let the oil stand in a warm place for approximately two weeks. Gently swirl the oil occasionally during the extraction period. Strain and press the oil out of the herbs into small medicine bottles with glass droppers. To use the oil, start by warming the bottle of oil in a small pan of warm water. Test a drop of oil on your wrist. When it is warm, take a few drops of the oil and massage gently in a circular and downward motion behind the ear and along the neck (following the eustachian tube). Then gently massage in front of the ear. Tip your head, pull the earlobe to open the ear canal, and drop the oil in the ear until you can feel it fill (about 4 drops). Place a cotton ball gently in the ear. Placing oil in the ear should not be done if the eardrum has ruptured and/or the ear is draining. Alternatively, place 2 drops of the oil on the corner of a cotton square and place in the ear. This remedy can be very helpful anytime the ear is sore or stuffy, particularly prior to and during colds and flu. I have had numerous students and clients over the years who are amazed that this simple remedy allays cold symptoms within minutes of application. Blocking the ear with cotton helps, too, but the garlic or garlic-mullein oil has kept many people well. I have a number of clients with serious chronic disease who report that while their family members are sick during cold and flu season, they have stayed healthy because they used the ear oil every time they felt the cold coming on. Some use it prophylactically and reported less or no colds. The ear is very sensitive to "wind." In TCM, colds are exterior wind conditions. Taking care of the ears by protecting them from actual wind and moistening them with oil makes good sense.

External applications of **echinacea** are used for hard-to-heal wounds, eczema, burns, psoriasis, and herpes simplex. It has been used topically for cleansing and deodorizing cancerous growths, for cleansing infected wounds, and to wash surgical sites postoperatively. Preparations of echinacea have been applied to eczema and psoriasis with good results.

Calendula possesses antispasmodic, diaphoretic, anti-inflammatory, wound-healing, and antiseptic properties. Calendula tea or extract can be used externally as an eyewash for conjunctivitis or as an ointment or compress for sore nipples, diaper rash, or wounds.

Plant constituents of **St. John's Wort**, hypericin and pseudohypericin, have been shown to inhibit encapsulated viruses such as *Herpes simplex* I and II and human immunodeficiency virus.

Chop one **onion** into small pieces. Place lightly cooked or raw onion in the center of flannel fabric. Fold over the edges and secure them so that the onion will not spill out. Place the compress over the inflamed area, such as the chest or on or behind the ear for ear infection, and leave in place for two hours, but do not secure the compress in place because this could lead to skin irritation. Check the skin every fifteen to thirty minutes.

Goldenseal is applied topically to conditions of the nose and throat. It is used for sore throat, rhinitis, inflammations of the tonsils, and in diphtheria. Powdered goldenseal used to be snuffed into the nostrils for nasal inflammation, and today some sinus sprays have goldenseal in them. Goldenseal and berberine do not have a systemic antibiotic-like effect unless coming in direct contact with some infected tissue such as in wound care. Goldenseal, while stimulating the mucous membranes to secrete, increases the IgA that naturally flows at the beginning of a cold or flu as the body attempts to shed the virus on its own. Therefore, goldenseal is not needed when the body is producing enough mucus and antibodies. Because goldenseal has become a very popular herb and is often over or misused because of misinformation, plant populations are at risk. The Convention on International Trade in Endangered Species (CITES), lists goldenseal as an Appendix II plant (www.wcmc.org. uk/CITES/eng/index.shtml). This means that although it may not be currently threatened with extinction, it may become so if the trade of the plant is not strictly regulated. Whenever a root of a plant is used medicinally, the risk of depleting plant populations is greater. It takes years to grow a root sufficient for harvest. Herb growers are being encouraged to cultivate goldenseal, and in the meantime, health practitioners and the public can help prevent the loss of goldenseal by becoming educated regarding the proper use of the plant.

In an in vitro study, an alcohol extract of **thyme** was found to be effective at killing head lice. It was most effective when the treatment was followed with a rinse of thyme essential oil, vinegar, and water.

Lavender essential oil is used to treat infections, including *Candida*. It is also used for laryngitis, asthma, insect bites, cystitis, inflammation, and to help boost immunity.

Because of its bacteriostatic and anti-inflammatory actions, **yarrow** tincture can be used instead of iodine for children's minor scrapes. The tincture is diluted 1:1 or 1:2 in water so that it will not sting infants and young children. Tea can be used also and that does not have to be diluted.

Environmental Remedies

For a **thyme** bath, prepare a strong infusion of thyme using 2 cups (227 g) of dried thyme and 2 quarts or liters of boiled water. Cover and steep for ten minutes. Strain and pour into a filled tub (98°F). Immerse yourself and breathe deeply. Plan to be in the tub for twenty minutes. People with strong hearts can submerge themselves so that the water level is above the heart; otherwise the water level should be below the heart. While in the tub, gently tap your sternum with your fingertips, alternating hands. This is called a "thymus tap" and is thought to stimulate the thymus and decrease stress. After the bath, wrap yourself in two big towels and a blanket and let yourself perspire for thirty minutes. I don't recommend doing this in bed unless you plan to change the sheets, because the body is shedding the toxins and virus/bacteria through the pores. Do not reuse the towels after this process without washing them first. Your heart may beat slightly fast as you go through this very important second part of the thyme bath experience. Do not skip this step. When your heart rate is back to normal and you are no longer perspiring, sponge off a little with a warm wash cloth and dress warmly. Remember to put on socks. Get into bed and rest well.

Chamomile steams of the infusion of the flower relieve sinusitis pain. Essential oils in the flower head are antibacterial and anti-inflammatory.

Lemon essential oil is used as a sedative and an antifungal and anti-parasitic agent. It is also used to reduce the frequency of bouts of chronic bronchitis. The oil is increasingly being used in hospitals to neutralize unpleasant odors, as a disinfectant, and to disperse stale air. It has been found to have a psychologically strengthening effect on clients, especially those with terminal illness.

Yarrow tea (inside and out) can be used to help increase perspiration in people who have viral illness such as cold or flu. Yarrow opens the pores and encourages sweating. In many traditions, the concept of sweating an illness out of the body is well known. In TCM, the herbs that have this action are said to "release the exterior" of the body. Native Americans use the sweat lodge. A classic sweating tea recommended by herbalists includes yarrow, peppermint, and elder flower. This release, or sweat, enables the body to shed the virus much as it does when the nose drips, shedding the virus through excess secretions. An old remedy for the common cold (and many chronic discomforts) in herbalism was to take a pint of strong yarrow tea on going to bed and then to put a hot brick at the feet wrapped in a cloth wet with vinegar. Today, people coming down with a cold can still benefit from a hot water bottle at their feet and a cup of yarrow tea before going to bed with lots of warm blankets. In the morning, they should bathe, dress warmly, and change the bed linen.

In ancient Greece, Arabia, and Rome, **lavender** was used as an antiseptic, a bactericide, and to disinfect hospitals and sick rooms. Lavender essential oil can be used as a disinfectant for the sick room when clients or their caregivers are chemically sensitive to synthetically fragranced or disinfectant products.

NURSE-HERBALIST ASSESSMENT

TCM	ROY MODEL*
Health Concerns	**Physiological Mode**
Thermal (Hot/ Cold)	
Resp/Breath Pattern (Rate, Quality)	Oxygenation
Intake (Thirst /Appetite)	Nutrition / Fluid and Electrolytes
Outflow (Urine and BM color quality consistency)	Elimination
Pain (Location, Quality, Better with touch or not)	
Skin (Dryness, Itching)	Protection
Senses (Hearing, Visual field)	(Skin Integrity and Sensitivity)
Sleep/Rest (Patterns, Insomnia, Dreams)	Senses
Motion (Gait, Speed, Forcefulness, Spasms)	Activity and Rest
Speech (Speed, Forcefulness, Loudness, Pitch)	Neurological Function
	Endocrine Function
Pulse Diagnosis	
(Quality, Rate, Depth, Rhythm, Profile)	
Tongue Diagnosis	
(Tissue Color, Shape, Fissures)	
(Tongue Coat Presence, Color, Thickness,	
Moisture)	
Behavior (Personality, Moods, Interactions)	**Self Concept Mode**
	Body Image (How does client view self?)
	Body Sensation
	(How does client feel in body?)
	Self-Consistency (Response to situation)
	Self-Ideal (What would client like to be?)
	Moral – Ethical – Spiritual – Self
	(What does client believe?)
Lifestyle (Work, Play, Habits)	**Role Function Mode**
	What roles does the client play?
	Age/sex/developmental stage.
	Sick Role?
	How does client feel about roles?
	Conflict?
Self-in-Relation to Others	**Interdependence Mode**
Environment (Home, Work, Global)	
	Close Relationships
	Sense of Belonging
	Support System
	Giving and Receiving

©1995 Martha Mathews Libster   *Andrews & Roy (1986). Essentials of the Roy Adaptation Model.

INDEX

NURSE-HERBALIST

Q

R

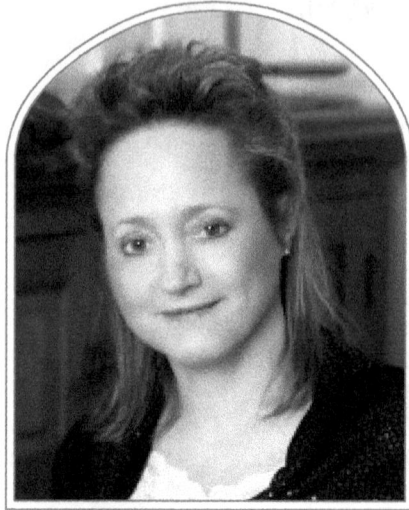

Dr. Martha Mathews Libster is an educator, Advanced Practice Nurse, healthcare historian, and Herbal Diplomat® known internationally for her work on the complementarity of nursing practice, technology, and healing traditions, in particular the use of botanical therapies. She is the author of numerous journal and book publications including: *Demonstrating Care, The Integrative Herb Guide for Nurses, Enlightened Charity*, and the award winning *Herbal Diplomats*, a history of nurses' botanical contributions to 19th century health care reform.

Dr. Libster is the Director and Chair of Nursing at Governors State University near Chicago, USA. She is also Director of Golden Apple Healing Arts, LLC, a consultation and education firm that promotes self-care and informed, holistic health decision making where she offers dynamic webinars and and seminars including Herbal Diplomat® - a comprehensive certification program preparing nurses for the next dimension of nurse-herbalism.

Dr. Libster is a Board-Certified Advanced Practice Holistic Nurse and Psychiatric Clinical Nurse Specialist specializing in the care of infants 0-3 and their families, people living with chronic illness, infertility, wounds that won't heal, anxiety disorders, and parapsychology. She has over 25 years of experience working in a variety of health care settings where she has developed the integration of conventional nursing and technology with the use of herbal remedies and other healing traditions. Dr. Libster has practiced as a clinician-consultant in Traditional Chinese Herbal Medicine and European and Western herbal therapies for over 25 years. Her first herbal teacher was her grandfather Arthur of the Cornish Celtic Rankin family. Dr. Libster focuses her botanical practice on the use of herbal and floral teas, syrups and topical remedies and teaching her clients to make their own simple "medicines" for use in self-care. She has also practiced and taught European Foot Reflexology with Herbal Applications since 1986. Dr. Libster is the Associate Editor for Botanicals for the Journal of Holistic Nursing and a member of the advisory board of the American Botanical Council. She is the founding director of The Bamboo Bridge international online community that promotes global health partnerships and cultural diplomacy between nurses and traditional, community healers through education and research. Dr. Libster has spoken for the World Health Organization, the Royal College of Nursing, the United States Botanic Garden, professional organizations, healthcare providers, and the public on integrative care, botanical therapies, health care reform, self-care, healing traditions, and the history of nursing.

For information about opportunities to study with Dr. Libster online and face-to-face please go to www.GoldenAppleHealingArts.com

www.ingramcontent.com/pod-product-compliance
Lightning Source LLC
Chambersburg PA
CBHW060018030426
42334CB00019B/2093